Nuclear Medicine Hybrid Imaging
for Radiographers & Technologists

Luca Camoni · Luigi Mansi
Editors

Nuclear Medicine Hybrid Imaging for Radiographers & Technologists

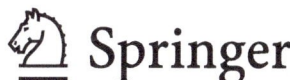 Springer

Editors
Luca Camoni
Department of Nuclear Medicine
University of Brescia and ASST
Spedali Civili di Brescia
Brescia, Italy

Luigi Mansi
Interuniversity Research Center for
Sustainability (CIRPS)
Rome, Italy

Medicina Futura
Acerra (NA), Italy

ISBN 978-3-031-86227-4   ISBN 978-3-031-86228-1   (eBook)
https://doi.org/10.1007/978-3-031-86228-1

This Springer imprint is published by the registered company Springer Nature Switzerland AG
The registered company address is: Gewerbestrasse 11, 6330 Cham, Switzerland

If disposing of this product, please recycle the paper.

Preface

Life, my friend, is the art of encounter

The first seed of this book was planted in 1895 by Wilhelm Conrad Roentgen and gave life in a very short time to a plant, that of radioscopy and X-ray radiography, which led him to receive the first Nobel Prize for Physics in 1901. Also of revolutionary importance was the discovery of radioactivity, which occurred the following year, thanks to Antoine Henri Becquerel, who shared the Nobel Prize for this discovery in 1903 with Marie Skłodowska-Curie (the first woman to have won it and the only woman to have won two) and Pierre Curie.

Yet the role of radioactivity in medical diagnostics (and therapy) would be clinically expressed only in the 1940s, when Iodine-131 became available, giving rise to the birth of the *good nuclear* as a positive epiphenomenon of the bad nuclear energy of the atomic bomb. Thus, for decades, diagnostic imaging was only X-ray radiology.

Thanks to Iodine-131, nuclear medicine was born at the clinical level both as a diagnostic and as a therapy, performed with a gamma- and beta-emitting radionuclide, which became the basis, varying the doses, both of scintigraphy and of the metabolic therapy of thyroid diseases. Already at birth, the seed of that plant that we call today theragnostic was planted which, having produced for decades only in the field of thyroid pathologies and in other areas of lesser importance, has recently started to provide new fruits, increasingly significant. After more than 50 years from the introduction of radioiodine, theragnostic is becoming, in the third millennium, one of the main fulcrums of our discipline.

Nuclear medical diagnostics was born even without images, based on analogical probes that counted radioactivity, differentiating normal from pathological according to the number of counts. The first great revolution in equipment, which led to the first images, not real but dependent on the concentration of the radiopharmaceutical, occurred with Cassen's rectilinear scanner (1950), which created scintigraphs on paper through the oscillation of a hammer that drew more or less intense lines (or of different colors) based on the intensity of the radioactivity. Thus was born the thyroid scintigraphy and then all the other scintigraphs performed, in addition to I-131, with radionuclides disappeared because they were inefficient and/or required high doses of irradiation, such as Au-198 and Hg-203, or were applied very little, such as F-18, used as fluoride in bone scintigraphy with rectilinear scanner, which would forcefully reappear in the 1980s with the entry into the field of PET-FDG.

Two great revolutions occurred, at the turn of the 1970s, thanks to the entry into the clinical field of Tc-99m and the gamma camera, developed by Anger starting from the second half of the 1950s. The premise was created to perform faster acquisitions, with "more photographic" images, and the possibility of performing dynamic exams was born. For many years, however, the scans were analog, because only in the 1970s did the computer begin to forcefully enter the field, giving life to computerized techniques. While in radiology, this led to the birth of CT and the Nobel Prize to Hounsfield and Cormack, in nuclear medicine, alongside the possibility of building SPECT and PET tomographs, computerized examinations were born, with immediately important applications at a clinical level in various fields such as cardiology and nephrology.

In the 1980s, a binary diagnostic world was created, made up of two separate monocular visions: (a) morphostructural imaging, based on anatomical and anatomo-pathological data, characterized by the possibility of high spatial resolution and of a regional analysis; (b) functional imaging, based on physiopathological assumptions, which through a biological resolution sees function and molecular metabolism. In this way, the diagnosis may be anticipated, individuating the alteration that precedes the structural damage, being also better characterized the lesion/disease in its relationships with prognosis and therapy. Since urography, many ultrasound techniques, functional MRI, and some CT methods are also functional imaging, nuclear medicine is the queen discipline, existing only as a functional method, applicable exclusively on living beings. But the enormous potential of our discipline, which is enhanced with the entry into play of PET, suffers from the inability to define well the morphological and spatial connotations of the identified pathology.

A great further revolution is therefore that of the birth of hybrid machines, which combine PET (or SPECT) and CT in the same scanner, transforming the two monocular visions into a splendid and effective binocular vision that increases sensitivity, specificity, and accuracy, creating the conditions for a new and extraordinary season of diagnostic imaging. To the hybrid machines with CT, after a complex technological work, has been also added the PET/MR scanner that opens up further applications not only linked to the different significance of the resonance images compared to the density's ones of CT but also for the possibility of adding to the morphostructural eye of the RM and the functional/molecular eye of PET, a third eye that sees the function also through fMRI.

This book wants to talk about the state of the art of hybrid machines and the methods connected to them and we therefore want to celebrate the meeting of different worlds. We wish to celebrate this convergence by guiding the reader on a journey that starts with the equipment and leads to the true focus of healthcare professions: the patient.

The first meeting is that of morphostructural with functional and molecular imaging. The second is the meeting of different skills that include not only those of the physician and the technologist/radiographer but also those of the physicist, the chemist, the psychologist, the nurse, the manager, and all those who contribute to a modern and sustainable healthcare, which preserves humanity, having the patient at its center.

This book is also and perhaps above all the meeting between two new friends, one differently young, who began to take an interest in nuclear medicine in 1972 and who worked with all the tools described above, from probes, to rectilinear scanner, the analog and computerized gamma camera, SPECT, PET, up to hybrid machines. The other, much younger, was born and grew up with computerized and hybrid imaging. Our dialectical collaboration has enriched us with a productive comparison between a vertical competence in exponential growth, structured on the state of the art of technologies, with the experience gained in over 50 years with almost a hundred different tools that have matured and grown a lateral thinking that can see what others look at but do not recognize.

We are very happy to share this editorial enterprise, for which we thank the splendid authors who have accompanied us on this magnificent journey, concluding with the phrase of Vinicius de Moraes that became Samba da Bênção with the music by Baden Powell: **Life, my friend, is the art of encounter**.

Brescia, Italy   Luca Camoni
Rome, Italy   Luigi Mansi

P.S. Editors' Note
For the purposes of this book and to facilitate a cohesive and accessible approach for both authors and readers, we have chosen to use the terms radiographer, technologist, and nuclear medicine technologist (NMT) interchangeably. We recognize that these titles may have different meanings, qualifications, and responsibilities in various healthcare systems around the world. However, we adopt a generalized use of these terms to represent professionals who are integral members of the healthcare specialist team, capable of undertaking the full spectrum of nuclear medicine procedures. This decision is intended to simplify communication and is not intended to overlook or minimize the distinct roles and qualifications associated with each title in their specific contexts or countries. Rather, it aims to unify the terminology internationally, acknowledging the contributions of different authors while respecting their cultural and organizational context.

About This Book

Nuclear medicine is a multidisciplinary specialty that requires close collaboration between radiochemists, technologists, medical physicists, nurses, and physicians. Hybrid imaging development reflects the nuclear medicine field's evolution, advancing due to the constantly increasing demand for more complex and precise diagnostic patients' management. Neither the field nor the methods would have become widely acknowledged as valuable without the professional workforce. Those groups of medical experts evolved through years to become a comprehensive team of professionals not only supporting but also leading the most advanced procedures, including studies performed in accordance with the theranostic management requirements, working hand in hand in their daily clinical practice.

Starting from the conventional radiography, technologists and radiographers developed along with the novel diagnostic imaging evolution. Escalating the basic and expanding the advanced sets of knowledge, skills, and competencies, these professionals gained wider responsibilities and fulfilled the demand for highly specialized hybrid imaging experts. Currently, the most recognized characteristics and obligations of nuclear medicine technologists are the direct communication with patients, participating in planning and performing both diagnostic and therapeutic procedures, as well as evaluating the initial study outcomes to deliver the best and most detailed set of the analytic, clinical data to the reporting nuclear medicine physician. Nuclear medicine technologists and physicians' direct cooperation is the pillar of modern hybrid imaging for which the broad and comprehensive knowledge, skills, and competencies are the mandatory requirements.

The collaboration between the interdisciplinary medical professionals is vital for the advanced hybrid imaging procedures' outcomes. The complexity of the methods' technical and physical basis, their advanced performance, and the detailed reporting algorithms make the elevated abilities of the medical professional partaking in the procedures essential. Modern nuclear medicine experts, despite their profession, are specialists operating hybrid imaging modalities with ease and the accurate level of awareness and responsibility that contemporary nuclear medicine demands.

Agata Pietrzak—EANM Technologists' Committee Chair (2023–2025).
Jolanta Kunikowska—EANM President (2021–2022).

Contents

Introduction to Hybrid Imaging Technologies: The Physician's Perspective

1

Francesco Dondi and Francesco Bertagna

1.1 Historical Evolution and Development of Nuclear Medicine and Hybrid Imaging

The birth of nuclear medicine is classically ascribed to George de Hevesy, a Hungarian physicist-chemist who worked with Ernest Rutherford in Manchester. The scientist lived in a boarding house where the landlady served a grand roast for dinner each Sunday and suspected that the dinner was turned up again in the hash and served on Wednesday. To confirm his idea he sprinkled a sample of a radium isotope on a bit of meat on Sunday and on Wednesday he found out that the hash was radioactive. This was the first application and the birth of the tracer principle. Notably, for his invention, de Hevesy received the Nobel Prize in 1943 [1].

Nuclear medicine is characterized by the use of radioactive tracers whose distribution in the body is imaged by different technological devices, and different landmarks helped to launch and establish this particular field of medicine, such as the production and the evaluation of different radiopharmaceuticals able to image and define different metabolic pathways. In addition, the evolution of nuclear medicine is strictly connected to the evolution of technology, and its clinical applications have been widening due to technological innovation in hardware and software. Initially, the detection of photon was performed using Geiger–Müller counters that were manually moved over the target of interest to measure the uptake and the concentration of the radionuclide, and one of the first field applications of this technique was the assessment of the rate of radioiodine uptake in the thyroid gland. Subsequently, in 1960, Benedict Cassen started to investigate and evaluate the use of metallic crystals as scintillation counters that could therefore enhance the sensitivity and the detection of photon emission by switching out the detectors in Geiger–Müller counters with calcium tungstate. Later, increased sensitivities were achieved by switching to thallium-doped sodium iodide crystals, adding photomultiplier tubes and automating the scanning system. Another important advance in the evolution of nuclear medicine imaging came with the development of the rectilinear scanner, which automated the positioning of the scanner and became the standard instrument used for nuclear imaging from the 1950s, with a variety of possible applications ranging from preoperative localization of brain tumours to determination of cardiac output or kidney function [2].

A fundamental breakthrough in the evolution of nuclear medicine imaging came, however,

F. Dondi (✉) · F. Bertagna
Department of Nuclear Medicine, University of Brescia and ASST Spedali Civili di Brescia, Brescia, Italy
e-mail: francesco.dondi@unibs.it; francesco.bertagna@unibs.it

with Hal Anger's invention of a gamma camera that incorporated collimation and had an array of photomultiplier tubes to improve detection efficiency. Anger in 1958 described the basic principles and components of scintillation cameras such as the detector, the collimator, image display and the position circuitry. In this setting, other important milestones of the evolution of this imaging modality were the multidetector produced by Brownell and Sweet that was developed in 1953 for the assessment of brain tumours and the first circular array of detectors by Yamamoto et al. for imaging the brain. In addition, in the 1960s Kuhl and Edwards developed their tomographic imaging device and also introduced the concepts of longitudinal and transaxial tomography, considered the predecessor of modern single photon emission computed tomography (SPECT) systems. In 1963, the first commercial scintillation camera was therefore manufactured in Chicago. Initially, tomographic reconstruction with a gamma camera was achieved by rotating the patient in front of a stationary camera. It was not until 1977 that Keyes et al. created the first camera that rotated around the patient, followed up by the introduction of the cantilever system by Larsson in the 1980s [2].

Several subsequent technological advances have led to the development of the modern SPECT modality. The main strength of this imaging technique is its potential to provide quantitative measurement of the three-dimensional distribution of radiopharmaceuticals, since the camera head rotates around the object to image and at each step the camera collects events. As a consequence, the data acquired from each angle provide a planar count distribution of the radiotracer, allowing the determination of the number of tomographic slices and the whole distribution on the injected tracer. In addition, several modifications of the basic collimator design have been proposed during the years in order to improve spatial resolution or sensitivity, such as the development of rotatory or converging collimators. At this point, it is worth underlining that the determination of the attenuation of the photon emission of the radiopharmaceutical is mandatory to achieve a clear and precise representation of its

distribution in the field of view. In this setting, as discussed later, the most accurate method to determine attenuation is by means of acquisition of computed tomography (CT) images, even though in the past external sources and different mathematical methods have been proposed [3].

Focusing on positron emission tomography (PET) imaging, two initial reports of the opportunities offered by the use of coincidence detection of positron capture were initially published independently in 1951 by Wrenn and Sweet, and subsequently the first clinical application of this technology in the diagnosis and treatment of brain tumours was reported in 1953 by Brownell and Sweet. Subsequently, in the late 1960s Brownell et al. developed a scanner by constructing static two-dimensional arrays of individual coincident detectors, and Burnham and Brownell allowed small sodium iodide crystals to be encoded by fewer, larger photomultipliers, thereby reducing cost and improving spatial resolution. In addition, the principle of Anger cameras was applied also in the field of positron imaging, with Chesler that rotated the positron camera to record multiple views, which were then filtered and back-projected to obtain transaxial tomographic images. Several technological improvements allowed the introduction of faster scintillators and the development of methodologies to correct for scattered coincidences, allowing the use of more open field of view and increased axial length, leading to the current state-of-the-art PET scanners [4]. In addition, the development and the improvement of reconstruction algorithms permitted better image quality, and notably one of the first PET instruments to employ filtered back projection was developed by Ter-Pogossian, Phelps and Hoffman in 1975 [2].

In recent years different technological advances have been introduced in the field of nuclear medicine, and in the current state-of-the-art scanners, spatial resolution has already improved by a factor of 10 and sensitivity by a factor of 40 in comparison to the scanners from the early 1970s [5]. Nevertheless, the introduction of hybrid imaging, which by definition is the fusion of different imaging modalities, has led to the development of multimodality configuration such as SPECT/CT, PET/CT or PET/magnetic resonance (MR).

1.1.1 Development of Hybrid SPECT/CT Imaging Modality

Initially, the transmission scanning used to assess body contours in planar scintigraphic studies and to correct for attenuation was performed by using 99mTc or 153Gd flood source. This was followed by the development of a variety of different transmission solutions that included multiple line sources, high-energy source that penetrated the collimator, rod source and fanbeam collimator implemented on a triple head system and the scanning line source. Despite these different technical innovations and settings, transmission scanning failed to be universally accepted, partly due to deficiencies in the commercial devices and associated reconstruction software that were sold [6].

Around the same time as the development of SPECT transmission, Hasegawa et al. in the mid-1990s proposed a combined SPECT/CT scanner that is considered the introduction of dual modality imaging as known today since this prototype formed the basis for the development of the first commercial SPECT/CT system, introduced in 1999. The introduction of CT images not only allowed for better attenuation correction but was also crucial to have a clear anatomical identification of the structure involved in the acquisition. This system was characterized by good contrast object detectability, and a high contrast-to-noise ratio was demonstrated at low doses using this system. Additionally it was later upgraded to a four-slice system with the possibility to have fully diagnostic CT options with a 16-slice or 64-slice system [6]. Interestingly, in 1996 Blankespoor et al. presented a combined SPECT/CT design comprising a clinical SPECT gamma camera in tandem with a clinical single-slice CT with a tandem acquisition of the two modalities, using the CT data to generate the SPECT attenuation correction factors. In this setting, nowadays SPECT and CT scans are acquired sequentially

but the two modalities are integrated in the same gantry and can also operate independently [7, 8].

In the last decades, the technical evolution of nuclear medicine equipment has led to the introduction and implementation of fully diagnostic multislice CT integrated in SPECT/CT systems, and in addition low-cost CT technology including flat-panel detectors has been introduced. In addition, focusing on the SPECT part of this hybrid technique, improvement in the energy and spatial resolutions have been proposed, allowing for lower radiation exposure of the patients and increased diagnostic accuracy. More recently, the introduction of solid-state detectors based on cadmium zinc telluride (CZT) has been one of the most important advances, leading to better energy and spatial resolution allowing therefore for an improvement of the performances of SPECT/CT devices with considerable clinical implications [5, 8]. Notably, the combination of two different modalities has been clearly demonstrated to be clinically worth more than the sum of the parts, and in the actual patient's management both functional and anatomical information are essential. In this setting, there is growing acceptance of the merits of SPECT/CT and growing confidence in the quantitative accuracy that can be achieved in SPECT utilizing CT information [6].

1.1.2 Development of Hybrid PET/ CT and PET/MR Imaging

As mentioned, during the 1990s there was a growing interest in combining and fusing different imaging modalities, and PET did not make any exception. In this scenario, in 1991 Townsend and Nutt proposed a combination of PET with CT even though they were unaware that in 1984 Nagai et al. developed the first hybrid design that comprised a PET and a CT scanner side by side with a single bed mounted on a platform that moved sideways transporting the bed from one scanner to the other. In contrast with these configurations, the idea of Townsend and Nutt combined the PET and X-ray CT modalities into a single device that would image both anatomy and function that, as a matter of fact, is the first application of modern PET/CT scanner. The results obtained from this early scanner were encouraging and impactful, and in 2001 two different hybrid scanners were commercially available. Interestingly in 2004, only 3 years later, PET-only scanners were not available from the majority of the vendors. From that point different design and technical innovations have been proposed to improve image quality and diagnostic accuracy, and as an example, one of the most clinically impactful was the introduction of a new photodetector [4].

The introduction of CT in conjunction with PET was fundamental not only to assess attenuation but also for the addition of complementary information from the same examination and the improvement of imaging quality of PET images. Nowadays, the commercial availability of hybrid PET/CT systems has led to widespread clinical use, and all major domains of human health are represented in current clinical and research applications [4]. Digital PET/CT systems are now using silicon photomultipliers (SiPMs) attached to the crystal instead of analogue photomultiplier tubes, allowing for enhanced sensitivity, higher spatial and energetic resolution leading therefore to enhanced performances. This technological innovation was fundamental to propose total-body PET/CT systems that allow for total body dynamic acquisitions simultaneously, facilitating application of kinetic models [5].

In view of the success and clinical impacts of PET/CT, the expectations for new hybrid combinations, such as PET/MR, have been very high. MR imaging (MRI) is known to be a more versatile technique than other radiological modalities, able to determine a number of physiological and metabolic characteristics of human tissue by going beyond plain anatomical imaging. In addition, it can offer a high capability to differentiate soft tissues with better contrast compared to CT, but it can also assess functional processes in living subjects by diffusion-weighted (DW) and functional MRI. Moreover, in contrast with CT, MRI does not add radiation

exposure to the patient [9]. Considering the advantages of MRI relatively to CT, PET/MR systems might have potentially higher diagnostic accuracy than PET/CT especially in some specific organs. In this scenario, around the mid-1990s considerable interest in the preclinical domain for the combination of PET with MRI was present. Unfortunately, PET detectors could not be operated inside or close to an MR scanner, precluding the possibility of a PET/CT-like approach without additional shielding or a different detector configuration, and throughout the 1990s the development of semiconductor photodetectors resolved this problem. In 2006, the first PET detector ring with photodiodes that could be inserted into a 3T clinical MR to acquire PET data simultaneously with the operation of the MR was produced. More recently, in 2010, the first whole-body PET/MR scanner with simultaneous imaging capability was launched, and in 2013 the first SiPM PET/MR scanner was produced [4].

1.2 The Role of Hybrid Imaging Within the Field of Diagnostic Imaging

As previously stated, the introduction of hybrid imaging systems was a breakthrough for nuclear medicine, allowing for higher diagnostic accuracy and spreading therefore its clinical applications. Nowadays, functional and anatomical information are essential for the current management of the patients, and a modality able to fuse and retrieve both these data has a significant role by providing comprehensive information on the state of the patient. In addition, patients can also benefit from a single examination able to give two fundamental data, reducing therefore the need to perform different scans. As a result, following their introduction into the clinical setting, combined PET/CT, PET/MR and SPECT/CT devices are now playing an increasingly important role in the assessment of human pathological conditions.

1.2.1 Clinical Application of SPECT/ CT

The interpretation of SPECT images has been significantly improved since the introduction of hybrid SPECT/CT devices, and the recent technological developments are well suited to organ-specific imaging with potential to provide enhanced performances adapted to a specific imaging task. Since its introduction in the late 1990s, SPECT/CT experienced a steady increase in the number of installed systems, accompanied by increasing evidence of clinical usefulness and therefore spreading its field of application.

Starting from the skeletal system, hybrid imaging has contributed to a further improvement of the diagnostic accuracy of pre-existing methods. Bone scintigraphy with 99mTc-labelled diphosphonates is known to have high sensitivity but low specificity for the assessment of a wide range of pathological conditions such as infection, joint prosthesis mobilization, Paget's disease, fibrous dysplasia, avascular necrosis and so on. The introduction of SPECT/CT systems led to an improvement of diagnostic accuracy, increasing the specificity of this examination even when compared to SPECT alone. This had a significant clinical impact also in the oncological field where bone scintigraphy is used to stage and eventually restage the presence of bone localization of disease, in particular for prostate and breast cancer. The same statements are true even when considering labelled white blood cell scintigraphy, with hybrid imaging that is able to correctly define the extension of infectious processes. Interestingly, with the introduction of CT, the clear involvement of soft tissue can be properly evaluated [10, 11].

Focusing on the heart, even in the clinical setting of the assessment of cardiac function and perfusion, SPECT/CT had a predominant impact. In terms of myocardial perfusion imaging in patients affected by coronary artery disease, it has been reported that the information obtained by the combination of anatomy and function can improve the evaluation of extent and severity of the disease, allowing for better diagnosis, improving risk stratification and guiding appropriate management strategies. In particular, the introduction of CT in combination with SPECT and the improvement of reconstruction techniques on the basis of anatomical imaging led to better attenuation correction with better definition and classification of areas of impaired perfusion. SPECT/CT helps to overcome heterogeneous photon attenuation in the thorax, which is one of the most notable limitations of myocardial perfusion scintigraphy [12]. Interestingly it has also been reported that the fusion of SPECT and CT acquisition in the specific setting of cardiac evaluation offers interesting different possibilities, such as, for example, the attractive possibility to combine the assessment of calcium scoring from CT and the information from SPECT in both cases of viability or perfusion evaluation [7, 13]. In addition, the assessment of cardiac amyloidosis can also be performed with bone scintigraphy with specific tracers, and even in this setting the introduction of hybrid imaging has led to higher diagnostic sensibility allowing furthermore the dynamic and functional evaluation of the left ventricle of these patients.

When using SPECT/CT hybrid imaging modalities in both ventilatory or perfusion pulmonary scintigraphy, they could help to enhance the diagnostic accuracy of planar images, allowing better diagnostic information on the presence of possible embolism since they can exactly contribute to the clear identification of the site of reduced uptake in terms of anatomical references. In addition, nuclear medicine is fundamental for the metabolic assessment of some specific neoplastic forms such as, for example, neuroendocrine tumours, neuroblastoma, paragangliomas and pheochromocytomas that can be imaged with both 123I-meta-iodobenzylguanidine (123I-MIBG) or 111In-pentetreotide. In this field the introduction of SPECT/CT has drastically improved the diagnostic ability of these examinations, allowing for better assessment and definition of the disease, but also leading to the possibility to evaluate response to therapy. Nevertheless, in a theranostic setting, since 131I-MIBG can be used for the therapeutic treatment of such patients in specific cases, a better definition of the disease by the introduction of hybrid SPECT/CT systems is mandatory for a clear planning of the best therapeutic regimen. Similarly, 131I is a fundamental therapeutic and diagnostic tool for the management and the treatment of patients affected by differentiated thyroid cancer, and even in this setting the evolution of SPECT/CT has led to improved diagnostic accuracy, aiming therefore for a more patient-centred therapeutic regimen with a possible prognostic impact. Lastly, the introduction of hybrid imaging devices has improved the diagnostic accuracy of other nuclear medicine examinations such as parathyroid scintigraphy and lymphoscintigraphy.

The combined use of CT was fundamental to achieve an improvement of absorption and scattering of emitted photons and also for attenuation correction. In parallel, this fact also led to important achievements in many aspects like image quality, quantitative accuracy and diagnostic confidence. As a consequence, most of the modern SPECT/CT systems are suitable for quantitative emission tomography, that is the in vivo quantification of the activity of an injected radiopharmaceutical in a specific organ, an operation that in the past was only achievable with PET/CT imaging and tomographs. Despite that, in this specific field of application a high standardization is required in order to reduce bias in quantitative measurements due to technical implementation and site-specific choices. Established clinical applications of this feature are still rare and need therefore to be implemented in practice, even though first evidence on their usefulness for the assessment of skeletal disease, dosimetry and thyroid diseases have been reported. In addition, targeted radionuclide therapy could take advantage of the introduction of SPECT/CT quantification and theranostic, that is by definition the combination of the terms therapeutic and diagnostic, since better diagnostic accuracy is strictly related to better and more personalized therapeutic approaches [8, 14, 15].

Recently, the possibility to achieve a clear quantification of tracer uptake in SPECT/CT imaging has emerged, and different researches have been proposed in this field. Robust clinical applications of quantification on SPECT imaging are, however, hard to achieve since they rely on standardized and defined processes for image acquisition. In this setting, it is clear that the value of hybrid imaging for the correct assessment of patients and the validation of these modalities is central. Interestingly, one of the main fields of research and application of quantification with scintigraphic imaging is the assessment of cardiac perfusion with 99mTc-labelled tracers and comparing it to the established evaluation made by PET/CT.

1.2.2 Clinical Application of PET/CT and PET/MR

MRI, CT and PET offer different and complementary views of a patient, and hybrid imaging devices, which combine these different modalities, have transformed the evaluation of a high amount of different clinical conditions. In this scenario, new PET radiopharmaceuticals are continuously produced and tested, and in parallel, the sensitivity and diagnostic accuracy of tomographs are increasing allowing for high resolution and specific imaging. PET is able to give fundamental and unique metabolic information; however, without a clear map of the body provided by conventional imaging methods such as CT or MRI, it is difficult to clearly pinpoint the anatomical source of these metabolic activities. In addition, it has been reported that the diagnostic accuracy of PET/CT imaging exceeds that of PET or CT alone [14].

The clinical application of PET hybrid imaging depends on the radiotracer used to perform it, and in this setting a wide variety of different radiopharmaceuticals have been produced and are continuously proposed. Starting from 18F-fluorodeoxyglucose (18F-FDG) that is the most diffused and used tracer worldwide, given its ability to image the glycolytic activity of different tissues. In particular, the value of 18F-FDG PET/CT has been historically demonstrated in oncology, since it can image different types of neoplasms. In this setting, its clinical applications are extremely wide, including, for example, the assessment of lung cancer, head and neck cancers, colorectal cancer, melanoma, lymphoma, breast cancer and a wide range of many different neoplastic conditions. The abilities of 18F-FDG hybrid imaging to diagnose, stage, restage, assess the response to therapy and also to determine the prognosis of patients affected by such neoplasms have been clearly demonstrated in the past. In addition, a role for this imaging modality for the evaluation of different non-neoplastic conditions has been underlined, since inflammatory cells are also characterized by enhanced glycolytic activity. For example, vasculitis, fever of unknown origin, spondylodiscitis, sarcoidosis, endocarditis and other similar clinical conditions can be imaged with 18F-FDG. Moreover, the use of 18F-FDG PET/CT imaging offers the unique possibility to assess the functional status of the brain, allowing therefore the diagnosis and the assessment of neurodegenerative conditions. Clearly, the introduction of CT coupled with PET has offered the unique advantage to enhance the diagnostic ability of this imaging modality, particularly for small structures and anatomical regions in which the physiological uptake of the tracer by some organs could mask the pathological uptake. In addition, the introduction of CT images allowed a precise correction for attenuation, which is a mandatory point to carry out a quantification of the tracer uptake that in terms of PET imaging is reflected by the calculation of standardized uptake value (SUV). The diagnostic value of SUV has been demonstrated in a different range of neoplastic and benign conditions, and its ability to aid diagnosis and to give some insights on the prognosis of the patients have been underlined. Different clinical criteria based on the SUV of 18F-FDG uptake have been proposed to evaluate the response to therapy of patients in different pathologies, and all of them can offer important diagnostic information. In addition, the use of anatomical information obtained with CT has also been used to perform motion correction, raising the diagnostic accuracy of PET systems, particularly in the clinical setting of small lesions' assessment.

Various positron emitters radiotracers different from 18F-FDG and suitable for PET/CT imaging have been proposed and introduced in the last years. One of the most interesting radiotracers is labelled prostate specific membrane antigen (PSMA) that has wide clinical application in the assessment of patients affected by prostate cancer. Again, the importance of hybrid imaging in this field has to be researched in the complementary anatomical information that CT can give, aiming therefore for a precise evaluation of small foci of tracer uptakes. As an example, this is particularly important in the case of unspecified bone uptake (UBU) that can be revealed with 18F-PSMA-1007 and in which the anatomical assessment of the bone is mandatory to give an interpretation of these uptake, with significant clinical implications in the management of these patients. Another widely used and important tracer that benefited from the hybrid imaging PET/CT is labelled DOTA-peptides for the evaluation and eventually the treatment of neuroendocrine tumours. In addition, several radiopharmaceuticals such as, for example, 11C/18F-choline, 11C-methionine, 18F-fluorothimidine, 18F-DOPA, 18F-NaF and many other agents have been studied and proposed, and as previously underlined, all of them benefitted from the introduction of hybrid imaging modalities, since they can offer a clear anatomical localization of the focus of uptake and allow a precise quantification of tracers uptake which, as mentioned, offers unique advantages for the assessment of these patients.

Recently the introduction of PET/MR is emerging as a powerful diagnostic tool in several infective, inflammatory or neoplastic diseases. This fact is due to the aforementioned high ability of MRI to image soft tissues and bones determining a number of physiological and metabolic characteristics of human tissue by going beyond plain anatomical imaging. In this setting, different clinical conditions can potentially benefit from PET/MR imaging such as, for example, brain tumour assessment that can be performed with different radiotracers, such as 11C/18F-choline, 11C-methionine, 18F-fluoroetilthyrosine, 18F-fluorothimidine and so on. In addition, the usefulness of PET/MR performed with 18F-FDG and other tracers for the evaluation of breast and prostate cancer has been reported in the past [16].

However, it is important to underline that the high cost of PET/MR technology and the high clinical impact that PET/CT has gained are limiting the use of the first imaging modality to the field of research, also reducing its applications in the clinical setting. Interestingly, some data in literature did not reveal a significant benefit from the use of PET/MR in comparison to PET/CT as long as MRI is only used to provide an anatomical framework. Nevertheless, PET/MR imaging could become more feasible and affordable in the future, resulting in an increase of its clinical applications and indications. As mentioned, prostate cancer has been reported as the first key application in oncology for PET/MR imaging and seemed to have potential applications in the diagnosis of primary tumour by fusing together anatomical and functional information, facilitating targeted biopsy, monitoring tumour aggressiveness, particularly during active surveillance approaches and the early detection of early recurrence. Different studies assessing the role of PET/MR in the field of neurosciences are starting to emerge in particular for functional activation studies, drug challenges and functional connectivity investigations. Similarly, the assessment of cardiac conditions is starting to emerge as a field of application of this hybrid imaging technique [4].

1.3   Challenges, Future Directions and Perspectives

As the previous pages pointed out, the field of hybrid imaging is constantly evolving, and the introduction of several technological advances has been experienced in the past and will probably continue in the future.

In the last few years, artificial intelligence (AI) has been gaining attention due to its increasing application in a variety of fields, including medicine. That said, in the particular setting of nuclear medicine and based on its current evolution, AI would probably have a profound impact in both technological aspects and image reading. In addition, this particular technology is already employed for improving imaging acquisition and

reconstruction, with better attenuation correction, better artefact-free image reconstruction and better anatomical landmarking. Hopefully, these developments would also lead to better image quality, shorter acquisition time and lower radiation exposures. Moreover, even if only in the specific setting of research, AI is already used for providing assistance in image reading, automated disease classification and automated metastases delineation. In this setting, hybrid imaging generates a large amount of multimodality medical data with high complexity and depth, and AI applications promise to facilitate the assessment of different diseases and conditions with high quality and efficiency for lesion detection, characterization and response assessment. Interestingly, oncological applications of AI beyond imaging based tasks will probably focus on a holistic integration of multi-source diagnostic data including radiomics, genomics and metabolomics to personalise diagnostics at the molecular, cellular and organism level. Future patients may therefore benefit from the combination of enhanced image quality and individualized image reporting [17, 18].

Related to the concept of AI, there are also other interesting branches that have emerged in the last few years: radiomics, machine learning and deep learning. The first one is a rapidly evolving field of research that uses the extraction of multiple quantitative metrics from medical images. Similarly, machine learning (ML) is a hot topic of recent clinical research and focuses on the development of algorithms that can use different combinations of features in order to predict a specific target. In addition, deep learning is a class of ML algorithms that use multiple neural networks to progressively extract higher-level features, possibly simulating human decision-making. These entities are starting to demonstrate their value for the assessment of a high amount of neoplastic and benign conditions, and they could hopefully help in the future to reach a more precise final diagnosis in some critical cases, to improve the diagnostic ability of nuclear medicine modalities and to better define some prognostic parameters of patients in order to tailor a specific and focused therapeutic management. In addition, deep learning might benefit from the application of AI in automated raw image pre-processing to refine image quality with promising applications in ultra-low radiation imaging, attenuation correction and denoising. Further areas of implementation include image reconstruction, image processing and automated image analysis by ML approaches. Despite these promising results, it is, however, necessary to underline that in the specific setting of nuclear medicine these fields of research are strictly connected to the technological evolution of the systems used to acquire images, and therefore hybrid imaging evolution will be fundamental for the correct evaluation of the pros and cons of AI, ML, deep learning and radiomics. As an example, several studies have addressed the fact that the extraction of radiomics features could be potentially influenced by the technology used for imaging acquisition, possibly limiting the standardization and the reproducibility of this field of research, reducing therefore its strength in the clinical scenario. In this setting, it is worth underlining that nowadays expectations regarding AI tools in medical imaging have become more critical, and discussions on its implementation focus on the limitations and weaknesses of the technology. Many hurdles remain therefore to be addressed before these branches of research could be implemented in daily routine [18].

One of the main clinical applications of hybrid imaging that in the future will probably require more attention is the field of theranostics. In the past decades a long path has been travelled to incorporate nuclear medicine into theranostics, demonstrating therefore the benefit and precision of personalized medicine. In this setting, there is an increasing understanding of the extensive cancer heterogeneity between different individuals and among cell populations in the same subject. Theranostic approaches are connecting imaging to therapy more than ever, and current nuclear medicine physicians need to focus their expertise in this setting. In addition, it is clear that the technological evolution of imaging devices and hybrid imaging is a fundamental point that could help in the correct assessment of patients in a theranostic setting, resulting therefore in more specific and personalized therapies that could therefore allow a more patient-centred therapeutic approach [19].

References

1. Bonte FJ. The evolution of nuclear medicine. J Nucl Med. 1995;36(10):26N–7N.
2. Anderson CJ, Ling X, Schlyer DJ, Cutler S. A short history of nuclear medicine. In: Radiopharmaceutical chemistry; 2019. p. 11–26. https://doi.org/10.1007/978-3-319-98947-1_2.
3. Brownell AL, Nikkinen P, Liewendahl K. The development of nuclear medicine imaging. Scand J Clin Lab Invest Suppl. 1990;201:119–25. https://doi.org/10.3109/00365519009085808.
4. Jones T, Townsend D. History and future technical innovation in positron emission tomography. J Med Imaging. 2017;4(1):011013. Epub 2017 Mar 31. PMID: 28401173; PMCID: PMC5374360. https://doi.org/10.1117/1.JMI.4.1.011013.
5. Vaz SC, Oliveira F, Herrmann K, Veit-Haibach P. Nuclear medicine and molecular imaging advances in the 21st century. Br J Radiol. 2020;93(1110):20200095. Epub 2020 May 13. https://doi.org/10.1259/bjr.20200095.
6. Hutton BF. The origins of SPECT and SPECT/CT. Eur J Nucl Med Mol Imaging. 2014;41(Suppl 1):S3–16. Epub 2013 Nov 12. https://doi.org/10.1007/s00259-013-2606-5.
7. Beyer T, Freudenberg LS, Townsend DW, Czernin J. The future of hybrid imaging-part 1: hybrid imaging technologies and SPECT/CT. Insights Imaging. 2011;2(2):161–9. Epub 2011 Jan 29. PMID: 23099842; PMCID: PMC3288981. https://doi.org/10.1007/s13244-010-0063-2.
8. Ritt P. Recent developments in SPECT/CT. Semin Nucl Med. 2022;52(3):276–85. Epub 2022 Feb 21. https://doi.org/10.1053/j.semnuclmed.2022.01.004.
9. Beyer T, Freudenberg LS, Czernin J, Townsend DW. The future of hybrid imaging-part 3: PET/MR, small-animal imaging and beyond. Insights Imaging. 2011;2(3):235–46. Epub 2011 Mar 25. Erratum in: Insights Imaging. 2012 Apr;3(2):189. PMID: 22347950; PMCID: PMC3270262. https://doi.org/10.1007/s13244-011-0085-4.
10. Glaudemans AW, Prandini N, Di Girolamo M, Argento G, Lauri C, Lazzeri E, Muto M, Sconfienza LM, Signore A. Hybrid imaging of musculoskeletal infections. Q J Nucl Med Mol Imaging. 2018;62(1):3–13. Epub 2017 Nov 22. https://doi.org/10.23736/S1824-4785.17.03045-X.
11. Palestro CJ, Love C, Schneider R. The evolution of nuclear medicine and the musculoskeletal system. Radiol Clin North Am. 2009;47(3):505–32. PMID: 19361673. https://doi.org/10.1016/j.rcl.2009.01.006.

12. Gaemperli O, Kaufmann PA, Alkadhi H. Cardiac hybrid imaging. Eur J Nucl Med Mol Imaging. 2014;41(Suppl 1):S91–103. https://doi.org/10.1007/s00259-013-2566-9.

13. Camoni L, Santos A, Attard M, Mada MO, Pietrzak AK, Rac S, Rep S, Terwinghe C, Fragoso Costa P. Technologist Committee of the European Association of nuclear medicine (EANM). Best practice for the nuclear medicine technologist in CT-based attenuation correction and calcium score for nuclear cardiology. Eur J Hybrid Imaging. 2020;4(1):11. PMID: 34191150; PMCID: PMC8218053. https://doi.org/10.1186/s41824-020-00080-0.

14. National Research Council (US) and Institute of Medicine (US) Committee on State of the Science of Nuclear Medicine. Advancing nuclear medicine through innovation. Washington, DC: National Academies Press (US); 2007.

15. Schober O, Kiessling F, Debus J, editors. Molecular imaging in oncology (Recent results in Cancer Research, 216). 2nd ed. Berlin: Springer Nature; 2020. ISBN3030426181, 9783030426187 Lunghezza 918 pagine.

16. Aboagye EO, Kraeber-Bodéré F. Highlights lecture EANM 2016: "Embracing molecular imaging and multi-modal imaging: a smart move for nuclear medicine towards personalized medicine". Eur J Nucl Med Mol Imaging. 2017;44(9):1559–74. Epub 2017 Jun 8. PMID: 28597119; PMCID: PMC5506106. https://doi.org/10.1007/s00259-017-3704-6.

17. Seifert R, Weber M, Kocakavuk E, Rischpler C, Kersting D. Artificial intelligence and machine learning in nuclear medicine: future perspectives. Semin Nucl Med. 2021;51(2):170–7. Epub 2020 Sep 12. https://doi.org/10.1053/j.semnuclmed.2020.08.003.

18. Feuerecker B, Heimer MM, Geyer T, Fabritius MP, Gu S, Schachtner B, Beyer L, Ricke J, Gatidis S, Ingrisch M, Cyran CC. Artificial intelligence in oncological hybrid imaging. Nuklearmedizin. 2023;62(5):296–305. English. Epub 2023 Oct 6. https://doi.org/10.1055/a-2157-6810.

19. Gomes Marin JF, Nunes RF, Coutinho AM, Zaniboni EC, Costa LB, Barbosa FG, Queiroz MA, Cerri GG, Buchpiguel CA. Theranostics in nuclear medicine: emerging and re-emerging integrated imaging and therapies in the era of precision oncology. Radiographics. 2020;40(6):1715–40. PMID: 33001789. https://doi.org/10.1148/rg.2020200021.

Hybrid Imaging Specialist: The Professional Evolution

Agata Karolina Pietrzak ⓘ, Luisa Roldão-Pereira ⓘ, Giorgio Testanera ⓘ, and Andrea Santos ⓘ

2.1 Introduction

Nuclear medicine (NM) is a multidisciplinary branch of medicine requiring a broad level of underpinning knowledge including basic, medical and health sciences. Since NM focuses on using various sources of radiation, even the core skills of the NM professional require in-depth knowledge regarding their practical applications. NM as a field carries a great clinical and scientific potential due to a rapid progress, particularly in recent years, focusing on novel technologies and drug development. Accordingly, with the complexity of the field, the broader knowledge, skills and behavioural capabilities are required to sustain more advanced competencies, expected from the contemporaneous NM professional.

Hybrid imaging (HI) originated from the NM and radiologic modalities, combined in one, complex technique. HI can be nowadays considered an advanced imaging modality, requiring a particular understanding of both methods included in the fixture used for diagnosis and inevitably in therapy [1–3]. The most common HI methods are single photon emission tomography/computed tomography (SPECT/CT), positron emission tomography/computed tomography (PET/CT) and positron emission tomography-magnetic resonance imaging (PET/MR) [1–4].

Since the beginning of NM, and HI as a consequence of the field's evolution, various medical professionals have been involved in the procedures and equipment operating. To ensure and maintain the HI efficacy and the highest standards of the procedures' performance, the HI professional is obligated to an extensive understanding of the anatomy, radiobiology, physics, engineering, radiation protection and radiochemistry in efforts to ensure the best patient care and comfort. In addition, the need for continuous improvement seems to be a pillar of the NM workforce routine [5, 6]. The great example of such professionals are commonly recognized NM technologists (NMTs) [4–7] or NM radiographers (NMRs) [6, 7].

A. K. Pietrzak (✉)
Electroradiology Department, Poznan University of Medical Sciences, Poznan, Poland

Nuclear Medicine Department, Greater Poland Cancer Centre, Poznan, Poland
e-mail: apietrzak@ump.edu.pl

L. Roldão-Pereira
Nuclear Medicine/Oncology Department, Maidstone and Tunbridge Wells NHS Trust, Maidstone, UK
e-mail: luisa.roldaopereira@nhs.net

G. Testanera
Faculty of Life Sciences and Medicine, King's College London and Guy's and St Thomas' PET Centre, School of Biomedical Engineering and Imaging Sciences, London, UK
e-mail: giorgio.testanera@kcl.ac.uk

A. Santos
Nuclear Medicine Department, Hospital Cuf Descobertas, Lisbon, Portugal

Some entities such as International Atomic Energy Agency (IAEA), recognized NMTs and NMRs as relevant medical specialists and a significant part of the NM-HI workforce, creating dedicated units focusing on the NMTs and NMRs international cooperation for the purpose of continuous improvement, exchange of experiences and best practices, as well as joint scientific and educational development. Several societies, such as the European Association of Nuclear Medicine (EANM) [8], the European Federation of Radiographer Societies (EFRS) [9], the Society of Nuclear Medicine and Molecular Imaging (SNMMI) [10], the Canadian Association of Medical Radiation Technologists (CAMRT) [11], the Australian and New Zealand Society of Nuclear Medicine (ANZSNM) [12] and many more, actively support this mission by providing a wide platform, thus ensuring international collaboration. The results of those frameworks' activities include developing a series of initiatives and documents, summarizing the entry-level and the advanced set of skills and competencies, reflecting the professional evolution of HI specialists in regards to the historical, geographic and technologic characteristics of the NM field and technologists' background.

2.2 Hybrid Imaging: The NM Professional Development's Catalyst

The imaging in the NM field consists of more than stand-alone functional imaging since the hybrid SPECT/CT and PET/CT scanner prototypes have been introduced to the medical market in 1990 and 2001, respectively [13–15]. Initially, the NM tools have been used to measure the activity of the radiotracers in small organs, such as thyroid glands [3], expanding to the scintigraphy techniques performed with gamma cameras [14], involving bone structures and multiple organ imaging, including the central nervous system or heart. In 1963, Kuhl and Edwards introduced the SPECT system which was then combined with the CT scanning into one complementary system between 1990 and 1992 [14, 16].

The first commercially available hybrid SPECT/CT scanner was released in 1999 [14]. Early transmission scans utilized for the purpose of attenuation correction became a complete and independent technique followed by the development of the PET/CT method [3, 14].

Starting from neuroimaging as initially separately performed PET and CT scanning, the PET/CT study came a long way to the daily clinical practice, gradually becoming an oncological essential and being applied to several other non-oncological diagnoses (i.e. neurological and neurodegenerative diseases' diagnosis) [17, 18]. The HI's introduction in daily clinical routine has not been, however, as swift and convenient as it may seem. Up to this point, the functional NM imaging still gets insufficient recognition [3] due to its complexity both in terms of performance and interpretation for the purpose of medical reporting.

The idea to combine PET and MRI methods arose in 1990 with the first literature mentioned in the doctoral thesis of Raymond Robert Raylman in 1991 [19, 20]. Although the initial PET/MR scans had been obtained in 1997 [21], it took several years to put into practice the idea of simultaneous PET and MRI scanning as an integrated technique (2010) [22]. Since its introduction, the PET/MR became a new HI variation for functional and anatomic imaging in NM, described by some authors as not only a novel option, but also the frontier in the hybrid technology era [20]. The availability of PET/MR scanners remains very low [19] when compared with not only other HI modalities (availability of which is nonetheless still insufficient compared with the demand). Furthermore, the high cost of the technique and its performance significantly impacts the future perspectives of the study accessibility. Compared with the PET/CT, the PET/MR study provides improved soft tissue contrast, better motion correction as well as decreased radiation exposure due to the lack of CT component [19]. Additionally, the possibility to implement the diffusion-weighted imaging (DWI) seems beneficial for the diagnosis and therapy of several diseases [19]. The limitation of the PET/MR method, apart from low availability and high costs, is the necessity to develop study protocols available for clinical applications which are not clearly specified despite the progressive development of the technique [19].

The rise of combined, targeted and personalized diagnostic and therapeutic patients' management approach, commonly recognized as theranostics [23], is inevitably tied with the advanced and modern HI as well as its workforce [23, 24]. Similarly to HI, theranostics came a long way since the first diagnostic/therapeutic compounds became available. The possibility to use and follow the theranostic protocols is ensured by monitoring disease progression and response through hybrid imaging methodologies, especially PET/CT. Although theranostics is not a latter discovery itself, the rapid drug development has been crucial and it has been observed in recent years with the introduction of novel compounds for targeted alpha therapy (TAT) [25–30], complementing or potentially replacing also seemingly novel lutetium-177, which validates the NM steady advancement rate [25–30].

The common denominator of all HI applications is the necessity to operate the advanced and complex equipment; therefore, it cannot be detached from the clinical contribution from the operator. Similarly to the rise and progression of the constantly evolving generation of equipment and protocols, proficiently utilizing techniques and dedicated radiopharmaceuticals, it calls for a reflection on the evolution of the professional capabilities of the NM specialists whose knowledge and expertise do not include solely basic concepts of singular method's characteristics. According to authors [4–7, 22, 23], a team of highly qualified technologists, knowledgeable in each separate element of hybrid technique, is mandatory to ensure service flow and high study efficiency.

2.3   NMTs, NMRs, Technologists: Many Names of One Professional Identity

The term "technologist" was shaped on the basis of the associated technological advancements [31] which is particularly relevant for NMTs who aim to operate the equipment sourced from the

engineering and medical progress combined for the purpose of satisfying the healthcare needs and demands. This correlates with the history of HI developing from the simple and predefined imaging, associated with the conventional roentgenography, up to highly advanced, complex modalities [3, 14, 16]. Since the beginning of radiologic imaging, the person performing the studies has always been present within the medical team. Nevertheless, the initial X-rays have been performed not by technologists but by X-rays inventor, Wilhelm Conrad Röntgen [32] (first mentioned by William Morgan, 1785 [33]), followed by the pioneer use of the invention in the clinical settings by John Hall-Edwards (Birmingham, United Kingdom; UK) on 11 January 1986 for the purpose of surgical operation monitoring [34]. The perspective and evolution of HI started with mentioning NM as a potentially independent field of medicine and science, in Sam Seidlin's report in the *Journal of American Medical Association* in 1946 [35], and its acknowledgement in 1971 by the American Medical Association (AMA) [35].

The medical imaging development dictated the necessity to involve a new, specialized workforce into the daily clinical practice. Initially, the professionals were commonly recognized as technologists, performing X-ray imaging or radiotherapy. In 1920, the American Society of Radiologic Technologists (ASRT) was founded, with the goal of gathering and representing medical technologists, trained in roentgenography, radiology and radiotherapy, willing to learn and develop their profession, aiming for a voice at national level [36]. The rapid development and commercialization of open sources of radiation, along with the evolution of NM modalities, resulted in reforming the existing profession, originating a new group of medical professionals who were assigned duties of study performance as well as radiotracer synthesis. A more defined position for the NMTs or NMRs began to gradually establish itself, often with technologists coming from a background of radiology as well as medical laboratory [37]. The first technologists, although graduated from sciences, have only been trained to perform medical imaging, with no college degree required from the employers. Gradually, the requirements developed along with the technical evolution, with two bodies offering certification: the American Registry of Radiologic Technologists (ARRT), which credentialed radiographers, and the American Society for Clinical Pathology (ASCP) focusing on medical technologists [37]. When NM was recognized as an independent discipline, the Nuclear Medicine Technology Certification Board (NMTCB) had been founded in 1977 [37]. NMTCB started to evaluate and represent professionals whose skills, knowledge and competencies have been considered different from those already established in radiology or radiotherapy—emphasizing the role of NMTs—specialized in NM procedure performance, participating in drug development [37], and eventually—in fusion imaging—key players in the HI evolution. Outside of the United States of America (USA), the profession also experienced its great evolution across the globe. Canadian technologists' certification, depending on the region, consisted of non-academic training (Quebec) and an undergraduate university degree (other parts of the country) [38]. Meanwhile, in Europe, technologists have been involved in medical imaging in Germany, with a professional title of Medical-Technical Assistant of Radiology, certified locally [38]. Furthermore, in the UK, radiographers or medical technical officers (MTOs) stepped into NM daily clinical practice [38] with the particularly relevant basic competencies for the NMTs being published in 1998 [39].

In 2002, the Society of Nuclear Medicine Technologist Section (SNMTS) and the ASRT organized a conference, aiming to establish a consensus in terms of specific regulatory system, recommendations and educational objectives necessary to be covered by the NMTs certification and training in the USA [40]. The leading objective of the meeting was to obtain an agreement between the participating parties: technologists, physicians, educators, several vendors' representatives and various states officials, ensuring the high HI performance standards by education, training and credentialing reached a consensus across the USA [40]. Although the consensus succeeded in the USA, the NMTs training across Europe remain highly heterogeneous [41]. EANM and EFRS released a series of documents aiming to harmonize the skills, knowledge and competencies of NMTs and NMRs as a reference for the local official regulations, ultimately establishing the European Qualification Framework (EQF [42]) benchmarks, proposing entry-level requirements obligatory to fulfil by the bachelors (BSc), master of sciences (MSc) graduates and recently evolving doctors (PhD) [6, 43]. The harmonization of competencies worldwide reflects the professional evolution of the workforce involving NMTs, NMRs, radiographers or technologists. Nevertheless, the title, along with the clear distinction between technologists involved in NM-HI and other medical disciplines, seems essential to develop and maintain the professional identity of this group of specialists [44], which is vital for shaping the direction of the technologists' future careers evolution perspectives.

2.4   EQF 6–8: A Consensus Serving the HI Professional Evolution

The rapid HI advancement in terms of both technical and drug development demands equally active evolution of the medical workforce capability to implement those novel applications in daily clinical practice. Each advancement shapes a new dimension of knowledge and skills necessary to be adapted by the medical professional willing to fulfil the new, advanced set of competencies in the expanding area of requirements and demands. The evolution of NM-HI modalities and resources can be understood as a response to the escalating healthcare needs regarding diagnosis and therapy, especially those observed in oncology. The role of technologists in the growing field of NM becomes more and more inevitable yet often underrepresented due to a non-harmonized curriculum and training worldwide, with the "European" model being highly heterogeneous, resulting in the competencies often relying strictly on the single-institutional protocol or local regulations.

Currently, there is no standardized training model dedicated to the NMTs that fully satisfies the technologists' capabilities in terms of their competencies or involvement in the HI procedures' performance. Nevertheless, the technologists/radiographers community organized in societies as EANM [4, 6, 8] or EFRS [9, 43] exercises certain skills-knowledge-competencies consensuses in efforts to provide a widely recognized and harmonized referential point as an updated regulatory framework proposal. Despite the fact that EANM [4, 6, 8] and EFRS [9, 43] operate on disparate procedural basis and differ considering their leading objectives, mainly due to the independent versus dependent from the national societies background, respectively, the EQFs [6, 42, 43] proposed by the entities seem comparable, depicting the reality observed in several highly developed European countries, with the difference of the document proposed by the EANM focusing on NMTs and EFRS on radiographers as a heterogenous group of professionals, inclusive of NMRs. A great example of such a focal point is the UK, with the reason being that UK NMRs are being offered the most expanded and rigorous advanced competencies when knowledge and skills necessary to obtain specific professional qualifications are considered. Additionally, Portugal with its comprehensive level 6 course, and highly complex credentialing system results in excellent training outcomes. On the other hand, countries such as Poland or those in the Central Europe area represent the most heterogeneous and multidisciplinary curriculum with no possibility to obtain NM-dedicated specialty [38, 45, 46]. The expression of the Polish NMTs evolutionary pathway in accordance with the medical technologies, including HI advancements, is progressing their curriculum and incorporating academic graduation into their training [38, 45, 46]. Starting from the 2-year schools for medical technologists/radiographers/radiotherapy technologists [38], the Polish technologists gained the opportunity to graduate and attain BSc, MSc [46] and—currently—PhD title as well. Nevertheless, the

nomenclature of this group of professionals significantly varies from the currently recognized technologists, NMTs or NMRs as the educational course and the specialists are called "electroradiologists," recognized also in France [38, 45–47]. Additionally, the Polish electroradiologists' graduation and post-graduation opportunities remain heterogeneous across countries with several universities offering BSc courses and only a few—MSc completion, which only enhances the need for the training standardization within the continent. Comparably, the Czech Republic NMTs developed from trained nurses through short-term schooling and finally academic credentialing [38].

The document prepared by the EANM Technologists' Committee in 2017 [6] and endorsed by the EFRS [43] considers all of the above-mentioned variations of curricula focusing on offering solutions that might be considered a well-balanced approach and the European reference for the entry-level set of NMTs' knowledge, skills and competencies. The database consists of several sub-chapters, developed on the basis of the international exchange of data and external revision to ensure the most appropriate consensus in offering the set of skills, knowledge and competencies organized in the entry-level requirements summary. The structure of each document involves the most relevant areas of consideration in accordance with the current state of the knowledge regarding NM-HI applications, shaping the NMT profile as professionally knowledgeable and skilled in 13 pillars of NM field (HI as its core) [6]: establishment of a nuclear medicine department and equipment installation, departmental organization, patient care and welfare, instrumentation quality assurance (imaging, non-imaging and radiation protection instruments), radiopharmacy including PET and SPECT, performance of imaging including PET and SPECT, HI, performance of in vitro tests, radiopharmaceutical therapy procedures, radiation protection, occupational health and safety, research and education. Published in 2017 as EQF for Level 6 (BSc) is now followed by the Level 7 (MSc) document. The EFRS proposed a joint document [43], presenting the knowledge, skills and competencies summary describing Level 7 (MSc) and Level 8 (PhD), defining the advanced practice requirements for radiographers in a variety of disciplines. Despite the obvious differences in scope and nomenclature of the above-mentioned documents, the fundamentals remain very similar: to translate the technical development into the modern technologists' professional profile and updated curriculum, and to propose the accord ensuring a factual competencies' harmonization across Europe.

2.5   Summary

The history of HI development accompanied by professional NMT evolution shows that the NMTs are adaptable, versatile and have adequately increased their scope of practice to meet the demand of the services and the field's evolution, continuously recognizing the need to learn about the adjoining disciplines, and proactively growing as professionals. The professional identity of NMTs is not stagnant, but it has matured along the expansion of capabilities in favour of more integrated care. NMTs and NMRs combine skills and tasks originated from a range of professions, from which they dutifully learned, and eventually morphed in a unique professional profile.

The NMT skillset extends from the production (on-site or in specialized industrial units) to the direct clinical duties, including being proficient in a variety of techniques for radiopharmaceuticals' preparation, quality control and administration, providing insightful day-to-day radiation advice in different contexts, preparing and positioning the patient to obtain high quality images, processing those images and data, presenting and discussing the results with the physicians and ascertaining the need for further imaging. NMTs are also involved in fulfilling the responsibilities regarding waste management, safety of sealed and unsealed sources, quality control of equipment, personal monitoring and operational run of the department. Moreover, the NMTs are the specialists partially or fully responsible for the appropriate communication with the patients and their caregivers.

Following the HI development, the technologists have evolved into being capable of operating PET/MR, different radiation detectors, manual and automated dose dispensers, performing dynamic stress tests, administering and managing side effects of adjuvant drugs such as diuretics, thyroid blockers and in some departments even using contrast agents [48]. Effectively, the technologist is by nature eager to partake in innovation but due to their limited position in staffing levels, they are often needed to maintain the standard functioning of the departments, which prevents them from taking part in many activities for which they are well equipped and versed (e.g. auditing, dosimetry, therapies).

The under-representation of technologists in the decision-making and strategic multidisciplinary medical team results from not only historical heterogeneity and "growing on the ground" of other professions but also due to a lack of well-established knowledge, skills and competencies harmonization worldwide, at times strictly depending solely on the local regulations. That results in the absence of the voice of an experienced technologist in patient advocacy in an era of a patient-centred healthcare system approach, prioritizing the patient's well-being over the technological evolution. That seems highly relevant as the NMT is the professional interacting directly with the patient in all stages of their diagnostic and therapeutic management, where an incredible amount of knowledge and sensitivity to patient's needs are attained. Therefore, continuing to develop documents, establishing the consistent, harmonized worldwide, minimal requirements for each particular stage of education became an essential pillar of securing the future professional evolution of NMTs and NMRs.

References

1. Salvatori M, Rizzo A, Rovera G, Indovina L, Schillaci O. Radiation dose in nuclear medicine: the hybrid imaging. Radiol Med. 2019;124(8):768–76.
2. Cal-Gonzales J, Rausch I, Shiyam Sundar LK, Lassen ML, Muzik O, Moser E, Papp L, Beyer T. Hybrid imaging: instrumentation and data processing. Front Phys. 2018;6:47. https://doi.org/10.3389/fphy.2018.00047.
3. Hicks R, Lau E, Binns D. Hybrid imaging is the future of molecular imaging. Biomed Imaging Interv J. 2007;3(3):e49.
4. Camoni L, Santos A, Attard M, Mada MO, Pietrzak AK, Rac S, Rep S, Terwinghe C, Fragoso CP. Technologist Committee of the European Association of Nuclear Medicine (EANM). Best practice for the nuclear medicine technologist in CT-based attenuation correction and calcium score for nuclear cardiology. Eur J Hybrid Imaging. 2020;4(1):11.
5. Mathews J, Grewal H, Gillan C, Menezes R, Cornacchione P, Catton J. Development of nuclear medicine image quality assessment criteria for use in a technologist peer review program. J Med Imaging Radiat Sci. 2021;52(1):29–36.
6. Fragoso-Costa P, Santos A, Testanera G. EANM Benchmark Document on Nuclear Medicine Technologists' Competencies—Version 1.0 (2017). Official EANM website: https://www.eanm.org/contenteanm/uploads/2020/05/EANM_2017_TC_Benchmark.pdf. Accessed 1 May 2024.
7. IAEA. International Atomic Energy Agency. Nuclear medicine resources manual. Vienna; 2006. Official IAEA website: https://www-pub.iaea.org/mtcd/publications/pdf/pub1198_web.pdf. Accessed 1 May 2024.
8. Official EANM website: Technologists Committee. https://www.eanm.org/about/organs/committees/technologist-2/. Accessed 10 May 2024.
9. Official EFRS website: https://www.efrs.eu/. Accessed 10 May 2024.
10. Official SNMMI website: Technologist section. https://www.snmmi.org/Research/Content.aspx?ItemNumber=5480. Accessed 10 May 2024.
11. Official CAMRT website: https://www.camrt.ca/. Accessed 10 May 2024.
12. Official ANZSNM website: Technologists. https://www.anzsnm.org.au/about-anzsnm/sigs/technologists/. Accessed 10 May 2024.
13. Lammertsma AA. On the origin of hybrid imaging. J Nucl Med. 2020;61(Suppl 2):166S–7S.
14. Hutton BF. The origins of SPECT and SPECT/CT. Eur J Nucl Med Mol Imaging. 2014;41(Suppl 1):S3–16.
15. Beyer T, Townsend DW, Brun T, Kinahan PE, Charron M, Roddy R, Jerin J, Young J, Byars L, Nutt R. A combined PET/CT scanner for clinical oncology. J Nucl Med. 2000;41(8):1369–79.
16. Lang TF, Hasegawa BH, Liew SC, Brown JK, Blankespoor SC, Reilly SM, Gingold EL, Cann CE. Description of a prototype emission-transmission computed tomography imaging system. J Nucl Med. 1992;33(10):1881–7.
17. Traub-Weidinger T, Arbizu J, Barthel H, Boellaard R, Borgwardt L, Brendel M, Cecchin D, Chassoux F, Fraioli F, Garibotto V, Guedj E, Hammers A, Law I, Morbelli S, Tolboom N, Van Weehaeghe D, Verger A, Van Paesschen W, von Oertzen TJ, Zucchetta P, Semah F. EANM practice guidelines for an appropriate use of PET and SPECT for patients with epilepsy. Eur J Nucl Med Mol Imaging. 2024;51:1891. https://doi.org/10.1007/s00259-024-06656-3.
18. Cotta Ramusino M, Massa F, Festari C, Gandolfo F, Nicolosi V, Orini S, Nobili F, Frisoni GB, Morbelli S, Garibotto V, European Inter-Societal Consensus on the Biomarker-Based Diagnosis of Dementia. Diagnostic performance of molecular imaging methods in predicting the progression from mild cognitive impairment to dementia: an updated systematic review. Eur J Nucl Med Mol Imaging. 2024;51:1876. https://doi.org/10.1007/s00259-024-06631-y.
19. Raylman RR. Reduction of positron range effects by the application of a magnetic field: for use with positron emission tomography. University of Michigan ProQuest Dissertation & Theses, 1991.
20. Musafargani S, Ghosh KK, Mishra S, Mahalakshmi P, Padmanabhan P, Gulyás B. PET/MRI: a frontier in era of complementary hybrid imaging. Eur J Hybrid Imaging. 2018;2(1):12.
21. Pollard AC, de la Cerda J, Schuler FW, Kingsley CV, Gammon ST, Pagel MD. Evaluations of the performances of PET and MRI in a simultaneous PET/MRI instrument for pre-clinical imaging. EJNMMI Phys. 2022;9(1):70.
22. Ehman EC, Johnson GB, Villanueva-Meyer JE, Cha S, Leynes AP, Larson PEZ, Hope TA. PET/MRI: where might it replace PET/CT? J Magn Reson Imaging. 2017;46(5):1247–62.
23. Herrmann K, Giovanella L, Santos A, Gear J, Kiratli PO, Kurth J, Denis-Bacelar AM, Hustinx R, Patt M, Wahl RL, Paez D, Giammarile F, Jadvar H, Pandit-Taskar N, Ghesani M, Kunikowska J. Joint EANM, SNMMI and IAEA enabling guide: how to set up a Theranostics Centre. Eur J Nucl Med Mol Imaging. 2022;49(7):2300–9.
24. Gambini JP. Theranostic hybrid molecular imaging. World J Nucl Med. 2014;13(2):73–4.
25. Radzina M, Saule L, Mamis E, Koester U, Cocolios TE, Pajuste E, Kalnina M, Palskis K, Sawitzki Z, Talip Z, Jensen M, Duchemin C, Leufgen K, Stora T. Novel radionuclides for use in nuclear medicine in Europe: where do we stand and where do we go? EJNMMI Radiopharm Chem. 2023;8(1):27.
26. Miederer M, Benešová-Schäfer M, Mamat C, Kästner D, Pretze M, Michler E, Brogsitter C, Kotzerke J,

Kopka K, Scheinberg DA, McDevitt MR. Alpha-emitting radionuclides: current status and future perspectives. Pharmaceuticals (Basel). 2024;17(1):76.

27. Alam MR, Singh SB, Thapaliya S, Shrestha S, Deo S, Khanal K. A review of 177Lutetium-PSMA and 225Actinium-PSMA as emerging theranostic agents in prostate cancer. Cureus. 2022;14(9):e29369.

28. Feuerecker B, Kratochwil C, Ahmadzadehfar H, Morgenstern A, Eiber M, Herrmann K, Pomykala KL. Clinical translation of targeted α-therapy: an evolution or a revolution? J Nucl Med. 2023;64(5):685–92.

29. Taunk NK, Escorcia FE, Lewis JS, Bodei L. Radiopharmaceuticals for cancer diagnosis and therapy: new targets, new therapies-alpha-emitters, novel targets. Cancer J. 2024;30(3):218–23.

30. Jang A, Kendi AT, Johnson GB, Halfdanarson TR, Sartor O. Targeted alpha-particle therapy: a review of current trials. Int J Mol Sci. 2023;24(14):11626.

31. Finkelstein L. Science and practice: the formation of technologists—past, present and future. Meas Control. 1980;13(8):285–93.

32. Obaldo JM, Hertz BE. The early years of nuclear medicine: a retelling. Asia Ocean J Nucl Med Biol. 2021;9(2):207–19.

33. Morgan WXIV. Electrical experiments made in order to ascertain the non-conducting power of a perfect vacuum. Phil Trans R Soc. 1785;75:272–8.

34. Solve K. Discovery of X-ray and Details. OMICS J Radiol. 2021;10(4):e110.

35. Official SNMMI website: https://www.snmmi.org/AboutSNMMI/Content.aspx?ItemNumber=4175. Accessed 2 Jun 2024.

36. Official ASRT website: https://www.asrt.org/main/about-asrt/museum-and-archives/asrt-history. Accessed 2 Jun 2024.

37. Neal K. History of the nuclear medicine technology certification board (NMTCB). J Nucl Med Technol. 2020;48(Suppl):67S–71S.

38. Lass P. Nuclear medicine technologists' training in different countries—a comparison. Nucl Med Rev. 2001;4(2):65–8.

39. British Nuclear Medicine Society Technology Group. Basic competencies for the nuclear medicine technologist. Nucl Med Commun. 1998;19(4):327–34.

40. PET-CT Consensus Conference; SNMTS; American Society of Radiologic Technologists (ASRT). Fusion imaging: a new type of technologist for a new type of technology. July 31, 2002. J Nucl Med Technol. 2002;30(4):201–4.

41. Matos AC, Massa RC, Lucena FM, Vaz TR. Nuclear medicine technologist education and training in Europe: literature and web-based findings. Nucl Med Commun. 2015;36(6):631–5.

42. Description of the eight EQF levels | Europass: https://europa.eu/europass/en/description-eight-eqf-levels. Accessed 1 Jun 2024.

43. The official EFRS website: https://api.efrs.eu/api/assets/posts/208. Accessed 2 Jun 2024.

44. Bailey DS, Harding D. Professional identity and role perception of radiographers and clinical technologists in nuclear medicine - an exploratory qualitative study. Radiography (Lond). 2024;30(1):73–9.

45. Official Jagiellonian University in Krakow website: Electroradiology: https://studia.uj.edu.pl/en_GB/kierunki/wnoz/elektroradiologia. Accessed 3 Jun 2024.

46. Official Poznan University of Medical Sciences website: Electroradiology: https://www.ump.edu.pl/rekrutacja/elektroradiologia. Accessed 3Jun 2024.

47. Larpin F. Les soins cliniques et la formation du manipulateur en électroradiologie médicale [clinical care and training of the medical electroradiology technician]. Rev Infirm. 2023;72(291):44–5.

48. Official British Nuclear Medicine Society website: Professional Standards Committee: https://cdn.ymaws.com/www.bnms.org.uk/resource/resmgr/guidelines/administration_by_non-medica.pdf. Accessed 1 Jun 2024.

Image Formation in Nuclear Medicine

3

Tadeu Takao Almodovar Kubo,
Ana Luiza Silva Lima Kubo,
Franciele Aquiles dos Anjos Silva,
Gustavo Tukamoto, Luíza Lucchesi Cabral de Mello,
and Monica Araujo Pinheiro

3.1 Introduction to Nuclear Medicine and Radiology

Image formation in nuclear medicine plays a fundamental role in diagnosing and monitoring a wide range of clinical conditions. Image formation in computed tomography (CT) and nuclear medicine fundamentally differ in how radiation is used to create images. In CT, images are formed through a transmission process, where X-rays are generated by an external source and pass through the patient's body, being detected on the other side after interacting with various tissues. This method produces images that reflect how different anatomical structures absorb X-rays. In contrast, nuclear medicine imaging relies on emission, where the patient becomes the radiation source. A radiopharmaceutical is administered, emitting radiation from within the body to create the image. This core difference affects both the type of images produced and the information they convey: CT is well suited for detailed anatomical visualization, whereas nuclear medicine excels at capturing physiological and molecular processes. By providing information about the functionality and anatomy of organs and tissues, these images enable radiologists and nuclear medicine physicians to identify pathological changes early and monitor the effectiveness of treatments [1, 2]. Technical concepts, such as resolution, contrast, noise, and image reconstruction, are not merely scientific terms; they directly influence the clarity and precision of the information that clinicians and the multidisciplinary team have at their disposal [3, 4]. For radiologists, understanding these elements is essential for accurately interpreting exams and ensuring that patients receive appropriate diagnosis and treatment. Through a clear understanding of the fundamentals and technologies of image formation, healthcare professionals can make informed decisions, enhancing the safety and effectiveness of patient care [5, 6].

Nuclear medicine is a medical specialty that employs radioisotopes for the diagnosis and treatment of various diseases. It is based on the principle of radioactivity, a natural phenomenon that allows unique visualization of organs and tissues within the human body [6].

The focus of nuclear medicine is the use of radioactive substances known as radiopharmaceuticals. Each of these substances consists of a radioisotope linked to a drug that carries the material to the desired organ or tissue. Radiopharmaceuticals are administered to the patient and emit radiation, which is detected by

T. T. A. Kubo (✉) · A. L. S. L. Kubo
F. A. dos Anjos Silva · G. Tukamoto
L. L. C. de Mello · M. A. Pinheiro
Medical Physics, PhysRAD,
Rio de Janeiro, RJ, Brazil
e-mail: tadeu@physrad.com.br;
analuiza@physrad.com.br; franciele@physrad.com.br;
gustavo@physrad.com.br; luiza@physrad.com.br;
monica@physrad.com.br

© The Author(s), under exclusive license to Springer Nature Switzerland AG 2025
L. Camoni, L. Mansi (eds.), *Nuclear Medicine Hybrid Imaging for Radiographers & Technologists*,
https://doi.org/10.1007/978-3-031-86228-1_3

specific diagnostic equipment. This equipment detects the emitted photons and generates images that provide critical information about the function and structure of the organs being studied [6].

Nuclear medicine has a broad range of applications in diagnostics and is increasingly advancing into the therapeutic area. It is used to diagnose and treat a variety of conditions, from heart disease and cancer to neurological and endocrine disorders. Additionally, nuclear medicine plays a crucial role in medical research, contributing to the development of new therapies [6].

One of the most significant advances in nuclear medicine is the emergence of theranostics, which combines therapy and diagnosis in a single management approach [6]. This approach enables image-guided therapy, assisting in the prospecting and estimation of treatment outcomes in areas that have received the material. For example, the radiopharmaceutical lutetium-177 PSMA (prostate-specific membrane antigen) is used in the treatment of metastatic castration-resistant prostate cancer, allowing both visualization of the treated area and targeted therapy [6].

Today, nuclear medicine is constantly evolving with technological advancements that improve image quality and patient safety [4]. New radiopharmaceuticals are being developed to specifically target different types of cells and tissues, allowing for more precise diagnostics and effective treatments [4]. Furthermore, the integration of nuclear medicine with other imaging modalities, such as CT and magnetic resonance imaging (MRI), is expanding the possibilities for visualizing and understanding the human body [4].

3.2 Fundamental Principles of Nuclear Medicine

Nuclear medicine is a specialty that is based on the use of radioisotopes to diagnose and treat a wide range of medical conditions. This field of medicine combines principles of nuclear physics with imaging techniques to obtain functional and anatomical information of tissues and organs, offering a distinct approach to patient evaluation.

These radioisotopes are carefully selected to bind to specific molecules that will target particular organs or tissues, depending on the purpose of the examination or treatment. Examples of widely used radioisotopes include technetium-99m (for single photon emission computed tomography—SPECT), fluorine-18 (for positron emission tomography—PET), and iodine-131 (for thyroid therapies). Depending on the administered radiopharmaceutical, the human body will naturally eliminate it through a biological half-life, and it will also undergo reduction due to the physical half-life of the material [1].

Half-life is a fundamental concept in nuclear medicine, as it indicates the time required for half of the unstable nuclei of a radioisotope to decay and emit radiation. The choice of a radioisotope for a specific examination depends largely on its half-life, which must be long enough to complete the examination but short enough to minimize the patient's radiation exposure. For example, technetium-99m, with a half-life of approximately 6 h, is ideal for diagnostic imaging exams as it allows for good image quality and relatively low exposure for the patient.

The combination of physical and biological half-life results in the effective half-life, (Eq. 3.1).

$$\frac{1}{T_{1/2\,effective}} = \frac{1}{T_{1/2\,physical}} + \frac{1}{T_{1/2\,biological}} \quad (3.1)$$

3.3 Radioactive Decay

The process of radioactive decay is the spontaneous transformation of unstable nuclei in radioisotopes into stable nuclei, accompanied by the emission of radiation in various forms, such as beta particles, alpha particles, or gamma photons. Each type of radiation has characteristics that determine its application in different exams and treatments. In nuclear medicine, gamma decay is widely used for diagnostic purposes, as gamma photons can pass through the body and be detected by specialized cameras, as seen in SPECT and PET, the latter through positron annihilation. The activity of a sample will decay according to the relation, (Eq. 3.2):

$$A_{final} = A_{initial}{}^* \exp^{-\lambda t} \qquad (3.2)$$

where:

A_{final} = Final activity of a sample or patient (unit MBq);
$A_{initial}$ = Initial activity of a sample or patient (unit MBq);
λ = decay constant specific to each radionuclide (s^{-1});
t = time (s)

and,

$$\lambda = \frac{Ln(2)}{T_{1/2}} \qquad (3.3)$$

$T_{1/2}$ = physical half-life of a sample or effective half-life of a patient according to the radionuclide or radiopharmaceutical, respectively.

3.4 Interaction of Radiation with the Patient

When administered to the patient, radioisotopes in a state of decay release radiation that interacts with body tissues. The emitted radiation reaches the imaging equipment, which detects the location and intensity of metabolic and functional activities in the organs. For example, in PET scans, the decay of fluorine-18 allows for the assessment of the metabolic activity of tumor cells, which generally exhibit higher metabolism.

These physical principles provide the foundation for conducting examinations and treatments in nuclear medicine, supplying nuclear medicine physicians with critical information for accurate diagnosis and effective treatment monitoring. Understanding these characteristics enables the selection of the most appropriate radioisotope for each type of exam or therapy, ensuring the safety and efficacy of the procedure [1].

3.5 Fundamental Concepts of Digital Imaging in Nuclear Medicine and Radiology

Nuclear medicine and radiology have transformed the way we visualize the human body through advanced technologies [5]. Digital images in Digital Imaging and Communications in Medicine (DICOM) format follow a set of standards that ensure secure exchange and storage of these medical data [5]. To work efficiently with these images and understand their limitations, it is essential to know some fundamental concepts, such as:

1. *Pixel*: A pixel is the smallest component of a digital image. It represents a small point of color or intensity. In nuclear medicine images, each pixel can display the amount of radiation detected at a specific point in the body [5]. It is important to note that the image sampling rate must be at least twice as large as the region of interest and appropriate to the system's resolution. For example, to visualize a structure of 1.2 cm, a resolution of less than 0.6 cm is required, according to the Nyquist-Shannon theorem. The pixel size can be adjusted when using tools such as Zoom and Matrix size in nuclear medicine images.

$$\text{Pixel size} = \frac{\text{FOV}}{\text{Matrix} * \text{Zoom factor}} \qquad (3.4)$$

FOV = Field of view
Matrix = One dimension of matrix
Zoom factor = Value adopted for zoom.

2. *Voxel*: A voxel is like a pixel, but in 3D. It represents a small volume instead of a flat area. In three-dimensional images, such as those produced by CT, MRI, or SPECT (in nuclear medicine), voxels form the final image and display information such as tissue density or the amount of radiation in a specific area [5].

3. *Matrix*: The matrix is a grid of pixels that forms the digital image. The matrix size, such as 256 × 256 or 512 × 512, influences image quality. Larger matrices create more detailed images, but require more memory to be processed [5]. In nuclear medicine exams, matrices of 64 × 64 are commonly used for cardiac exams, and 128 × 128 for neurological exams, for example.

4. *Resolution*: Image resolution defines the level of detail it can display. In nuclear medicine, resolution depends on pixel size and equipment characteristics, such as the size of the detector crystal [5].

5. *Contrast*: Contrast is the difference between the light and dark areas of an image. It can be adjusted to highlight important features, such as the presence of tumors, in nuclear medicine images [5].

6. *Noise*: Noise in an image is any unwanted variation in pixel intensity that can distort image quality. Noise may be caused by the equipment or the image capture process, but noise reduction techniques help to improve image quality [5].

7. *Image reconstruction*: Image reconstruction is the process of forming an image from data collected from different angles around the patient. In nuclear medicine, this is done to transform the captured projections into a useful image for diagnosis [1, 5]. We will discuss the available algorithms in more detail below.

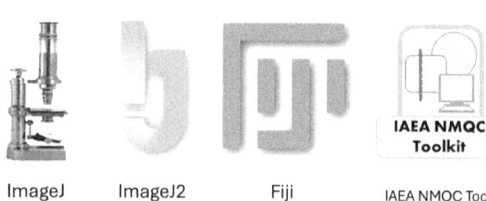

ImageJ   ImageJ2   Fiji   IAEA NMQC Toolkit

Fig. 3.1 Free programs available: ImageJ, ImageJ2, Fiji, and IAEA plugin: IAEA NMQC Toolkit

These concepts are essential for understanding the variables in imaging and how they can be used in nuclear medicine and radiology processing. They form the basis for generating high-quality images that can be used for both diagnosis and treatment planning and follow-up [5].

There are some DICOM medical image repositories that can be accessed for educational purposes and knowledge consolidation. One of the most well-known free programs for working with images is ImageJ (https://imagej.net/), where it is possible to open a DICOM image and study all its parameters. In addition to the ImageJ program, there are nuclear medicine–dedicated plugins, such as those created by the International Atomic Energy Agency—IAEA (IAEA-NMQC-Toolkit), for quality control (QC) assessments of equipment.

In Fig. 3.1, some versions of the available programs are shown, and in Fig. 3.2, some images with extractable variables and available processing options are displayed.

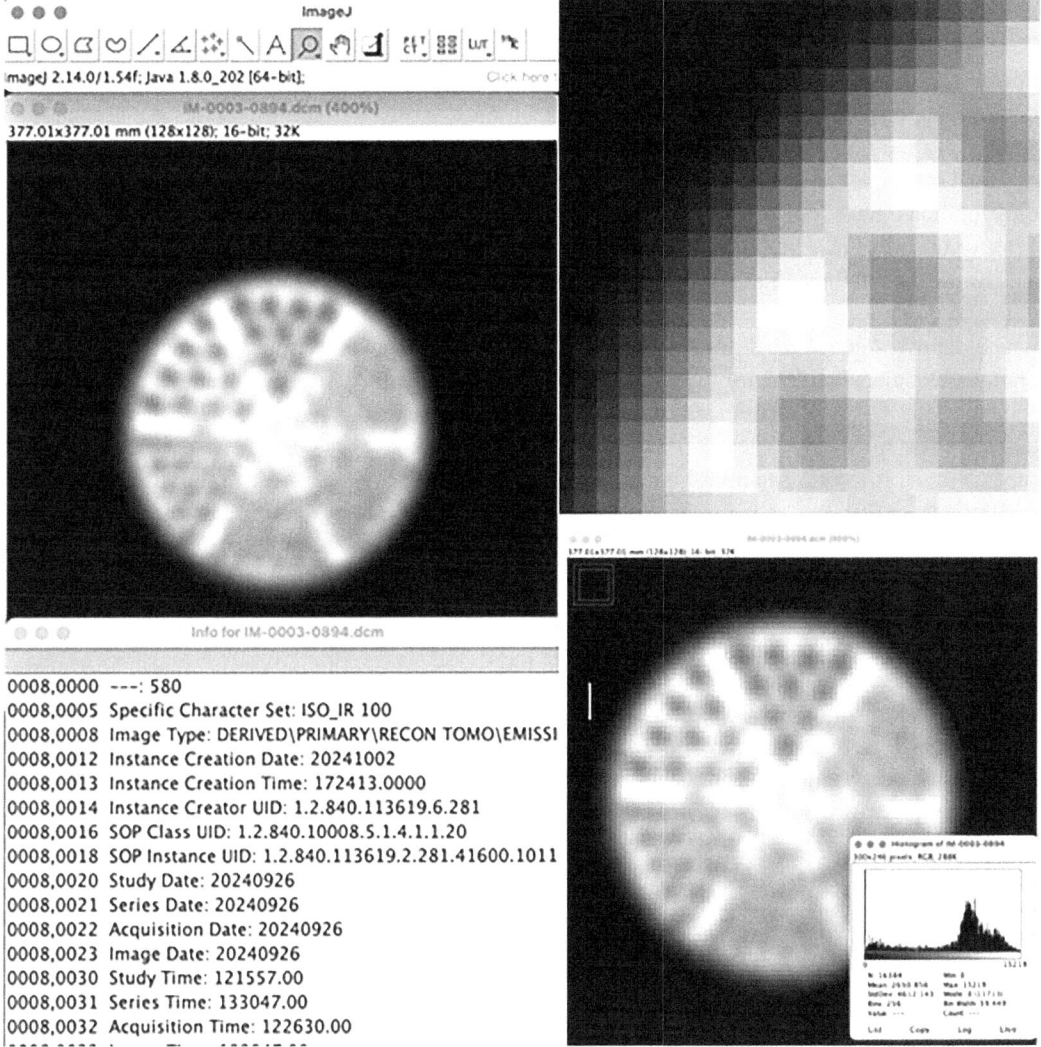

Fig. 3.2 Images from the ImageJ software showing the DICOM header content, image zoom, and pixel distribution histogram

3.6   Steps for Image Formation

After understanding the imaging elements, it is important to learn about the image formation process in nuclear medicine and CT in hybrid equipment. The first step involves administering a radiopharmaceutical to the patient, which, after a few minutes or hours, depending on the type of exam, concentrates in the organs or tissues of interest. The patient is then directed to the imaging equipment, which is typically either a SPECT

or a PET system. These nuclear medicine devices can be dedicated or hybrid, meaning they are combined with CT or even MRI (SPECT/CT, PET/CT, and PET/MR).

3.6.1   SPECT

In SPECT, the image formation process begins when photons emitted from the patient's body reach the equipment. These photons result from the radioactive decay of the radiopharmaceutical. To ensure a higher resolution image, the photons must be collimated before reaching the scintillation system, passing through the first part of the equipment, the collimator. The collimator is an essential component as it acts as a filter, allowing only photons traveling perpendicularly to the detector to reach the scintillation crystal.

The most common collimator in nuclear medicine facilities is the parallel-hole collimator, which improves image resolution by limiting the photons reaching the detector [1]. Additionally, some nuclear medicine equipment use solid-state detectors (such as CZT detectors) and pinhole-type collimators to enhance image quality [7].

While the collimators absorb the photons that come from other directions, the perpendicular photons hit the scintillation crystal, usually made of sodium iodide doped with thallium (NaI(Tl)), which converts the energy of the photons into visible light. The more photons reach the crystal, the more light is generated. This light is then transmitted through an optical connection with optical grease to the photomultiplier tubes, which receive the light and convert it into an electrical signal.

Not all photons received by the system are used for image formation. Depending on the radionuclide used in the study, an energy acceptance window is set by a multichannel analyzer that filters energy pulses, determining which ones can be included in the final image. The approved signals are then converted into digital format and sent to the acquisition station, where the image is generated according to the specific parameters of the study and the radionuclide used.

Finally, this image is transferred to the processing workstation and can be stored in the cloud for redundancy and easy access (Fig. 3.3).

3.6.2 PET

In PET, image formation begins with the administration of a positron-emitting radiopharmaceutical, such as fluorine-18 combined with a glucose analogue (FDG), which is widely used to assess metabolic activity in tissues. This radiopharmaceutical accumulates in specific body regions depending on its affinity for certain tissue types. After a short uptake period in the organs, the

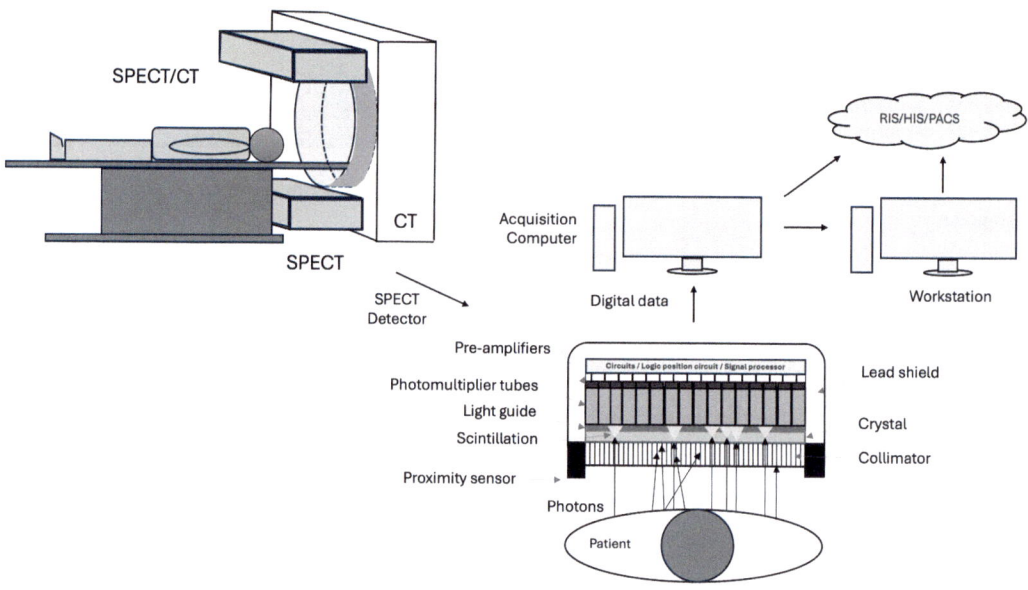

Fig. 3.3 Photon exit from patient, detector collimation, image processing, and cloud storage

patient is positioned in the equipment. The decay of the radioisotope through positron emission occurs inside the body of the patient.

When a positron encounters an electron in the patient's tissue, an annihilation event occurs, generating two high-energy photons (511 keV) that are emitted in opposite directions, forming a 180-degree angle between them. These photons are responsible for image formation in PET.

The annihilation photons are detected by a ring of detectors surrounding the patient, called the gantry. Unlike SPECT, PET does not use collimators; instead, it relies on an electronic system called the coincidence system. When two photons are detected simultaneously on opposite detectors, the system records a coincidence, indicating the line along which the annihilation occurred, known as the line of response (LOR), as shown in Fig. 3.4. This process allows for mapping the approximate location of the emission within the patient's body. It is important to note that some processes can interfere with coincidence image formation:

- Trues (or true coincidences): These are coincidence events that occur when two annihilation photons from a single annihilation reach opposite detectors simultaneously. These are the desired events, as they accurately represent the emission location in the body and contribute to the correct image formation.
- Randoms (or random coincidences): These are coincidence events that occur when two photons from independent, unrelated annihilations reach opposite detectors simultaneously. These events create false information and add noise to the image, reducing its quality. Corrections for these events are necessary to improve image accuracy.
- Singles (or single events): These are photons detected individually without coincidence with an opposite photon. While they do not directly contribute to PET image formation, they are used to calculate and correct random coincidences.

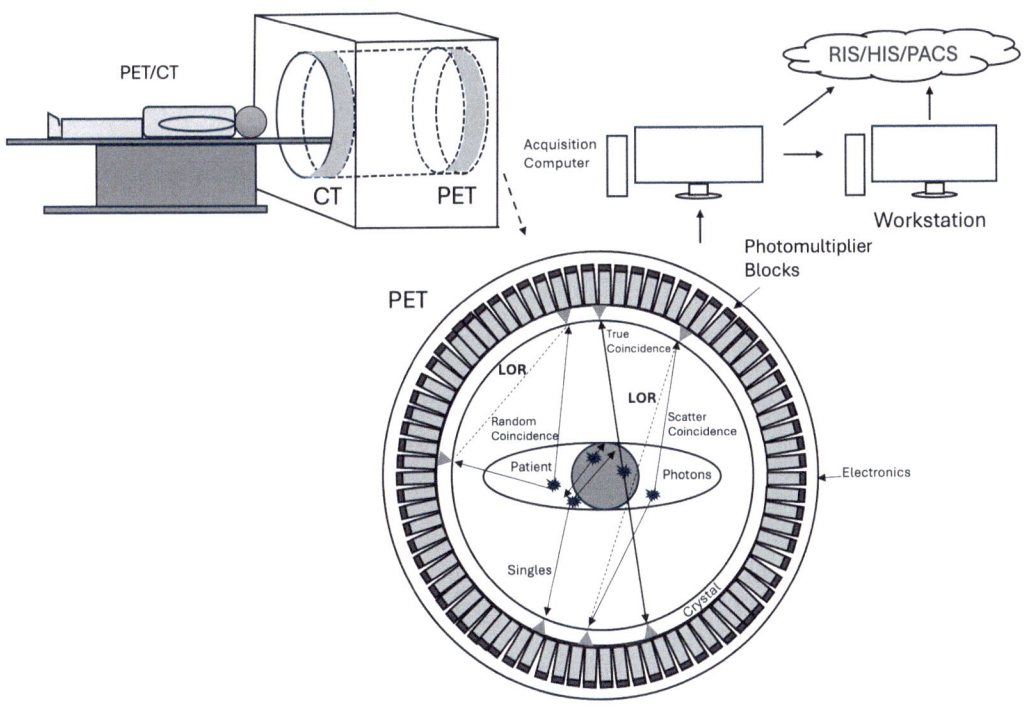

Fig. 3.4 Image formation workflow in PET/CT

To ensure image accuracy, attenuation corrections (to compensate for photon loss while passing through tissues) and scatter corrections (to adjust for photons that change direction) are applied. These corrections are essential to ensure that the detected photons accurately correspond to the emission's point of origin. Some PET systems also detect the temporal difference in the coincidence system. This application is known as time of flight (TOF) [1].

With the registered coincidence information, the system uses reconstruction algorithms, such as iterative reconstruction, to create a three-dimensional image of the radiopharmaceutical's distribution in the body. The result is an image that shows metabolic activity, making it particularly useful for detecting areas with abnormal metabolism, such as tumors.

As with SPECT, the final PET image is processed and sent to a processing workstation, where it can be analyzed, compared with other images, or stored for future reference.

In hybrid systems, such as PET/CT and PET/MR, the functional capabilities of PET are combined with the high-resolution anatomical images of CT or MRI. This combination improves diagnostic accuracy by precisely locating areas of interest and distinguishing them from adjacent structures.

3.7 Introduction to Image Reconstruction Algorithms

In nuclear medicine, image reconstruction is a fundamental process that transforms raw data into diagnostic images. In tomographic systems like SPECT and PET, the detector acquires data from different angles around the patient, creating a series of projections. To transform these projections into usable images, two main reconstruction methods are widely used: filtered back projection (FBP), which is an analytical method, and iterative methods such as maximum likelihood expectation maximization (MLEM) and ordered-subset expectation maximization (OSEM) [8, 9].

3.7.1 Filtered Back Projection (FBP)

FBP is a traditional analytical method that combines projections from each angle to form an image of the organ under study. This process involves applying a filter (usually a ramp filter) to attenuate image artifacts, such as the "star artifact," which can occur due to uneven distribution of counts. FBP has been popular for its speed and simplicity: projections are quickly converted into an image by back-projecting the data onto the image plane [8].

However, FBP is more sensitive to noise, and under conditions of low counts (such as in imaging small organs or patients with high attenuation), it can result in lower quality images, as is often the case in nuclear medicine. The simplicity of FBP remains advantageous for quick exams, but its precision is limited compared to more modern methods, especially in clinical applications that require higher image resolution [9].

3.7.2 Iterative Methods

More advanced iterative methods were developed to overcome the limitations of FBP, particularly in terms of noise reduction and improved image quality. These methods work through a continuous refinement process: an initial image is estimated and then compared to the acquired data. With each iteration, the image is adjusted to better align with the real data, resulting in a more accurate representation with fewer artifacts [8].

- MLEM: This algorithm is based on statistical principles and calculates the likelihood that the reconstructed image is consistent with the collected data. With each iteration, the image is updated, reducing discrepancies between measured data and the estimated image. This process is accurate but relatively slow, as each iteration adjusts all data [9].
- OSEM: A faster variation of MLEM, OSEM divides the projections into subsets, processing them independently before combining

them to refine the image. This technique reduces processing time, making it ideal for modern PET and SPECT systems. OSEM is widely used in tomography as it is more efficient and simultaneously produces high-quality images [10].

3.7.3   Corrections and Image Quality

In addition to reconstruction algorithms, applying corrections for attenuation and scatter is essential to ensure that detected photons accurately correspond to the emission's point of origin within the patient's body. In hybrid systems (such as PET/CT and PET/MR), CT or MRI provides an anatomical reference that can be used for attenuation corrections, improving the accuracy of localization and the sharpness of the final image [8].

Iterative methods also facilitate the use of correction parameters such as TOF, which considers the time difference in photon arrival to more precisely locate the emission area. These corrections are critical for obtaining high-quality diagnostic images, reducing noise and enabling better clinical interpretation, particularly in oncology and cardiology [9].

3.7.4   Choosing the Reconstruction Method in Clinical Practice

The choice between FBP and iterative methods depends on the type of exam and the required image quality. FBP is a practical option for routine exams that require speed and where detailed precision is less critical. Conversely, iterative methods, especially OSEM, are better suited for complex studies that require more detailed resolution and less susceptibility to artifacts, such as myocardial perfusion scans or tumor evaluation.

FBP remains useful for fast applications, but iterative methods are the standard for cases requiring high image quality. The incorporation of corrections and technologies like TOF in modern PET systems further strengthens the preference for iterative methods in current practice.

3.8   Gating Techniques and Their Importance

Patient movement, whether voluntary or involuntary, can significantly affect image quality. SPECT images, for instance, often require relatively long acquisition times, which increases the likelihood of voluntary patient movement. To minimize these movements, physical restraints can help reduce motion artifacts. However, for involuntary movements, such as cardiac and respiratory motion, gating techniques are employed [11].

Gating is an imaging acquisition technique used in nuclear medicine that synchronizes data capture with the patient's heartbeat or respiratory cycle, reducing inconsistent images and other movement-induced artifacts. To perform gating, monitoring devices are needed, such as electrocardiogram (ECG) electrodes for cardiac monitoring or an abdominal band that generates an electrical signal during respiration, or a camera-based fiducial marker system [1].

Data acquisition can then be controlled by physiological signals, such as cardiac or respiratory signals. In cases of repetitive signals, data from multiple cycles are combined and summed to achieve a sufficient count for image reconstruction. A cycle refers to the period in which a movement completes one full repetition, often comprising several images in the same phase of the movement [3].

For cardiac gating, synchronization is achieved based on specific cardiac events and cycle length. The duration of systole (contraction) and the initial phase of diastole (relaxation) varies according to cycle length, with the most variation occurring between the initial relaxation phase and atrial contraction (diastasis) [3].

Respiratory gating, in contrast, is based on methods such as measuring lung air volume (plethysmography), changes in chest or abdominal position, or imaging data. Plethysmography can be measured by airflow rate or by temperature changes in the air during inhalation and exhalation. Corrections may be required to avoid accumulated errors from cycle to cycle, caused by chest impedance and thoracoabdominal motion. Although complex, respiratory gating is becoming more common in high-resolution, quantitative PET imaging [3].

Gated imaging can be performed in frame mode or list mode. In frame mode, movement signals initiate the acquisition cycle, capturing images at specific phases of the cycle, such as cardiac or respiratory cycles, assuming the movement is consistently repeated in each cycle. In list mode, however, the system continuously records movement signals along with detector data, enabling retrospective synchronization and image creation in various phases of the movement. This approach offers greater flexibility by allowing motion synchronization adjustments after data acquisition. In both modes, images obtained over multiple cycles are combined to ensure a sufficient total count, resulting in statistically reliable images for diagnostic interpretation [12].

As highlighted by Kesner et al., real-time motion correction is essential in PET imaging to improve image quality and accuracy, especially in cases of significant patient movement, such as cardiac and respiratory exams [12]. The study explores correction methods that occur simultaneously with data acquisition, which is advantageous because it reduces the need for re-acquisitions and increases diagnostic efficiency. Additionally, as noted by Kesner et al., this dynamic correction enables more precise image quantification by capturing motion signals concurrently with emission data, resulting in clearer and more detailed images, which are critical for high-precision diagnostics [12].

Movement is a factor that can affect the quality of tomographic images, particularly for small objects, such as tumors, and less so for larger structures, like the liver. Gating is a crucial tool to minimize image degradation caused by movement, ensuring more accurate and reliable images [11].

3.9 Critical Components in Creating High-Quality Nuclear Medicine Images

The quality of an image must always align with the clinical purpose, whether for diagnosis or therapy. In nuclear medicine, for example, a CT image can be used as an anatomical reference for patient positioning and attenuation correction mapping, typically at a lower dose, thus limited in value for comprehensive clinical diagnosis. In this case, the CT image is primarily used for anatomical localization and planning, rather than for a detailed clinical report. However, if a full diagnostic CT scan is required, it can also be performed on the same hybrid nuclear medicine equipment, using parameters optimized for radiological diagnosis [11].

With advancements in semi-quantitative and quantitative techniques, such as in internal dosimetry, it is essential to distinguish between images processed solely for diagnostic visualization and those intended for detailed quantification. A low-resolution image may suffice for identifying the general location of organs, but an image intended for quantification requires higher quality processing, as it will be segmented and analyzed to extract data that will directly impact clinical management decisions [13].

Critical variables such as matrix size, scan speed, number of projections, acquisition time or statistics per projection, frames per second in dynamic studies, and the type of reconstruction algorithm applied directly influence the accuracy and reproducibility of quantitative data. Additionally, factors such as differences in FOV, equipment calibration, and operator technique variations can introduce significant uncertainties in quantitative assessments, such as standardized uptake value (SUV) and internal dosimetry. Alongside technical parameters, patient-specific clinical factors can also compromise high-quality assessments (Table 3.1) [14–16].

Achieving high-quality nuclear medicine images requires a balance between technical and biological factors that influence both image quality and quantitative accuracy. Parameters such as

Table 3.1 Biological and technical factors affecting SUV measurements in PET/CT assessments (adapted from [16])

Factor type	Factor	Description	Impact
Biological	Body composition	Higher body fat in heavier patients leads to higher SUV	SUV up to double in heavier patients
	Body size calculation	Body weight may fluctuate during treatment; body surface area or lean body mass is more stable	Corrections remove weight dependence on SUV
	Blood glucose level	High blood glucose levels competitively inhibit FDG uptake	SUV drop by more than 50% after glucose loading; corrections rarely needed
	Postinjection uptake time	FDG clears faster in normal tissue; longer scan times can increase SUV	SUV up to 30% higher for 4-h vs. 1-h uptake times
	Respiratory motion	Breathing can cause attenuation correction errors and SUV bias	SUV changes up to 30%
Technical	Scanner variability	Differences in detector design and TOF capability affect SUV	SUV differences up to 22.6% between scanners
	Reconstruction parameters	Matrix size, FOV and TOF impact SUV, especially for small lesions	SUV differences up to 12% for 1 cm spheres
	Calibration between scanner and dose calibrator	Improper calibration results in SUV errors	SUV errors up to 10%
	Timing mismatch	Decay correction errors between injection and scan time affect calculated SUV	SUV error up to 5% for an 8-min timing difference
	Use of contrast in PET/CT	Incorrect attenuation correction between contrast and noncontrast studies affects SUV	SUV differences up to 5.9%
	Interobserver variability	Different observers may define ROIs and voxels differently	SUV variation up to 17% in some measurements

matrix size, acquisition timing, reconstruction algorithms, and calibration must be optimized to minimize uncertainties. Additionally, biological variables, such as body composition and glucose levels, can impact SUV measurements and must be accounted for during interpretation. By understanding and controlling these critical factors, radiologists and nuclear medicine professionals can ensure that SPECT/CT and PET/CT assessments provide reliable and clinically valuable data, supporting more precise diagnoses and treatment planning, which fundamentally contribute to a better care for the patients.

To fully realize these goals, however, a focus on technical and biological factors alone is not sufficient; robust QC processes are also essential to maintaining image accuracy and reliability. Regular QC checks help ensure that equipment, calibration, and software are functioning optimally, minimizing variations and errors that could compromise both image quality and SUV precision. Comprehensive QC protocols—such as daily calibration, uniformity checks, and periodic validation of dose calibrators—play a critical role in maintaining consistency across exams over time. By adhering to rigorous QC standards, radiology and nuclear medicine teams can further reduce uncertainties in measurements and consistently provide high-quality images that enable accurate diagnoses and effective treatment planning, providing a better approach to patient care.

References

1. Cherry SR, Sorenson JA, Phelps ME. Physics in nuclear medicine. 4th ed. Philadelphia: Elsevier Saunders; 2012.
2. Powsner RA, Palmer MR, Powsner ER. Essentials of nuclear medicine physics, instrumentation and radiation biology. 4th ed. Hoboken, NJ: Wiley; 2022.
3. Bailey DL, Humm JL, Todd-Pokropek A, Aswegen A. Nuclear medicine physics: a handbook for students and teachers. Vienna: International Atomic Energy Agency; 2014.
4. Echavidre W, Fagret D, Faraggi M, Picco V, Montemagno C. Recent pre-clinical advancements in nuclear medicine: pioneering the path to a limitless future. Cancer. 2023;15(19):4839.
5. Kotina E, Ploskikh V, Shirokolobov A. Digital image processing in nuclear medicine. Phys Part Nucl. 2022;53:535–5401.
6. Weber WA, Czernin J, Anderson CJ, Badawi RD, Barthel H, Bengel F, et al. The future of nuclear medicine, molecular imaging, and theranostics. J Nucl Med. 2020;61(Supplement 2):263S–72S.
7. Imbert L, Poussier S, Franken PR, Songy B, Verger A, Morel O, et al. Compared performance of high-sensitivity cameras dedicated to myocardial perfusion SPECT: a comprehensive analysis of phantom and human images. J Nucl Med. 2012;53(12):1897–903. https://doi.org/10.2967/jnumed.112.107417.
8. Pan T, Mawlawi O. Image reconstruction in PET/CT and SPECT/CT. J Nucl Med Technol. 2019;47(4):295–304.
9. Reader AJ, Verhaeghe J. Comparison of PET iterative reconstruction algorithms: a review. J Nucl Med. 2020;61(5):1015–24.
10. van Sluis J, de Jong J, Schaar J, et al. Performance characteristics of the digital biograph vision PET/CT system. J Nucl Med. 2019;60(7):1031–6.
11. IAEA—International Atomic Energy Agency. Quantitative nuclear medicine imaging: concepts, requirements and methods. In: Human health reports, no. 9. Vienna: IAEA; 2014.
12. Kesner AL, Schmidtlein CR, Kuntner C. Real-time data-driven motion correction in PET. EJNMMI Phys. 2019;6(3):1–6.
13. Bailey DL, Willowson KP. An evidence-based review of quantitative SPECT imaging and potential clinical applications. J Nucl Med. 2013;54(1):83–9.
14. Lee JS, Lee DS, Kim HJ, et al. Quantitative evaluation of PET/CT image quality for attenuation-corrected PET reconstruction. EJNMMI Phys. 2015;2:7.
15. Dewaraja YK, Ljungberg M, Green AJ, et al. MIRD Pamphlet No. 23: quantitative SPECT for patient-specific 3-dimensional dosimetry in internal radionuclide therapy. J Nucl Med. 2012;53(8):1310–25.
16. Adams MC, Turkington TG, Wilson JM, Wong TZ. A systematic review of the factors affecting accuracy of SUV measurements. Am J Roentgenol. 2010;195(2):310–20.

Fundamentals in SPECT/CT

4

David Gilmore, Daniel Tempesta, Roberto Rinaldi, and Luca Camoni

4.1 Introduction

Single photon emission computed tomography (SPECT) has offered greatly improved resolution over nuclear medicine planar imaging as well as tomographic (three-dimensional) data. The basic principle of SPECT works by acquiring many planar images (x and y planes) called projections and reconstructing them into a three-dimensional image (x, y, and z planes). SPECT helps to solve several problems of planar imaging including low resolution, overlaying anatomy, and shine-through. The creation of hybrid systems partnering SPECT and computed tomography (CT) imaging together has further improved SPECT imaging because CT data can provide attenuation correction and anatomical correlation.

D. Gilmore (✉)
Nuclear Medicine Technology, Massachusetts College of Pharmacy and Health Sciences, Boston, MA, USA
e-mail: David.Gilmore@mcphs.edu

D. Tempesta
Department of Nuclear Medicine, Dana-Farber Cancer Institute, Boston, MA, USA
e-mail: Daniel_Tempesta@DFCI.harvard.edu

R. Rinaldi · L. Camoni
Department of Nuclear Medicine, University of Brescia and ASST Spedali Civili di Brescia, Brescia, Italy
e-mail: roberto.rinaldi@unibs.it;
luca.camoni@unibs.it

4.2 Gamma Camera Design

Manufacturers have developed many different styles of gamma cameras capable of performing SPECT and SPECT/CT. Despite this variety, a conventional gamma camera is composed of several typical components: a collimator, a scintillator crystal plate connected to an array of photomultiplier tubes (Fig. 4.1), and a data acquisition and processing electronics system, collectively known as the "head" of the gamma camera. The most traditional design is the typical lay-down gamma camera fitted with one, two, or three heads (detectors). As a general rule, increasing the number of heads will increase resolution of the images and also decrease the overall scan time [1].

In the gamma camera, the scintillator crystal is essential for detecting γ-rays by absorbing their energy, with the likelihood of interaction influenced by the crystal's thickness and material properties. Sodium iodide activated with thallium (NaI(Tl)) is the preferred scintillator material due to its effectiveness and cost, though it requires sealing to prevent moisture damage and shielding from light because of its hygroscopic nature. When γ-rays excite the scintillator, it emits light in the visible or near-ultraviolet range. After the scintillator produces a flash of light, photomultiplier tubes capture the total energy, which corresponds to the incident photon's energy, and generate amplified electrical signals proportional

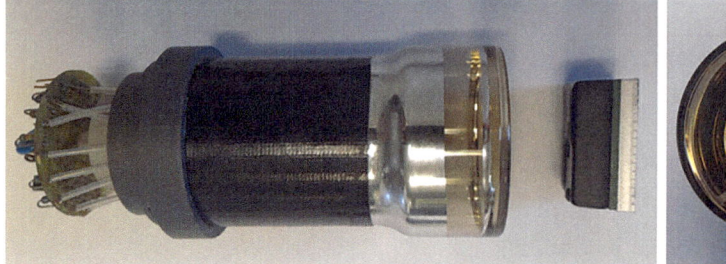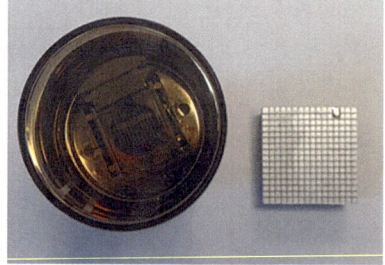

Fig. 4.1 The left side of the image shows lateral and frontal views of a traditional NaI(Tl) photomultiplier, while the right side displays an example of a modern digital detector used in last generation gamma cameras

to the light received. The electrons generated by the photomultiplier tubes are accelerated by a negative potential difference within the tube. A series of dynodes, metal plates at increasing potentials, amplify the number of electrons. Each dynode emits secondary electrons when struck, creating a cascade effect that further amplifies the electrical signal output.

The sum of the signals from the photomultipliers provides a measure of the energy deposited by the γ-ray. This data is processed electronically and sent to a computer for analysis. The γ-ray's impact point on the crystal is determined by calculating the centroid of the light distribution based on the spatial distribution of the signals from the photomultipliers. The summed signals are used to select photons with energies within specific energy windows, while others are discarded. This process, known as energy windowing, is specific to each isotope used in the imaging procedure. The energy window is defined by the photopeak energy and its width, typically expressed as a percentage of the photopeak. For example, when using 99mTc, the energy window is centered on the 140 keV photopeak with a 10% width, allowing the camera to accept photons with energies between 126 and 154 keV. This selective process ensures that only photons emitted by the source of interest, which have not undergone Compton scattering, are utilized for image formation.

A crucial aspect of gamma camera design for managing Compton scattering and determining image resolution and sensitivity is the collimator [2]. The collimator blocks gamma photons that are not aligned with the intended trajectory,

ensuring that the detected photons accurately represent the distribution of activity within the patient. To minimize the effects of Compton scattering, collimators are constructed from materials with high γ-ray absorption capabilities, favoring those with high atomic numbers and densities, such as lead or tungsten alloys.

The performance of a collimator is characterized by parameters such as hole diameter, septal thickness, and the distance between the collimator and the patient. For example, smaller hole diameters and thicker septa enhance spatial resolution but reduce sensitivity, as fewer photons are captured. Conversely, larger hole sizes increase sensitivity at the expense of spatial resolution.

Collimators are categorized based on their geometry, hole shape, and size. The geometry of a collimator defines the acceptance criteria for photons incident on the gamma camera. Common types include parallel-hole, pinhole, and converging or diverging collimators.

Parallel-hole collimators, the most commonly used type, consist of a block with parallel holes aligned perpendicular to the detector. This geometry offers a wide field of view and provides a true-to-scale projection of the activity distribution within the patient. Ideally, parallel-hole collimators allow only γ-rays traveling orthogonally to the detector to pass through. However, due to the finite size of the holes, the collimator also accepts photons within a specific angular range, with larger holes or shorter lengths reducing spatial resolution. Parallel-hole collimators are classified by their spatial resolution, efficiency, and energy application range. Examples include LEHR (low energy, high-resolution) for high spatial resolution with low-energy γ-rays, LEGP (low energy general-purpose) for a balance between resolution and efficiency, MEGP (medium energy general-purpose) for intermediate-energy γ-rays, and HEGP (high energy general-purpose) for high-energy γ-rays.

Pinhole collimators are specifically designed for high-resolution imaging of small objects. They consist of a single, double-cone-shaped hole that provides an inverted and either magnified or reduced image depending on the distance between the object and the collimator. Pinhole collimators achieve high spatial resolution, especially with smaller pinholes, although their efficiency decreases rapidly as the object-to-pinhole distance increases. The field of view also depends on this distance, with efficiency being higher for closer objects. Using multiple pinholes (multi-pinhole designs) increases both the field of view and overall sensitivity, making pinhole collimators ideal for high-resolution imaging in clinical gamma cameras.

Converging hole collimators magnify the image on the detector, making them suitable for imaging objects smaller than the detector. Due to their geometry, these collimators are more efficient than parallel-hole collimators, offering either higher sensitivity or better spatial resolution for small objects, although they reduce the field of view.

Historically, divergent collimators were also used, though they are now rare and seldom seen. Divergent collimators were designed for imaging larger objects than the detector itself. Both converging and diverging collimators, however, introduce image distortion, with magnification depending on the distance between the source and the collimator. This distortion is particularly significant in planar imaging but can be corrected in tomography through accurate collimator modeling in the reconstruction algorithm.

Collimators are integrated with position sensitive devices (PSDs). PSDs are designed to detect and respond to any contact or undue pressure between the gamma camera's head and the patient. These sensors are strategically placed on the surface of the collimators or head and are sensitive enough to halt the movement of the camera

in case of unintentional contact, thereby preventing any potential injury to the patient. This system acts as a safeguard, ensuring that the heavy and delicate equipment used in imaging does not cause harm, especially during close-proximity imaging required for optimal results. In addition, some systems use light rails on opposite sides of the detector heads to detect any object that passes between them, such as the patient, to prevent collisions with the collimator before they happen.

4.3 Image Acquisition

Understanding the design of the gamma camera makes it clear why the most common exam performed with this device is called "scintigraphy." The etymology is directly linked to the camera's design: scintillation + -graphy, a name derived from the scintillation crystal and the images produced using this technology. This nuclear medicine technique measures the local concentration of radiopharmaceuticals that emit γ-rays within the body. Scintigraphy is an "emission" technique, a single-photon emission imaging, where photons are emitted from within the body following the γ decay of an injected radioisotope. The γ-rays are then collected and converted into images, as previously described. This technique provides functional images that display the spatial distribution and intensity of biological, metabolic, or molecular processes.

Single-photon emission imaging can be performed in two primary modes: planar and tomographic. Planar imaging, often referred to as scintigraphy, captures a single projection of the radiopharmaceutical distribution and includes several submodalities such as static planar acquisition, dynamic acquisition, gated acquisition, and whole-body acquisition. In contrast, tomographic imaging, known as SPECT, allows for the three-dimensional reconstruction of radiopharmaceutical distribution by visualizing it across various sections, which are derived from a set of planar projections acquired at different rotational angles around the patient. When necessary, gated imaging can also be integrated into this process. Both planar and tomographic techniques are widely employed in clinical practice, with the gamma camera serving as the detector for both methods. The selection of the imaging mode is influenced by the specific diagnostic requirements, the area of interest within the patient's body, and the level of detail needed for accurate diagnosis.

In a static planar acquisition, the detector remains stationary relative to the patient, capturing all photons that reach the detection plane. This technique produces a single projection image by superimposing multiple depth planes, often necessitating several projections—such as anterior, posterior, and lateral views—to accurately distinguish between different anatomical structures.

Dynamic acquisition expands upon static planar imaging by capturing a series of images over time, which enables the observation of changes in radiopharmaceutical distribution. The acquisition is divided into frames, with the duration and number of frames carefully adjusted to match the biological process being examined.

Gated acquisition is a specialized mode predominantly used in cardiac imaging, where the timing of image capture is synchronized with the patient's ECG, specifically using the R-wave as a trigger. This approach produces a sequence of images representing different phases of the cardiac cycle, which are then combined to create an averaged depiction of the cycle. The most commonly used method in this context is frame mode, where the cardiac cycle is segmented into a predetermined number of frames, capturing the heart's motion across multiple cycles to ensure detailed and accurate functional cardiac assessments.

Whole-body acquisition is employed for imaging that covers regions beyond the axial field of view (FOV) of the gamma camera, typically needed in studies like bone scintigraphy or metastasis detection. Modern gamma cameras facilitate this by moving the patient table at a constant speed during scanning, allowing for the continuous capture of the entire body. Dual-detector systems further enhance this process by enabling simultaneous anterior and posterior projections, thereby improving both the efficiency of the procedure and the quality of the resulting images.

SPECT represents a tomographic acquisition mode where the gamma camera rotates around the patient, capturing images from multiple angles to enable the 3D reconstruction of the radiopharmaceutical distribution. SPECT is particularly valuable for providing detailed spatial information, surpassing the capabilities of planar imaging alone. Gated SPECT combines SPECT with gated acquisition, allowing for the capture of cardiac cycle data from multiple angles. This technique is particularly useful in cardiac imaging, as it provides both functional and structural information, significantly enhancing diagnostic accuracy and reliability.

4.4 SPECT-CT Imaging

SPECT offers improved resolution and three-dimensional imaging. A SPECT tomograph typically consists of two or three rotating heads, each equipped with its own collimator, that move around the patient. The system is connected to a computer that controls both data acquisition and detector rotation. During rotation, the number of planar images acquired during a SPECT acquisition are called views or projections, typically with dimensions of 64 × 64 or 128 × 128 pixels [3], representing a single section of the object, and their number depends on the orbit and resolution level desired. Tomographic acquisition is considered complete when projections are acquired from sufficient angular positions over at least 180°.

The path which the detectors take during acquisition and the mode of rotation can influence the image quality. The two modes in which the detectors move around the patient are known as continuous SPECT and step-and-shoot SPECT. As their names suggest, step-and-shoot SPECT works by acquiring each projection with the detector stationary until it moves to the next projection while continuous SPECT works by acquiring data around the patient without stopping.

There are three types of orbits, named circular, elliptical, and body contour, that can be used to acquire SPECT images. As the name suggests, the detectors move around the patient in a circle during a circular orbit. Elliptical orbits offer better contouring to the patient's body, especially around the chest and torso, if the patient is lying prone or supine. Lastly, body contour orbits move in as close as possible to the patient and end up creating a path around the patient that resembles the contour of the patient's body. Body contour orbits, and sometimes others, take advantage of light rail technology where the detectors are fitted with light beam sensors or an electromagnetic field-based technology allowing the detectors to move in very close to the patient without touching them. The organ of interest and body habitus of the patient should be taken into account when selecting the type of orbit to maximize resolution and prevent detector collisions with the patient.

Nevertheless, SPECT alone often lacks the detailed anatomical context needed to accurately localize functional abnormalities. This is where CT becomes invaluable, providing the morphological detail that SPECT cannot. By fusing SPECT with CT images, clinicians can obtain a broad view, combining both functional and structural information. This fused imaging is particularly beneficial in fields such as oncology, cardiology, and neurology, where precise localization and characterization of lesions are critical. The integration of CT into SPECT not only enhances anatomical correlation but also plays an important role in overcoming one of SPECT's major limitations: gamma-ray attenuation. Attenuation is particularly pronounced in SPECT, especially with 99mTc, a commonly used radionuclide, following an exponential law.

CT operates on the principle of X-ray attenuation, where X-rays passing through the body are absorbed by different tissues to varying degrees, depending on their density. The data collected from multiple angles around the patient are reconstructed into cross-sectional images, providing a detailed view of the body's internal structures. In a typical SPECT/CT system, the CT component usually employs a third-generation scanner equipped with a fan-beam X-ray source and a curved, multirow detector array. This configuration allows for the simultaneous acquisition of multiple slices, a process known as multislice or volume CT. During a spiral or helical acquisition, the X-ray tube continuously rotates around the patient while the table moves through the gantry, resulting in a spiral data collection path. This method is highly efficient and produces high-quality images, essential for accurate anatomical correlation with SPECT data.

The raw data from a CT scan are stored as sinograms, which graphically represent the attenuation values of X-rays at various angles and positions. These sinograms are processed using reconstruction algorithms, such as filtered back projection (FBP) or iterative reconstruction, to generate the final CT images. Each pixel in these images corresponds to a voxel in the patient's body, with its intensity reflecting the attenuation of X-rays, expressed in Hounsfield units (HUs). In a SPECT/CT system, the attenuation correction map is obtained directly from the CT image, with the values rescaled from CT X-ray energy to the γ-ray energy used in SPECT.

The Hounsfield scale, central to CT imaging, is directly linked to tissue density, with air typically at -1000 HU, water at 0 HU, and dense bone around $+3000$ HU. Due to the wide range of Hounsfield units in human tissues, it is often impossible to clearly visualize all tissue types in a single image. To address this, CT windowing is employed, allowing a specific range of HU values to be selected and mapped to the grayscale levels of the image. This technique enhances the visibility of certain tissues by focusing on a narrow band of HU values. For example, a soft tissue window (typically with a window width of 400 HU and a window level of 40 HU) optimally displays structures such as muscles and organs. In contrast, a lung window might use a width of 1000 HU and a level of -700 HU to better visualize air-filled structures.

4.5   Imaging Correction Parameters

To ensure optimal image quality and accurate diagnostic information in SPECT imaging, it is crucial to combine the careful selection of acquisition parameters with the application of essential correction parameters. These corrections are designed to address distortions inherent in the gamma camera system, which includes the scintillator, photomultipliers, and associated electronics, thereby enhancing the reliability of the scintigraphic data. It is essential to preset specific correction parameters. Despite the differences in design and operation across various gamma camera systems, the most commonly used correction parameters are the energy correction map, spatial linearity correction map, and uniformity correction map.

For a monoenergetic source like 99mTc with a peak energy at 140 keV, the ideal situation would have consistent centroid values of the photopeak across all x, y coordinates. However, variations in the scintillator crystal and differences in the efficiency of photomultipliers can cause nonuniform photopeak values across the detector. This inconsistency is corrected by applying an energy correction map, which is periodically generated and used during scintigraphic examinations. Depending on the gamma camera's design, this correction might be managed with a single map for all isotopes or multiple maps specific to different energy ranges or isotopes.

Photomultipliers do not respond uniformly to light across the entire crystal surface, potentially leading to spatial distortions in the acquired image. To correct these distortions, a spatial linearity correction map is created using a phantom with known geometric properties. This map adjusts for deviations by comparing the measured distances in the image with the phantom's known values. The creation and application of this correction map are integral to the routine maintenance of the gamma camera, ensuring spatial accuracy for all isotopes or tailored to specific ones as needed.

Uniformity correction maps address variations in counting efficiency across the detector's field of view (FOV). These maps can be intrinsic (without a collimator) or system-based (with a collimator) and are typically generated for each isotope and collimator combination. By uniformly irradiating the detector and calculating correction factors for each pixel, these maps ensure consistent image quality across the entire FOV during the acquisition process.

By integrating these correction maps with carefully selected acquisition parameters, such as the energy window, matrix size, and zoom factor, the SPECT imaging process can be significantly optimized. This broad approach ensures that the resulting images are not only of high quality but also provide precise functional and anatomical information when fused with CT data in hybrid imaging systems. The ability to correct for system distortions while finely tuning imaging parameters makes SPECT/CT a powerful tool in modern diagnostics, allowing for detailed visualization and accurate localization of pathophysiological processes.

4.6   Processing

Filtered back projection and iterative reconstruction are the two primary ways to process SPECT projection data. In filtered back projection, simple back projection is applied first which gives a basic processed image that is often blurry and contains streak artifacts. In order to reduce the artifacts from simple back projection, filters including Butterworth, Hanning, and Shepp-Logan are applied. Iterative reconstruction is also an option, and it often leads to improved image resolution compared to filtered back projection.

The primary benefit of filters is the removal of high-frequency components, which are sharp changes in image intensity between an area of interest and background. Filters that remove high-frequency components are referred to as low-pass filters, while filters that remove low-frequency components are referred to as high-pass filters. While high-pass filters help sharpen organ boundaries, they also have the undesired effect of increasing image noise.

One of the most common high-pass filters is the ramp filter. The ramp filter plays an important role in SPECT processing because it eliminates the blurring (low frequency) caused by simple back projection [4]. Another benefit of ramp filters is the removal of the star artifact. The main disadvantage of ramp filters is the increase in image noise which typically requires that a low-pass filter be used in conjunction with a ramp filter.

Hanning filters work by changing the cutoff frequency, with a lower cutoff frequency resulting in a smoother image due to more high-frequencies being removed. On the other hand, Butterworth filters have two parameters that can be adjusted. The power (order) factor defines steepness of the cutoff while the critical frequency represents the midpoint of the filter.

The fusion of SPECT and CT data is a powerful tool, but care must be taken to ensure that the data are fused correctly. CT data can help adjust the SPECT data to take into account attenuation in the body and it can also provide anatomical correlation to increase specificity. Most SPECT/CT systems will fuse data automatically which typically works well if the patient does not move. A misregistration, shown in Fig. 4.2, can occur if the patient moves between the SPECT and CT acquisitions. After acquiring a SPECT/CT exam, the technologist should make sure that the CT and SPECT images line up correctly. This is a fairly easy process when using radiopharmaceuticals that have easily recognizable landmarks on both the CT and SPECT, such as myocardial perfusion and skeletal imaging, but could be more difficult with radiopharmaceuticals that do not always have clear and consistent accumulation.

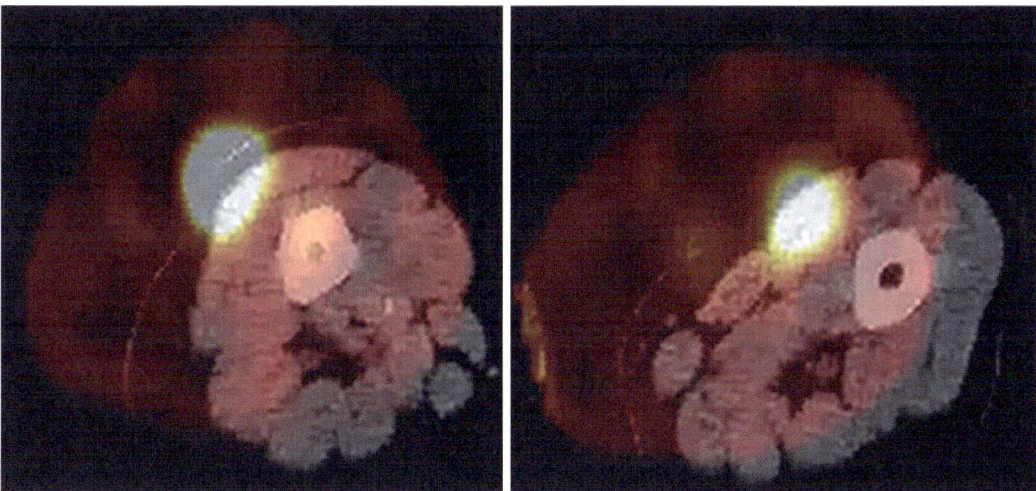

Fig. 4.2 Transverse fused slices of a skeletal SPECT/CT showing a misregistration between the SPECT and CT image. (Image from Dana Farber Cancer Institute, Boston, MA USA)

4.7   SPECT Limitations

While SPECT and SPECT/CT offer advantages over traditional planar imaging, there are some limitations and challenges with SPECT. Many of these limitations and characteristics of SPECT are also true of planar imaging; however, they are often more pronounced in SPECT because they affect an additional plane. While SPECT does not offer the same resolution as positron emission tomography (PET), it does offer a great improvement over planar imaging. SPECT offers an intrinsic resolution of 3–4 mm versus 2–4 mm with PET and SPECT having a reconstructed resolution of 10–15 mm versus 5–8 mm for PET [5].

The partial volume effect occurs when you have a voxel that lies between two different types of tissue and thus contains two different intensities of tracer accumulation. When this occurs, the intensity, or count density, is average for that voxel. The result is a loss in detail for that area of the image, which can be particularly problematic when performing oncological SPECT and imaging small lesions.

A common source of error for all hybrid imaging systems, including SPECT/CT, is misregistration. Misregistration occurs when the images acquired by the two modalities do not line up correctly and thus the same anatomy is shown in two different places. Two common causes of misregistration are patient movement between SPECT and CT acquisitions and misalignment during processing. As shown in Fig. 4.2, skeletal uptake of the radiotracer is being shown in the soft tissue because the SPECT and CT images are not aligned. Misregistration is problematic because it can cause attenuation correction issues as well as show uptake of radiotracer in areas of the body that are not a true representation of what is going on inside the patient. Improper attenuation correction can also lead to incorrect uptake values on systems performing quantitative SPECT/CT.

Scatter, attenuation, and noise are problems associated with nuclear medicine in general, but SPECT can often compound these issues making them more pronounced. Body attenuation as well as external attenuators can restrict photons from being detected by the system leading to less photons contributing to the image. Attenuation of photons can also cause them to scatter and be detected by the system not representative of where the photons originated which can contribute to image noise. Attenuators like large body habitus and metal are also responsible for causing artifacts on the CT images.

4.8   Clinical Applications

4.8.1   Liver/Spleen

SPECT and SPECT/CT are very useful for a variety of different indications involving the liver and spleen. Although not performed very often anymore, liver/spleen SPECT using Tc-99m sulfur colloid can be useful for identifying structural and morphological abnormalities. When imaging for splenules, accessory spleens, or ectopic spleen tissue, Tc-99m heat damaged autologous red blood cells may be beneficial. SPECT/CT is especially useful in these situations to provide CT correlation of any findings on the SPECT images. Lastly, SPECT can help provide better detail on hepatic hemangioma imaging of the liver using Tc-99m autologous red blood cells.

4.8.2   Renal

Morphological renal abnormalities, such as scarring, pyelonephritis, and polycystic disease, can be imaged using Tc-99m DMSA. Three-dimensional imaging is useful for providing better anatomical localization of the abnormality, and SPECT has been shown to identify more renal abnormalities compared to planar imaging [6]. Since these scans are typically performed on pediatric patients, SPECT is usually preferred over SPECT/CT due to the added dose of the CT portion of SPECT/CT.

4.8.3 Brain

Brain perfusion imaging can be performed using Tc-99m ECD or Tc-99m HMPAO. Perfusion imaging can be performed for a wide variety of indications including dementia, epilepsy (ictal and inter-ictal), cerebral ischemia, and brain death. Dopamine receptor imaging can be performed using I-123 Ioflupane to aid in the diagnosis of Parkinson's disease. Since the area of interest, the caudate and putamen, are small structures located in the interior of the brain, SPECT/CT helps improve image quality. Brain perfusion imaging with SPECT or SPECT/CT can be performed to evaluate dementia, epilepsy, brain death, and other neurological diseases. Due to the three-dimensional nature of brain anatomy, SPECT is very useful in looking at specific areas of the brain in greater detail than planar imaging would provide. This can be especially useful when trying to look at perfusion defects in specific areas, such as in the case of epileptic foci.

4.8.4 Myocardial Perfusion

The development of SPECT and SPECT/CT has had a huge impact on myocardial perfusion imaging. Coupled with exercise of pharmacological stress testing, myocardial perfusion imaging provides a noninvasive way to detect coronary artery disease with relatively low risks. In fact, using SPECT for myocardial perfusion imaging has become so popular and effective, manufacturers have developed SPECT cameras specifically designed for imaging the heart. Gated SPECT and SPECT/CT can also be performed which allows the SPECT images to be synchronized with the patient's heartbeat, providing additional information such as the detection of wall motion and the calculation of ejection fractions.

4.8.5 Parathyroid Imaging

Due to their small size and varying location, parathyroid adenomas can be difficult to detect and localize. Functioning parathyroid adenomas will take up Tc-99m sestamibi and imaging should include the neck and chest. When parathyroid adenomas are ectopic (not in their normal position behind the thyroid gland), SPECT/CT can be helpful in providing anatomical detail to exactly where the adenoma is located, helping surgeons locate and resect the adenoma. SPECT/CT can also be useful in differentiating an ectopic parathyroid adenoma from a lymph node that has taken up the tracer due to a partial infiltration of the dose during injection.

4.8.6 Pulmonary

SPECT and SPECT/CT are becoming more and more popular compared to planar imaging for lung V/Q imaging for the detection of pulmonary emboli. The main reason for this is that SPECT imaging of the lungs offers improved sensitivity, specificity, and accuracy [7]. Lung perfusion imaging can be accomplished using Tc-99m macroaggregated albumin (MAA) while several agents can be used for lung ventilation imaging including Xe-133 gas, Tc-99m DTPA aerosol, Kr-81m, and Tc-99m Technegas.

4.8.7 Sentinel Node Imaging

SPECT/CT may be beneficial in providing anatomical correlation for lymph nodes seen on planar imaging during sentinel node imaging. Three-dimensional images with CT correlation may be particularly useful to surgeons, especially when the sentinel node lies in areas of complex anatomy, such as the head and neck.

4.8.8 Y-90 Microsphere Planning and Treatment

SPECT can be useful for Y-90 microspheres pre-treatment planning using Tc-99m MAA as well as imaging after the treatment is performed. With the MAA mapping, SPECT/CT can be helpful with anatomical localization so that physicians can see in detail which parts of the liver will accumulate the Y-90 microspheres when they are given. SPECT images of the chest and liver can also be used to calculate the lung shunting value before treatment. After the Y-90 microspheres are administered, Bremsstrahlung SPECT images of the liver can be acquired to confirm proper administration of the therapy.

4.8.9 Post-therapy Imaging

Imaging of therapeutic radiopharmaceuticals has become more popular with the development of several new radiopharmaceuticals. While post-therapy imaging in nuclear medicine using I-131 sodium iodide has been around decades, imaging other agents such as Lu-177 DOTATATE (Lutathera) and Lu-177 vipivotide tetraxetan (Pluvicto) is becoming more popular. Performing SPECT and SPECT/CT scans of these patients helps to confirm that the lesions took up the therapeutic radiopharmaceutical as well as show any new lesions that may have developed since the patient's last imaging exam. Figure 4.3 shows a SPECT/CT of a patient after they received a dose of Lu-177 vipivotide tetraxetan (Pluvicto).

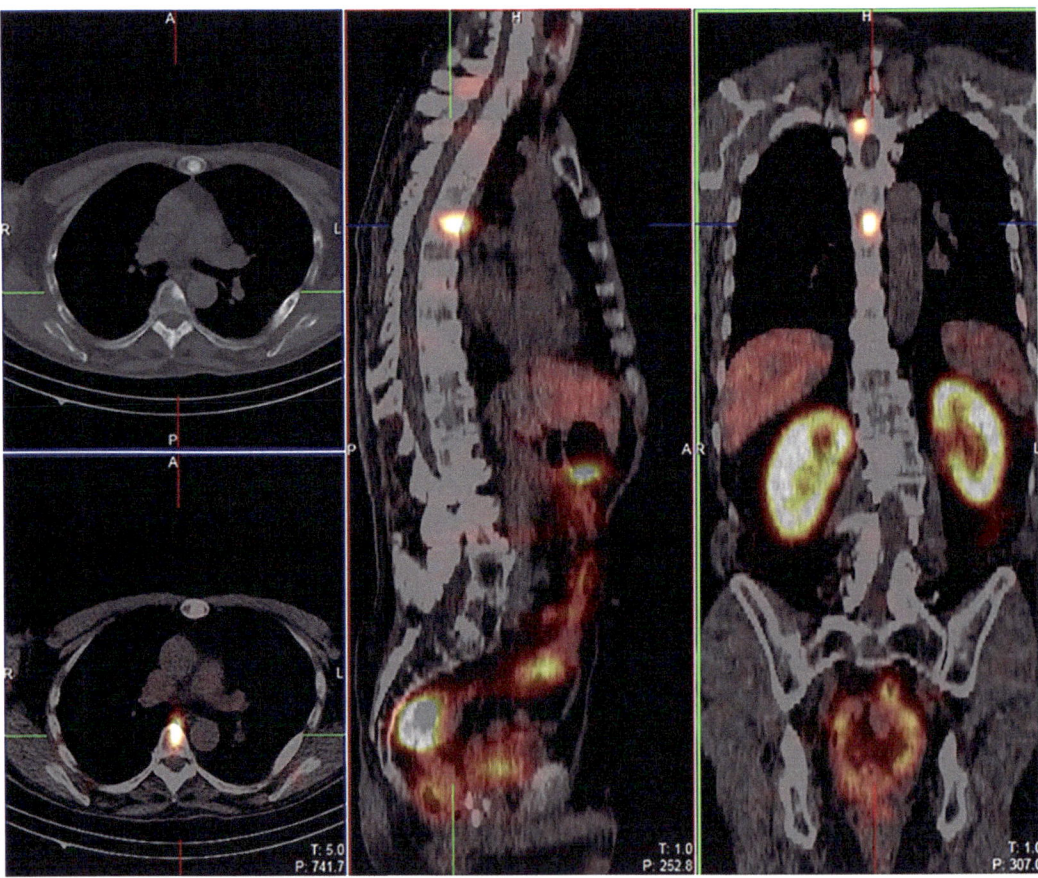

Fig. 4.3 Fused SPECT/CT images acquired after the administration of Lu-177 vipivotide tetraxetan (Pluvicto) demonstrating spine metastases. (Image from Dana Farber Cancer Institute, Boston, MA USA)

4.9 Conclusion

While SPECT and SPECT/CT do not reach the resolution power of PET, they do provide superior image quality over gamma planar imaging. In addition to improved resolution, SPECT/CT can provide attenuation correction benefits as well as anatomical correlation. For many years SPECT has been a useful tool in neurology and cardiology applications, and SPECT will continue to be important for posttherapy imaging as more therapy radionuclides are developed.

References

1. Khalil MM, Tremoleda JL, Bayomy TB, Gsell W. Molecular SPECT imaging: an overview. Int J Mol Imaging. 2011;2011:796025.
2. Van Audenhaege K, Van Holen R, Vandenberghe S, Vanhove C, Metzler SD, Moore SC. Review of SPECT collimator selection, optimization, and fabrication for clinical and preclinical imaging. Med Phys. 2015;42:4796–813.
3. Delbeke D, Chiti A, Christian P, Darcourt J, Donohoe K, Flotats A, Krause B, Royal H. SNMMI/EANM Guideline for Guideline Development 6.0. J Nucl Med Technol. 2012;40(4):283–9.
4. Gilmore D, Waterstram-Rich K. Chapter 10. Instrumentation. In: Nuclear medicine and molecular imaging: technology and techniques. 9th ed. St. Louis, MO: Mosby; 2023. p. 316.
5. Weissleder R. Molecular imaging: principles and practice. Shelton, CT: People's Medical Publishing House–USA; 2010.
6. Yen T, Chen W, Chang S, Liu R, Yeh S, Lin C. Technetium-99m-DMSA renal SPECT in diagnosing and monitoring pediatric acute pyelonephritis. J Nucl Med. 1996;37(8):1349–53.
7. Roach PJ, Schembri GP, Bailey DL. V/Q scanning using SPECT and SPECT/CT. J Nucl Med. 2013;54(9):1588–96.

Principles in Conventional PET/CT

5

Alfredo Palmieri, Marco Maccagnani, Valentina Mautone, and Federica Fioroni

5.1 Principles of PET System Acquisition

Positron emission tomography (PET) is a powerful imaging technique used in nuclear medicine to visualize and measure metabolic processes in the body. It involves the use of a radioactive tracer, typically a radiopharmaceutical labelled with a positron-emitting isotope such as fluorine-18.

PET is a versatile imaging technique that provides valuable insights into various physiological and pathological processes, making it an essential tool in modern medicine. It is used in various fields of medicine for diagnostic (oncology, neurology, cardiology, and infection imaging), research, and therapeutic purposes.

A. Palmieri (✉)
Nuclear Medicine Unit, Azienda Unità Sanitaria Locale di Reggio Emilia – IRCCS, Reggio Emilia, Italy
e-mail: palmieri.alfredo@ausl.re.it

M. Maccagnani
Medical Physics Department, IRCCS Azienda Ospedaliero-Universitaria di Bologna, Bologna, Italy
e-mail: marco.maccagnani@aosp.bo.it

V. Mautone
Nuclear Medicine Unit, Istituto Romagnolo per lo studio dei Tumori "D. Amadori", Meldola, FC, Italy
e-mail: valentina.mautone@irst.emr.it

F. Fioroni
Medical Physics Unit, Azienda Unità Sanitaria Locale di Reggio Emilia – IRCCS, Reggio Emilia, Italy
e-mail: fioroni.federica@ausl.re.it

5.1.1 Physical Principles

Unlike SPECT, PET uses radioisotopes that emit positrons as a result of β^+ decay. After travelling a short distance, these positrons annihilate with an electron in the surrounding medium. As a result of the annihilation process, two γ-rays of energy equal to 511 keV are simultaneously emitted. The two photons are emitted simultaneously along the same line but in opposite directions, and their flight direction is defined using a series of time-coincident detectors placed around the patient. The emission angle between one γ-ray and the other is about 180°, so it can be assumed that they travel along the same flight path [1].

The physical process used to obtain information about the distribution of unknown activity can be divided into several distinct phases: the emission of the positron, its annihilation, the interaction of the emitted γ-rays with the surrounding biological tissue, and their detection.

5.1.1.1 Positron Emission

The positron is the antiparticle of the electron: these two particles are identical in all their characteristics (including their mass) and differ only in the sign of their electric charge (and magnetic moment). Therefore, the positron is a particle with a positive charge. For these reasons, the positron is often indicated by the symbol e^+ or, more frequently, by β^+.

Positrons are naturally produced through the decay of various nuclei, whose instability is caused by the presence of an excessive number of protons compared to neutrons. These nuclei reach a more stable state by transmuting a proton into a neutron through a process called β^+ decay. In this transformation, a nucleus X characterized by a number Z of protons and N of neutrons transforms into a nucleus with Z-1 protons and N+1 neutrons, through the emission of a positron and an electron neutrino, namely:

$$_z X \rightarrow _{z-1} X^* + \beta^+ + \nu_e$$

As it traverses the tissue, the positron loses its energy through a series of collisions (Coulomb interactions) with electrons, following a tortuous trajectory, and moving away from the emission point. The positron's range depends on the energy with which it is emitted, as well as the electron density of the surrounding material. In water, which is a good approximation of biological tissue, the average range of a positron emitted by a typical radioisotope used in PET (for example, ^{18}F) is about 1–2 mm [2].

5.1.1.2 Positron Annihilation

When colliding with an electron of the surrounding matter, the positron gives rise to a phenomenon called annihilation. In this process, the positron and the electron (each with a rest mass of 511 keV) transform their mass into energy, which is equally divided between the two γ-rays, namely:

$$E_\gamma = \left(m_e c^2 + m_\beta c^2 \right) / 2 = 511 \text{ keV} + 511 \text{ keV}) / 2$$
$$= 511 \text{ keV}$$

where m_e and m_β are, respectively, the rest mass of the electron and the positron.

The two γ-rays are emitted along the same line but in opposite directions (180° apart from each other).

5.1.1.3 Detection of γ-Rays

Therefore, a PET system consists of instrumentation capable of measuring the flight paths of a pair of annihilation photons. To this end, the γ-rays are detected through a system of time coincidence between the detectors surrounding the patient; that is, two γ-rays are recognized as belonging to the same annihilation event when two opposite detectors have detected them with a temporal difference less than a certain value Δt, called the "time window." Coincident detection, which typically occurs within a time window of about 10 nanoseconds (ns), defines the line of response (LOR) and thus the direction along which the annihilation occurred (electronic collimation). Coincidence events are only a fraction of those "observed" by the detectors. In most cases, only one of the annihilation γ-rays is detected, while the other either does not reach the detectors or passes through one of them without interacting. These events are called "singles" and are not acquired as they are not significant for image reconstruction. Once the LORs are recorded, appropriate reconstruction software uses the acquired information at various angles and for certain positions along the axis to obtain an image of the radioisotope concentration within the organ under examination [1].

5.1.2 PET Scanning Systems

The PET acquisition system consists of a set of ring detectors surrounding the patient, needing to capture events comprising a pair of γ-rays emitted at a 180° angle to each other. Today, all clinical PET systems consist of one or more (multiring) rings of detectors placed around the object under observation. Each detector is coincident with those located on a diametrically opposite arc of the circumference. The tomographic acquisition is achieved by recording lines of response (LORs) at various angles. PET scanners are typically engineered with detectors (block detectors) arranged in an array of full rings, typically with a diameter ranging from 80 to 90 cm.

5.1.2.1 PET Detectors

The detection system of a PET scanner is one of the key elements that crucially influences the performance of the entire machine. Photon detectors can be divided into two major families depending on the technique employed in the detection process, which can be indirect or direct. In the first case (conventional systems), the detector consists of two main components: a scintillating material, the part sensitive to the photons to be detected, and the photodetector that detects the secondary photons produced by the scintillator (often called optical photons as they have a wavelength falling within the visible range) by producing a measurable electrical signal. The second case (digital systems) essentially involves semiconductor detectors with a high atomic number Z in which the sensitive part constitutes the detector itself. In this case, we have the direct conversion of γ-rays into a signal [3].

5.1.2.2 Characteristics of the Detection Crystals

The approach typically used in PET detectors is to divide the scintillator into small crystals. The most commonly used solution is that of the so-called block detector. Although the process of detecting gamma photons is similar to that exploited by gamma cameras, the photons emitted from annihilation events are much more energetic. For effective photon detection, materials with high electron density are necessary. Some characteristics of the main PET crystals are shown in Table 5.1. Another important parameter is the light output; indeed, such materials must be able to produce a lot of light per event. Materials with higher electron density can allow for the use of a thinner thickness, making the definition of the position of the event detected by the crystal more precise. A short decay time instead allows for the reduction of the time window (and therefore the probability of detecting random events) and is necessary to perform time-of-flight correction. Bismuth germanate (BGO) has long been the most commonly used material for building

crystals and is therefore present in many tomographs still in use. It has a high linear attenuation coefficient, high electron density, and therefore high detection efficiency, but it is burdened by a low light output and a long decay time, resulting in worsened spatial and energy resolution. Lutetium oxyorthosilicate (LSO) boasts high light output and efficient density, but its primary advantage lies in its very short decay constant. This superior time resolution of LSO has empowered PET scanners to measure the time disparity between the arrivals of the two annihilation photons, a technique known as "time of flight" (TOF). TOF furnishes previously unattainable positioning information, allowing us to pinpoint an annihilation event within a few centimetres. Lutetium yttrium orthosilicate (LYSO) is currently employed in the latest TOF-PET scanners due to its marginally improved light output and energy resolution compared to LSO. Some manufacturers have chosen to replace BGO with gadolinium orthosilicate (GSO). GSO's principal advantage lies in its enhanced energy resolution, offering an alternative to LSO in certain applications [4].

5.1.2.3 Photomultiplier Tube

Photomultiplier tubes (PMTs) have historically been the primary photodetectors utilized in PET scanners. PMTs are vacuum tubes encased in glass, comprising three essential components: a photocathode, dynodes, and an anode (Fig. 5.1). Their operation is grounded in the photoelectric effect, whereby light interacting with a photoelectric material induces the emission of electrons. Within PMTs, the photoelectric element is referred to as the photocathode. Upon stimulation by scintillation photons, electrons are emitted

Table 5.1 Characteristics of the main PET crystals

Property	NaI (Tl)	BGO	GSO	LSO	LYSO
Z_{eff}	51	74	59	66	60
Density (g/cm³)	3.67	7.13	4.89	7.4	7.2
Light output (ph/keV)	41	9	10	31	30
Wavelength (nm)	410	480	440	420	420
Decay time (ns)	230	300	60	40	41

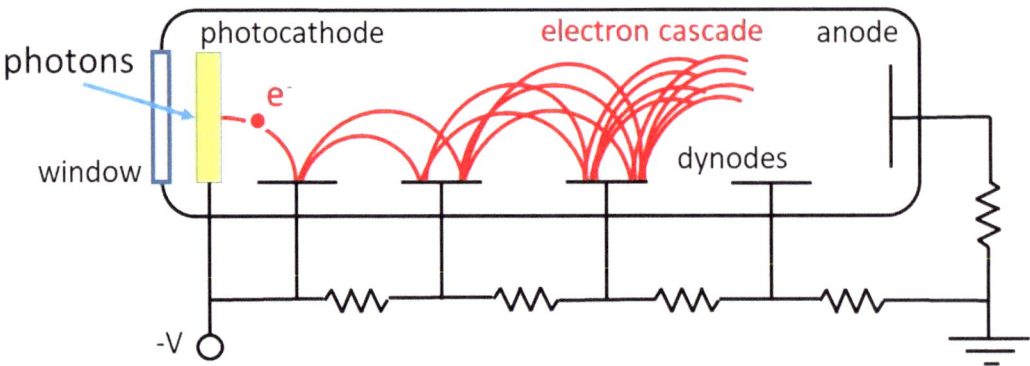

Fig. 5.1 Representation of a PET photomultiplier and its operation

from the photocathode and subsequently drawn toward the anode by the electric potential generated. Along their path to the anode, electrons collide with the dynodes, triggering secondary electron emissions upon collision. The resulting electrical current is directly proportional to the initial scintillation photon count and is converted into an electrical signal. Recent developments in the physics and construction technologies of semiconductor materials have enabled semiconductor photodetectors to become a valid alternative to PMTs, which have been (and in some respects still are) the premier photodetectors for many years. Among the main advantages of solid-state detectors over PMTs are high quantum efficiency (down to single photon detection), compact size, significantly lower operating voltages (below 100 V), and the ability to operate in the presence of magnetic fields [1].

5.1.2.4 Electronic System of a PET Detector

The signal from each detector follows two distinct paths: one for signal measurement and one for timing. The signal passes through timing discriminators that generate temporal signals containing information about the arrival time of the gamma ray. At this point, a temporal window of about 10 ns is opened. If during this interval a second γ-ray hits an opposing detector, a coincidence is registered, and the system

captures the event. At the same time, a suitable amplitude discriminator inhibits acquisition if too small an energy is measured. In the measurement path, when an event is involved in a coincidence, the signal from each photomultiplier is measured and digitized. This process takes some time. During this interval, the detector is in a state of the so-called dead time, during which it cannot accept other events. This fact results in the loss of a certain fraction of events, which must be appropriately corrected (dead time correction).

5.1.2.5 Time of Flight

The detection and acquisition system of a standard PET scanner cannot determine the position along the LOR at which the annihilation process occurred, so a uniform probability distribution is assigned to the segment of LOR intersecting the object under examination. However, if a detector system and its associated electronics are fast enough, it is possible to determine this position by measuring the time difference of arrival of both photons. This time difference is called time of flight (TOF). The main advantage of TOF-PET systems that also utilize this information for image reconstruction lies in a reduction of background variance and, consequently, an improvement in the signal-to-noise ratio. As a result, it is equivalent to an increase in the sensitivity of the equipment.

5.2   Multimodality Imaging

5.2.1   PET/CT Scanner

As described for SPECT/CT, the combination of a PET scanner with a computed tomography (CT) system shows significant advantages compared to using the two techniques separately. The main advantage consists in obtaining almost simultaneously functional PET and morphological CT images. The fusion of PET functional information with CT morphological images allows spatial localization, useful, for example, to identify the anatomical site of an area with high uptake. CT also allows for lesion characterization, resolving many diagnostic doubts and increasing the sensitivity of the method. Finally, CT can provide information that complements the clinical picture, such as tumor dimensions, and visualization of small lesions otherwise not visible in PET. Another important aspect of using CT is the ability to use attenuation coefficient information to perform attenuation correction of PET data [5].

The characteristics of scanners vary depending on the vendor, although the basic elements of design are largely similar. PET scanners have "full-ring" geometry and are integrated with CT scanners in a single device. From a hardware perspective, a PET/CT system typically consists of a PET scanner and a CT scanner aligned one behind the other, inside the same gantry, with the axes of the two tomographs lying on the same line (Fig. 5.2). From a construction standpoint,

the main complexities of a PET/CT system are related to the mechanical combination of the two systems. The two scans occur autonomously and sequentially. During the examination, the patient lies on the patient's table. The table moves through the scanner gantry during the CT acquisition and subsequently moves further into position for the PET scan to the rear of the housing. However, the two scanners must be perfectly aligned with each other, at a known distance, to overlay the images in the fusion process. Finally, to ensure accurate image registration, any vertical bed deflection must be minimized as the pallet extends into the field of view [4].

5.2.2   Overview of CT Technology

In a CT, volumetric anatomical images are obtained from information acquired by measuring the attenuation properties of an X-ray beam at various angles, evaluating the distribution of linear attenuation coefficients of tissues.

The essential components of a CT scanner are the X-ray source (radiation tube) and the detection system, mounted diametrically opposite each other on a motorized mechanical ring capable of rotating around the patient. The CT system combined with PET is similar to diagnostic ones used in radiology departments. Today, PET/CT systems are equipped with CT scanners with even more than 128 slices, which can also be used for diagnostic purposes and with the use of contrast agents. Over the past years, the two main goals of CT scanner development have been improved image resolution and reduced radiation exposure for the patient. This has been made possible also by improved iterative methods of CT image reconstruction [6].

Generally, at least two sets of CT images are reconstructed: diagnostic images, used for anatomical correlation in fusion images, and images used as CT attenuation maps for PET data correction. The latter serve no diagnostic purpose and therefore are not stored in the PACS.

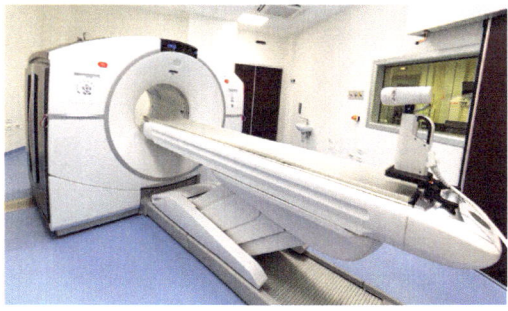

Fig. 5.2 Example of a modern PET/CT scanner

5.2.3 Image Display

Postprocessing refers to the manipulation of the resulting image by the operator. PET/CT operators have access to a diverse range of postprocessing functions, including windowing, which adjusts the image contrast to highlight specific structures or tissue types, and multiplanar reconstructions (MPRs), which generate 2D images in the sagittal, coronal, or axial planes.

Modern PET/CT processing workstations allow for the visualization of individual and fused images using multiple modalities, enabling nuclear physicians to accurately report on the examination. Some systems are also equipped with artificial intelligence–based tools that provide helpful assistance in recognizing tracer distribution anomalies and various pathologies.

5.3 Data Acquisition and Corrections

5.3.1 Data Acquisition

Acquisition data in PET involves detecting two photons with an energy of 511 keV resulting from the annihilation of an electron, as well as a β^+ particle originating from the source, occurring on opposite sides. These photons are captured within an electronic time window set for the scanner, aligned along the line connecting the two detectors (LOR).

To enhance sensitivity and photon detection, the scanner is encircled by a ring of detectors. Data are acquired simultaneously by all detector pairs, which are arranged in blocks in 2D arrays (Fig. 5.3). Each block consists of one detector encircling the ring (along the X-axis) and one detector positioned axially to the ring (along the Y-axis).

Behind each detector, an array of photomultipliers (PMs) captures the scintillation light (the 511 keV photons) to identify the detector in which the event occurs. In block detectors, each is coupled with four PMTs, with two connected detectors detecting a coincidence event within a time window and collecting the scintillation data [4].

During the absorption of annihilation photons, a random delay process of response occurs, leading to occasional missed coincidences. This uncertainty in response is influenced by various parameters such as: detector characteristics, primarily scintillation decay, light output, and the varied arrival times of photons caused by differences in annihilation site distances. To address this issue, logic pulses have a finite width, ensuring overlap despite timing resolution differences.

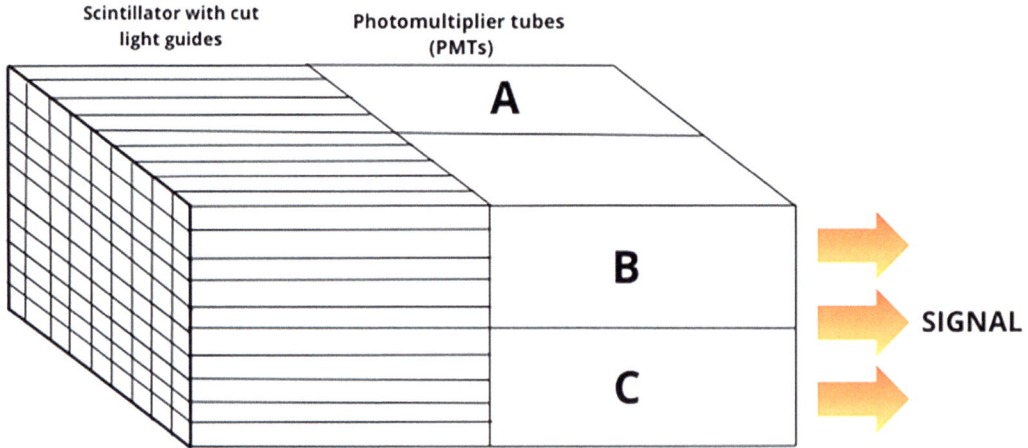

Fig. 5.3 PM transmission signal in PET/CT crystals

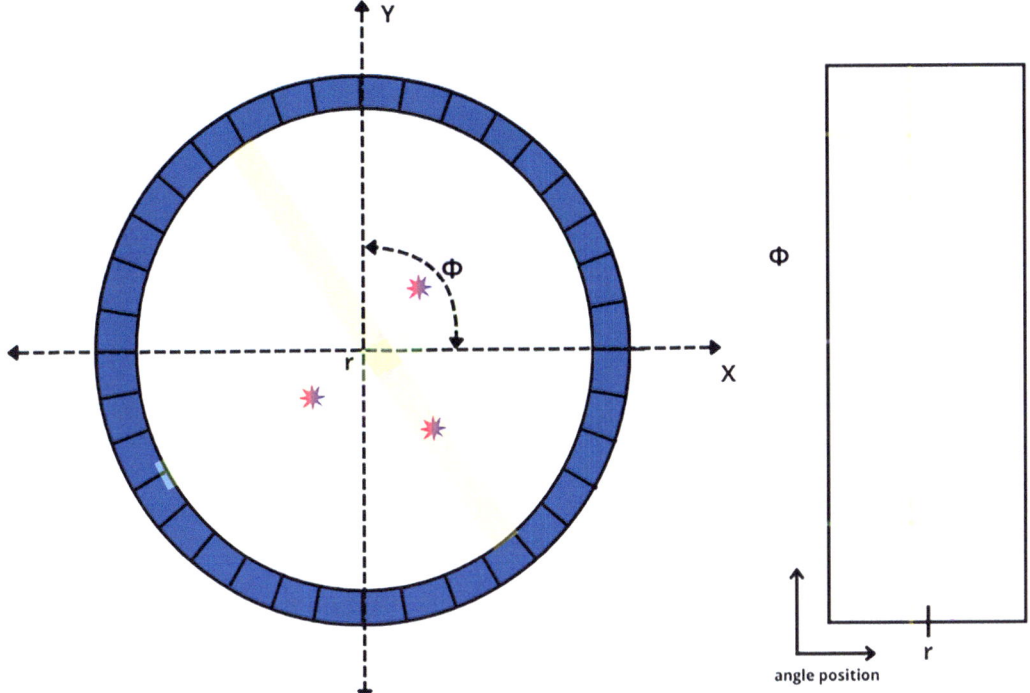

Fig. 5.4 PET data acquisition and recalculation in sinogram, every LOR data is evaluated in coordinates that give the exact position of the sinogram in the space

Pulses produced in PMTs are utilized to determine the location of the two detectors. An algorithm estimates the weighted sum of each pulse, normalized with the total pulse obtained, with the weighted factor depending on the tube's position in the array.

Collected data are stored in sinograms, where each detector pair represents a particular pixel with a specific orientation angle and distance from the gantry's centre. For each detection, the associated LOR determines the pixel location in the sinogram, with the value in the pixel incremented based on the number of coincident detections (Fig. 5.4). Each slice produces a distinct sinogram, which, when summed, generates raw PET data [7].

Raw PET data can be presented in two modalities: a series of sinograms with a separate sinogram for each slice or a series of projection views with a separate view for each projection angle (Fig. 5.5).

5.3.2 Factors Affecting Acquired Data

In order to accurately depict tissue activity concentration within each voxel, the raw sinogram data must account for variations in detector efficiency among detector pairs, as well as factors such as random and scattered coincidences, photon attenuation, dead time, and radial elongation. Each of these elements influences the sinogram in PET imaging, albeit with varying degrees of significance.

Fig. 5.5 Sinogram in 3D PET acquisition. The cross represents the angle of coincidence between two blocks

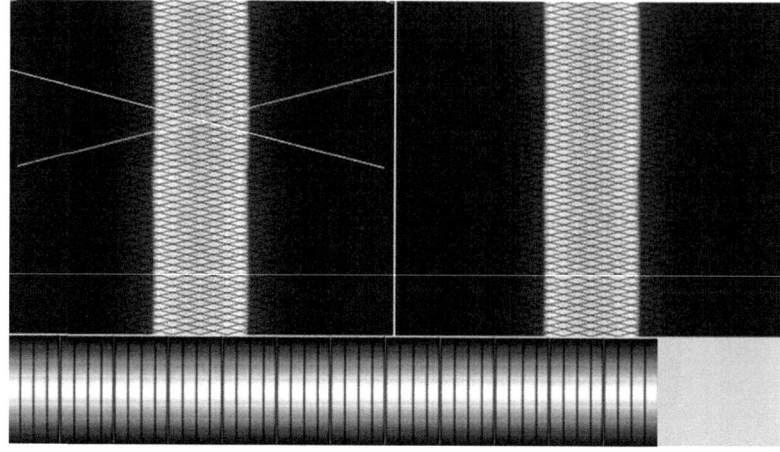

5.3.2.1 Normalization

Nonuniformities in raw data result from various factors such as individual detector efficiency (physical dimensions), geometrical variations, and detector electronics. All of these factors contribute to variations in coincidence detection due to the different LORs in the system.

These problems are corrected using a normalization method. This method corrects all individual LORs using a multiplication factor that compensates for the nonuniformities. The generation of normalization correction is based on measuring all the geometrical efficiency variations of each detector, as well as any variations in plane-to-plane measurements.

The normalization method involves collecting data from a uniform plane source of activity positioned at 6–8 equally spaced projection angles. The goal is to collect a sufficient number of counts per LOR to provide accurate estimates of efficiencies while minimizing statistical noise to obtain the final image [8].

Another method for determining the normalization matrix is the component-based method. In this approach, the individual detector efficiency for the entire system is determined from a scan of a uniform cylinder centered on the scanner. The sum of coincidences is determined for each detector and its complement. This sum is then corrected for scatter and random coincidences and is directly proportional to the individual detector efficiency. This method provides an estimate of the normalization factor with virtually no

statistical noise due to the large number of detector elements.

5.3.2.2 Attenuation Correction (AC)

There is a high likelihood that a 511 keV photon, generated through annihilation or both processes, undergoes attenuation as it traverses tissue before reaching the detector and interacting with the subject, resulting in another form of effect (Compton scattering). This phenomenon, known as attenuation, leads to irregularities in images due to the increased loss of coincidence events from the central tissue to the periphery.

Furthermore, as photons pass through various types of tissue and organs along the LOR, attenuation contributes to additional irregularities. Attenuation can be corrected using mathematical models or a combination thereof. The correction process involves eliminating scattered events from LORs and then adjusting each LOR for the proportion of events scattered from that specific LOR [4].

The calculated attenuation correction assumes that the object's outline can be approximated as an ellipse and that attenuation remains constant. To generate the attenuation correction, the chord length (Di,j) is determined for each LOR using the equation:

$$Ai,j = \exp\left(\mu Di,j\right) = I\left(0\right)/I\left(Di,j\right)$$

This model is useful in imaging phantoms where attenuation is uniform and can also be applied in brain studies. However, this method is

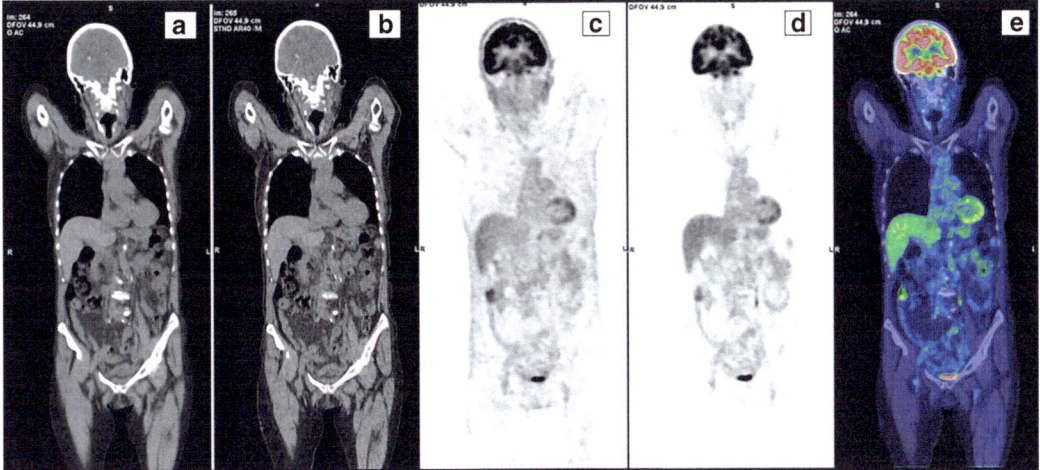

Fig. 5.6 Coronal images of ^{18}F-FDG PET CT: (**a**) CT map for attenuation correction, (**b**) CT for fused images, (**c**) PET uncorrected for AC, (**d**) PET corrected for AC, (**e**) fused PET/CT images

labor-intensive, particularly in systems that generate a large number of images.

Where attenuation is nonuniform due to the variety of tissue structures, the theoretical method is challenging to apply. In PET/CT systems, attenuation is corrected through a CT transmission scan (Fig. 5.6). With this method, an image of the attenuation coefficient is first reconstructed by taking the natural log of the attenuation correction of the sinogram and then reconstructing the sinogram using CT techniques. Typically, the image information is sufficient to allow image segmentation into fixed categories of attenuation correction (such as soft tissue, bones, etc.). Each image can be traced along each LOR to calculate an almost noiseless estimate of the attenuation correction [3].

5.3.2.3 Random Coincidences

Random and scatter coincidences increase the background in the images. Specifically, random events occur when two unrelated annihilation events are detected and recorded by a detector pair simultaneously as valid coincidences. This type of coincidence increases in frequency with wider energy windows and coincidence timing windows, along with increasing activity.

Random coincidences do not convey any spatial or physiological information but cause image artifacts and a loss of image contrast, particularly posing more significant challenges in low-efficiency detectors such as NaI(Tl) crystals and 3D counting.

The rate of random events depends on the formula:

$$R = 2_\tau \times C_i \times C_j$$

where τ is the windows nanosecond and C_i and C_j are the single count rate in counts/s of each detector on the same LOR.

The most common method to reduce random coincidences involves the use of two types of windows: standard (e.g., 5 ns) and delayed (50 ns), employing identical energy windows. The standard window encompasses both standard and random coincidences, while the delayed window contains only random coincidences. Assuming that random events are consistent in both windows, they can be subtracted from the standard window using the delayed window.

5.3.2.4 Scatter Coincidences

Scatter coincidences occur when one of the annihilation events, instead of directly reaching the detector, undergoes Compton interaction, changing direction before reaching the detector. These scattered radiations increase the background image while degrading image quality. Typically, the number of scatter coincidences increases with the density and depth of body tissue, the density

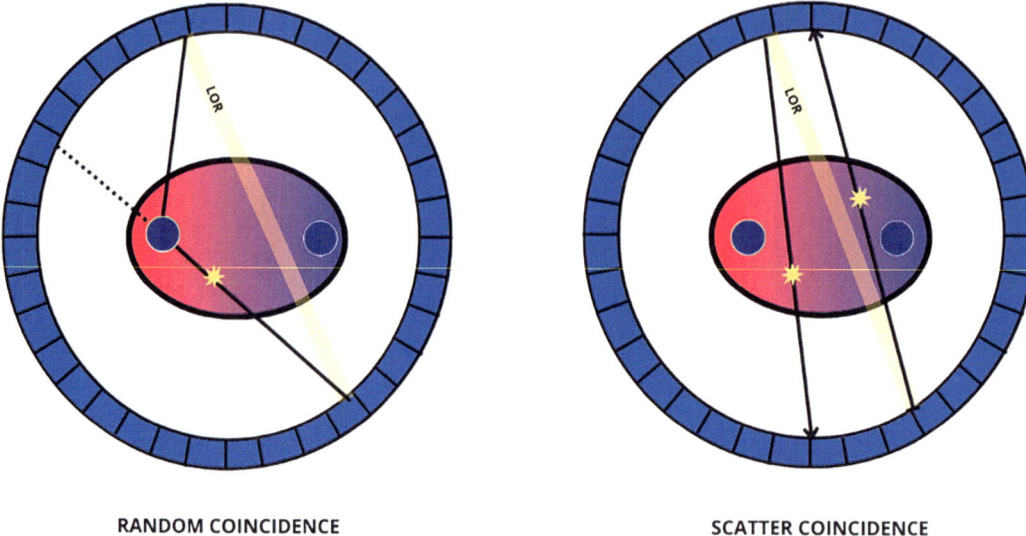

Fig. 5.7 Random coincidence and scatter coincidence in PET/CT acquisition

of detector materials, activity injected into the patient, and the window width of PHA (pulse height analyzer) in PET systems.

The scatter-true ratio remains constant and does not fluctuate with activity due to their rates, which remain linearly variable with administration. Typically, the fraction of scatter events ranges from 15% (2D) to 40–50% (3D) in PET systems [4].

The correction of scatter typically involves measuring counts outside the field of view (FOV) where no true coincidences occur (Fig. 5.7). After subtracting both random and scatter counts, the remaining count represents only true coincidences. This correction assumes uniform scatter distribution throughout the FOV and is widely regarded as one of the most challenging aspects of PET imaging.

5.3.2.5 Dead Time

The dead time is the duration required to process a coincident event, from detection to registration, during which a second event cannot be registered and is consequently lost. This loss poses a significant problem at high count rates and varies depending on the PET system used.

Dead time loss can be reduced by employing detectors with shorter scintillation decay times and faster electronic components in PET sys-

tems. Dead time correction is performed through empirical measurements of count rates as activity concentration increases. Based on these data, the dead time is calculated and corrected to offset the loss caused by dead time [2].

5.4 PET Image Reconstruction

Image reconstruction for positron emission tomography has been developed over many decades, with advances coming from improved modelling of the data statistics and improved modelling of imaging physics.

5.4.1 Conventional PET Image Reconstruction

Conventional PET image registration methods, such as filtered back projection (FBP) and iterative reconstruction (IR) algorithms, have been widely used for several decades.

FBP is a traditional algorithm that involves back-projecting the measured data after applying a filter to remove noise and artifacts.

FBP is appreciated for its simplicity and predictability due to its linearity, although it often results in noisy images. This noise is typically mitigated by postreconstruction smoothing, which only requires adjusting one parameter. The primary drawback of FBP is its inability to account for varying noise levels in the data, which are particularly significant in count-limited PET data. This results in limited spatial resolution and reduced lesion detection [9].

Although FBP is the standard algorithm in tomographic reconstruction in the analytical approach, it is not routinely used in PET reconstruction due to the low signal-to-noise ratio.

Iterative image reconstruction algorithms aim to determine the radioactivity distribution that most accurately corresponds to the acquired emission data, considering the statistical characteristics of the Poisson-distributed raw data resulting from radioactive decay.

The approach involves iteratively updating the image estimate based on the measured data and a mathematical model of the imaging system, taking into account physical effects, such as the decay properties, radiation transport and detection processes including radiation interaction within the patient, detection efficiency, detector geometry, and intrinsic resolution of PET scanner.

The widely adopted iterative algorithms in image reconstruction, maximum likelihood expectation maximization (MLEM) and its faster variant, ordered subset expectation maximization (OSEM), are the most commonly used iterative algorithms.

Noise suppression is certainly a fundamental aspect of PET reconstruction for clinical use. To address the noise issue, penalized iterative reconstruction, also known as maximum a posteriori reconstruction (MAP) methods, was investigated.

These advanced iterative reconstruction techniques further improved image quality by integrating a model of expected image types through priors or penalties. These methods combine an improved noise model, better imaging physics, and a prior model that assigns probabilities to candidate images, preferring smoother images over noisier ones. This results in reduced noise and more accurate images, even with shorter scan times or lower radiotracer doses.

Overall, iterative methods like MLEM and OSEM, and their advanced regularized forms (MAP), offer significant improvements over traditional methods like FBP by providing better noise handling and more accurate image reconstructions [9].

5.4.2 AI-Based PET Image Reconstruction

The emergence of artificial intelligence (AI) has inaugurated a novel era in medical imaging. Deep learning–based methods have revitalized the field of image reconstruction.

Deep learning-based reconstruction methods are data-driven models that can learn intrinsic information and features from big data sets, unlike traditional reconstruction methods where models are designed based on mathematical characterizations.

The deep learning-based reconstruction methods have shown empirical performance improvement over traditional reconstruction methods [10].

Deep neural networks (DNNs) have been shown to effectively enhance PET image quality through both image-to-image and sinogram-to-sinogram mapping, utilizing supervised learning, transfer learning, or unsupervised learning approaches. In addition to denoising, DNNs can also facilitate PET image reconstruction by translating sinograms into images. This combination offers two main advantages over denoising alone: first, neural networks can leverage more information from raw sinogram data; second, the constraints of PET physics help reduce potential mismatches between training and testing data.

The integration of AI into positron emission tomography image reconstruction presents significant opportunities for enhancing clinical practice. However, several key challenges must be addressed to ensure successful implementation.

Effective AI models require large, diverse, and representative datasets. Acquiring such datasets involves extensive efforts to compile PET data from various sources, considering different scanners, acquisition protocols, anatomical regions, and potential variabilities.

The complexity of DL models often renders them as black boxes, complicating the understanding of their decision-making processes. This lack of interpretability can impede trust and acceptance in clinical settings, where transparency is crucial [11].

Rigorous clinical validation and translation of AI-driven PET IR techniques are critical. This requires comprehensive studies and multicenter clinical trials to establish the utility, generalizability, and impact of these methods across diverse patient populations and imaging protocols.

Each algorithm has its strengths and weaknesses, and the choice of algorithm often depends on factors such as the specific imaging system, the desired image quality, and the computational resources available [12].

5.4.3   Partial Volume Effect

The partial volume effect (PVE) in positron emission tomography arises due to the finite spatial resolution of PET imaging. It is a recognized challenge in accurately quantifying PET images, resulting in underestimated activity concentration in small tissue volumes and elevated activity concentration relative to surrounding tissues; it involves an ambiguity in the definition of tissue boundaries.

Because of this, particularly before the quantitative evaluation of metabolism and physiology of the organs/lesions, partial volume correction should be desirable in PET studies.

PVE has been extensively studied, prompting numerous efforts to devise effective correction techniques.

Most of these methods involve postprocessing of raw data and/or additional imaging data, producing regional or global corrections to address the issue of PVE.

Although the partial volume effect is well known, its correction is not generally available for PET/CT scanners currently in clinical use.

Some of the common algorithms used for PET/CT partial volume correction (postreconstruction methods) include the geometric transfer matrix (GTM) method which involves creating a system matrix to model the blurring effect and correct for it in the image reconstruction process.

The Muller-Gartner method applies a mathematical model to estimate the true activity concentration within a voxel by considering the effects of partial volume blurring.

Iterative deconvolution algorithms iteratively estimate and correct for the blurring effect by deconvolving the measured PET data with the point spread function of the scanner.

The most widely used approach is the recovery coefficient (RC) method. RC curves are generated to guide the correction of measured PET signals to account for partial volume effects. The method is region based and can be applied retrospectively to reconstructed PET images without the requirement of raw data or supplementary images from different modalities. PVE is scanner specific and thus a dedicated RC model had to be developed based on experimental measurements at the PET. Deep learning (DL) approaches have recently been proposed to perform PVC for PET images with and without employing anatomical information [9].

These algorithms are implemented to help mitigate the partial volume effect in PET images and enhance the accuracy of quantitative measurements, particularly in small structures or lesions. Each method has its advantages and limitations based on the characteristics of the imaging data and the specific application.

5.5   Performance Characteristics of PET Scanners

A variety of PET systems are currently available on the market, all of which are now hybrid, with various configurations. It is therefore necessary to understand the parameters that describe their main characteristics.

5.5.1 Sensitivity

Refers to the system's capability to detect photons generated by positron annihilation. It depends on various factors such as the geometry of the detection system, crystal efficiency, and efficiency of data acquisition/management electronics. This parameter can be expressed as a detection percentage or more commonly as a sensitivity coefficient, measured in counts per second per activity concentration (kcps × kBq/ml).

5.5.2 Spatial Resolution

Refers to the system's ability to accurately position the positron emission point. However, the PET system does not detect the positron emission point but rather the point of its annihilation. This detection depends on several factors:

- Range effect: The positron travels a short distance in tissues before annihilation. This effect is directly dependent on the energy of the emerging positron and the medium traversed (Fig. 5.8)
- Angular deviation: Photons emitted from annihilation do not travel with separate 180° trajectories. This occurs because the positron–electron combination happens in motion, altering the trajectories of the emerging photons. However, the PET system assumes a 180° trajectory, introducing a localization error (Fig. 5.8).
- Detector size: The size of individual crystals contributes to spatial resolution in PET imaging by determining the precision of LORs. Larger crystals increase the uncertainty of the annihilation position, thereby degrading spatial resolution. Conversely, smaller crystals reduce this uncertainty, although decreasing crystal size can diminish detection efficiency, necessitating a balance between spatial resolution and sensitivity. This contribution is minimal at the centre of the FOV and worsens toward the edges, with additional impacts from crystal pitch and parallax error.
- Parallax error: This error arises from the fact that some photons interact with detectors at an oblique angle. When a photon interacts within a detector, it is presumed that the annihilation event occurred along a line of response originating from the front of the detector, as the interaction depth in the crystal is not recorded. This component increases with distance from the detector's isocenter (Fig. 5.9).
- Sampling error: This error is associated with the discrete nature of photon detection. Since PET detectors sample space at discrete intervals (determined by the size of the crystals),

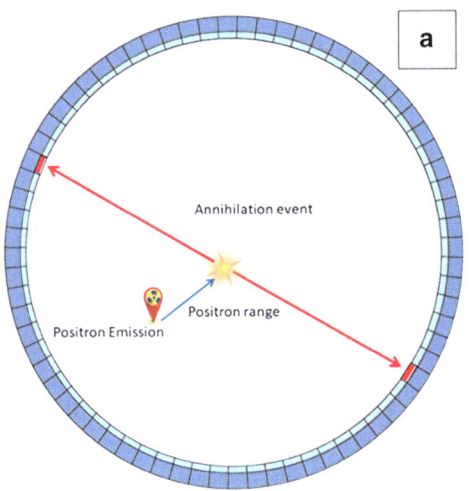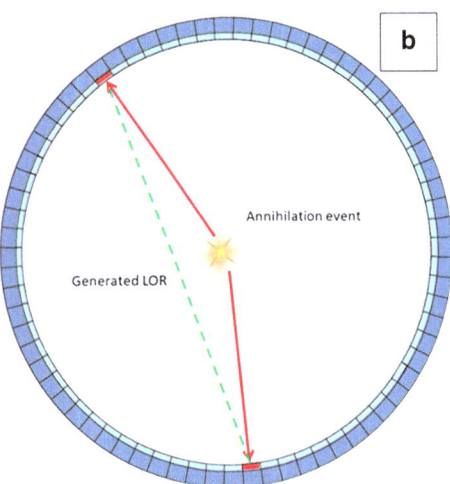

Fig. 5.8 Representation of the range effect component (**a**) and angular deviation component (**b**)

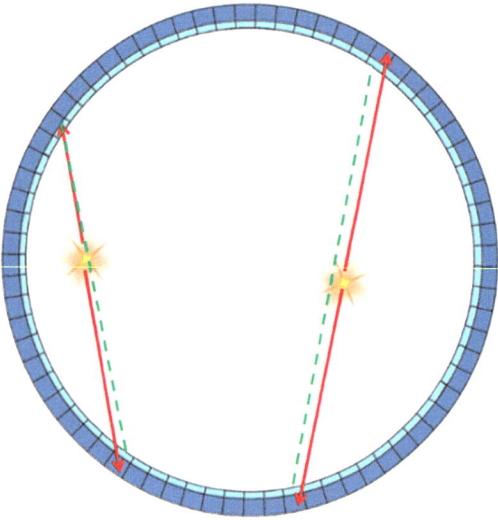

Fig. 5.9 Representation of two different contributions due to parallax error near the periphery of FOV

not all annihilation positions can be detected with infinite precision. The sampling error introduces a discrepancy between the actual annihilation position and the detected position, degrading spatial resolution. This effect is more pronounced when the crystals are larger or when the detection system has a less dense sampling grid.

- Decoding error: This error occurs during the interpretation of data collected by the detectors. In the process of decoding photon coincidence events, errors can arise due to the limited temporal and spatial resolution of the detection system. For instance, inaccuracies in determining the TOF of photons can introduce errors in the localization of annihilation events along the LOR. Additionally, the lack of precise information about the depth of interaction (DOI) within the crystals can contribute to decoding errors, further degrading spatial resolution [1].

5.5.3 Scatter Fraction (SF)

This is an estimate of the system's ability to recognize scatter events (S) from true events (T). SF is calculated as the ratio between the number of scatter events and the total number of events detected during a PET acquisition. It is usually expressed as a percentage or as a decimal fraction (Fig. 5.10).

$$SF = \frac{S}{T+S}(\times 100)$$

5.5.4 Noise Equivalent Count Rate (NECR)

Represents an indirect measure of the quality of acquired data concerning the presence of random events (R) and scatter. It measures the system's ability to select and acquire true events. It is defined as the ratio between the square of true events and the total recorded events (true, scatter, and random)

$$NECR = \frac{T^2}{T+S+kR}$$

where k represents a factor that depends on the method used for random coincidence correction. Procedures for calculating the NECR are defined in the NEMA UN2 protocols. It is typically measured for various activity concentrations and different radionuclides, thus creating NECR curves as functions of them (Fig. 5.10). These curves usually exhibit a peak at a certain activity concentration, known as the peak NECR activity, and this data is used for optimizing PET acquisition parameters [2].

5.5.5 Quality Control (QC) for Hybrid PET Systems

Due to their complexity, hybrid PET systems are subject to a strict quality control program that can be divided into two types: daily quality controls (DQAs) and periodic quality controls (PQAs). Both involve the PET scanner and the associated radiological imaging system (CT or MRI) and must be performed according to the instructions provided in the PET manual and current regulations.

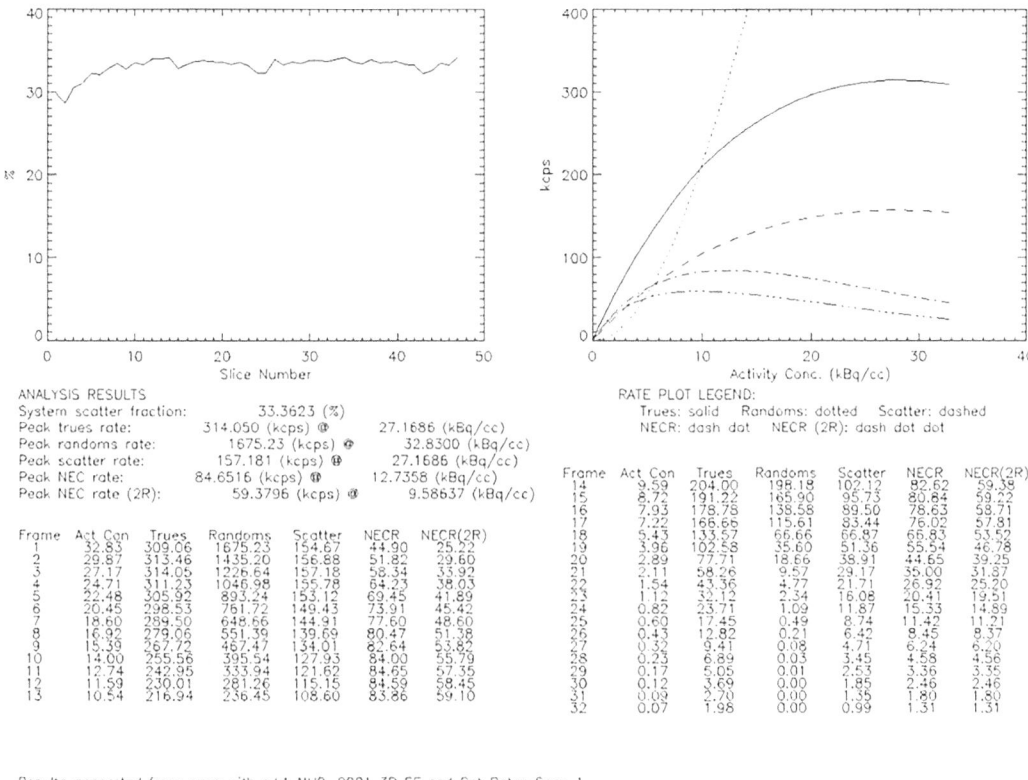

Fig. 5.10 Example of scatter fraction and NECR curves generated by a PET system during the acceptance test

5.5.5.1 DQA PET

It represents an important tool for system management due to the frequency with which it is performed. These are automatic or semiautomatic routine procedures, practical and simple to execute, using a Germanium 68 source to verify the correct functioning of the main components of the system, identify significant response variations of individual detectors or the system, and optimize performance. Among the typically verified parameters are coincidence time, photomultiplier tube gain, energy discrimination, and verification of detector response [13]. The result of this quality assurance (QA) can be displayed graphically and/or textually, always with colored indicators that show the compliance (green) or a mild (yellow) to strong (red) deviation from the tolerance range (Fig. 5.11).

These procedures need to take place before the start of diagnostic activity to avoid inappropriate exposures. Other checks not strictly related to the PET system that should be performed daily include verification of the environmental conditioning system, as significant temperature and humidity variations can affect PET detector performance, and the system clock, which must be synchronized with that of other systems (e.g., RIS, automatic injectors) with a maximum deviation of 1 min.

5.5.5.2 PQA PET

These checks allow for a more precise evaluation of the same parameters verified in the DQA through automatic or semiautomatic routines, and to save the baseline tables to which these refer. In addition, there is the normalization cali-

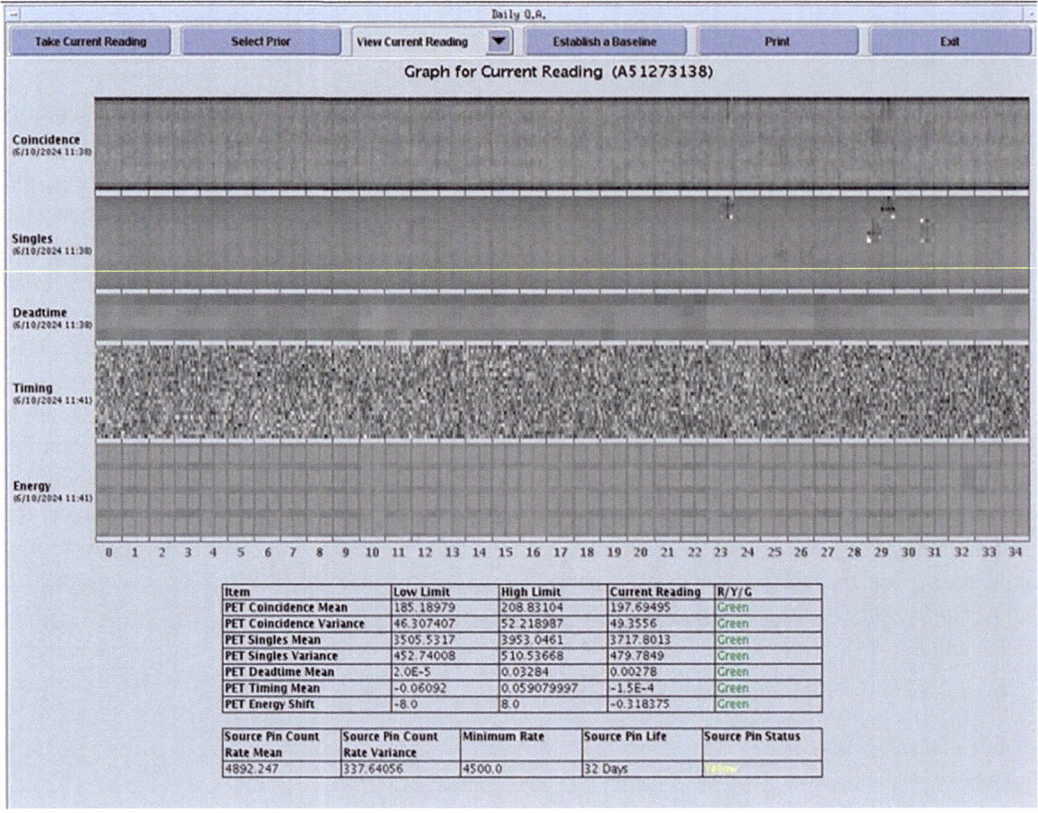

Fig. 5.11 DQA report generated by a PET system

bration necessary to correct the PET emission acquisition data for variations in the efficiency of the different LORs in each sinogram. To measure any efficiency differences, it is necessary to expose each detector pair to a radioactive source under the same measurement time and geometry conditions. This calibration generates the correction files necessary to eliminate sensitivity variations among the different acquisition planes and establish a correspondence between counts and activity concentration to obtain absolute quantification of the PET data [14].

5.5.5.3 CT Scanner
DQA procedures utilize tools and protocols specified in the equipment manuals, conducted after routine system initialization or start-up and before the first patient. These typically could involve tube conditioning, air calibration, and rapid CT quality assessments based on HU and noise metrics measured in water. Additionally, PQA, which differs depending on the manufacturer, generally entail supplementary image quality evaluations, CTDI measurements, slice thickness calculations, artefact assessments, and examination of scanner, gantry, and table functionalities.

5.5.5.4 MRI Scanner
Daily quality control procedures are conducted using manufacturer-provided phantoms after routine system initialization or start-up and before the first patient. Additionally, daily safety checks for PET/MR devices must be performed, including monitoring room temperature and humidity, checking the oxygen sensor, verifying the patient alert system and intercom systems, assessing coil status, and monitoring helium levels.

5.6 PET Acquisition Setting

PET offers the possibility to use different acquisition modalities, chosen based on the clinical question and desired parameters, by the hardware and software of the tomograph. Before the acquisition, there are several common phases for all modalities: entering patient and exam data, setting the patient's position on the bed, and positioning them on the tomograph bed. The choice of body position, arm placement, and the use of a headrest vary depending on the body segment being examined. Subsequently, the examination table is positioned for scanning with the tomograph's laser lights centered on the starting position, and parameters for scout, CT/MRI, and PET acquisition are set. The use of predefined protocols saves time and ensures quality exams with consistent results, maintaining consistent execution methods [14].

5.6.1 Data Recording

As we have seen, PET data is complex and can be demanding in terms of system requirements. There are two modes in which data is recorded for subsequent reconstruction:

- *Binned mode:* In this mode, data related to each LOR is saved after preprocessing and organization, allowing for structurally simple storage;
- *List mode:* In this mode, each detected event is recorded in a matrix called a sinogram, where every characteristic of the γ photon that generated it can be saved without any preprocessing.

Data in list mode can then be processed to obtain different sinograms by differentiating the acquisition parameters, excluding the duration of the acquisition. This mode has demanding requirements in terms of storage space and computing power, which can limit the duration of the acquisition. Both data recording modes can be applied to any type of PET acquisition.

5.6.2 Static Acquisition

This method is an acquisition with an extension equal to one PET axial field of view (commonly called bed), typically used for studying a single organ (e.g., brain) or a single body district (e.g., completing a total body study). The goal is to obtain an image of the highest possible quality by acquiring sufficient coincidences to reduce statistical error. However, the duration of this acquisition must be compatible with clinical practice and patient compliance. Some parameters to consider in defining the duration include the type and activity of the administered radiopharmaceutical, patient size, and body district of interest.

5.6.3 Dynamic Acquisition

This acquisition unfolds over time for the duration of a physiological/biological process of interest, typically performed in experimental settings and less frequently in clinical practice. The acquisition, with an extension of 1 bed, involves a sequence of frames with variable temporal frequency and appropriate timing (frame mode). The number and duration of frames depend on the kinetics of the radiopharmaceutical at the organ/tissue under examination and must cover the entire duration of the process under study. Recording events in list mode allows for overcoming the limitation of presetting frame data. For this acquisition, recording data related to the administered radiopharmaceutical activity may not be essential since quantitative data can be calculated based on the tracer distribution over time.

5.6.4 Total Body Acquisition

Is the most commonly used acquisition mode in clinical practice, requiring extensive study coverage, up to the entire body. During the acquisition, the patient bed moves axially in successive steps. At each step, a portion of the field of view equal to 1 bed is acquired. Individual beds are not acquired contiguously but with some overlap, necessary to correct artefacts generated in the outermost bed planes. The number of overlapping planes is determined based on the scanner characteristics, radionuclide, and administered activity. The overall duration of the acquisition is the sum of the acquisition times of the individual beds.

5.6.5 Gated Acquisition

This acquisition unfolds in frequency, synchronized to an external signal to the PET generated by a physiological signal (e.g., cardiac cycle). The synchronized acquisition is divided into frames or bins, the number of which is decided based on the desired counting statistics and the frequency of the phenomenon to be observed (frame mode). This serves the dual function of describing a phenomenon temporally and having the ability to reduce motion artefacts. Increasing the number of bins into which the phenomenon is divided increases temporal resolution but decreases counting statistics for each bin. This necessitates the acquisition of a greater number

of cycles, thus increasing the total acquisition time. Recording events in list mode allows for overcoming the limitation of presetting the number of bins.

5.7 Radiopharmaceutical Overview

The radiopharmaceuticals used in PET/CT typically consist of a pharmacophore labelled with a specific positron-emitting radionuclide. The most common radionuclides include ^{11}C, ^{15}O, ^{13}N, ^{18}F, ^{68}Ga, and ^{82}Rb (Table 5.2). The advantage of these isotopes lies in their short half-life (ranging from 78 s to 110 min) and their widespread availability, which is crucial for routine clinical applications. The pharmaceutical molecule can target cancer biomarkers such as enzymes, receptors, and transporters, or biological processes like energy metabolism, hypoxia, acidosis, and oxidative stress. Despite differences in composition, all these molecules share a set of attributes necessary to become effective imaging radiopharmaceuticals:

Table 5.2 Characteristics of the main PET radioisotopes

Isotope	Production	Half-life min	Type of emission	Max energy (MeV)
^{82}Rb	Generator	1.3	β^+	3.15
^{15}O	Cyclotron	2	β^+	1.70
^{13}N	Cyclotron	10	β^+	1.19
^{11}C	Cyclotron	20.3	β^+	0.96
^{68}Ga	Generator	68.1	β^+/electron capture	1.9
^{18}F	Cyclotron	110	β^+	0.64
^{64}Cu	Cyclotron	762	β^+/electron capture	0.66
^{76}Br	Cyclotron	972	β^+/electron capture	4
^{124}I	Cyclotron	60,192	β^+/electron capture	2.14

- High specificity
- High binding affinity
- Rapid clearance from nontarget tissues
- Stability in vivo
- Low immunogenicity and toxicity
- Accessibility and cost-effectiveness

Every pharmaceutical product relies on a pharmacopoeia, which serves as a national compendium of drug quality standards. Examples of well-known pharmacopoeias include the U.S. Pharmacopeia (USP) and the European Pharmacopeia (EP). These standards are always recognized through an official compendium [15].

In each state, regulatory authorities refer to the relevant monographs from the USP (in the U.S.) and the EP (in Europe) to ensure that pharmaceuticals meet consistent quality criteria. This practice helps prevent the marketing of inconsistent drugs and reduces potential risks to public health.

5.7.1 ^{18}F-Labelled Radiopharmaceuticals

The ^{18}F, for its physical and chemical characteristics, is the most widely used in the manufacture of PET tracers. Due to the high electronegativity of the fluorine atom, its incorporation significantly impacts the physicochemical properties of the vehicle molecule. When fluorine is included in the structure of biological compounds, it extends their half-life within the organism, affecting the molecules' metabolism, biodistribution, and protein binding kinetics (Table 5.3).

The ^{18}F radionuclide has a half-life of 109.7 min, and its compounds are utilized in imaging for almost all types of cancer, inflammation, cardiovascular disease, and brain studies [16].

Table 5.3 Characteristics of the most common radiopharmaceutical labelled with ^{18}F

Radiopharmaceutical	Target/target category	Function	Excretion via	Normal biodistribution
[^{18}F] Fluoro-2-deoxy-2-D--glucose FDG	Glucose transporters and hexokinases	Oncology, inflammation, cardiovascular disorder, central nervous system disorders	Renal	Bladder, kidneys, heart, brain
3′-Deoxy-3′-[^{18}F] fluorothymidine FLT	Thymidine kinase-1	Breast cancer, B-cell lymphoma, metastatic melanoma thoracic sarcoma	Renal	Bladder, liver, kidney, and bone marrow
O-(2-[^{18}F] Fluoroethyl)-L-tyrosine FET	L-type amino acid transporter system and Na$^+$-dependent system B0	Primary brain tumor, brain tumor metastases	Renal	Bladder
16α-[^{18}F] Fluoro-17β-estradiol FES	Estrogen receptor	Breast cancer	Renal	Liver, bladder
[^{18}F]Fluorocholine FCH	Choline kinases	Prostate cancer, breast cancer, brain tumor, liver cancer	Renal	Kidneys, liver, spleen
L-3,4-Dihydroxy-6-[^{18}F] fluorophenylalanine F-DOPA	Aromatic L-amino acid decarboxylase; L-type amino acid transporter system enzyme	Brain study, neuroendocrine metastatic lesions in bone	Renal	Bladder, kidneys, brain, liver, lungs
Fluorine [^{18}F] PSMA-1007	Prostate-specific membrane antigen CARBOSSIPEPTIDASI II (GCPII) antibody	Tumor with increased PSMA expression	Nonurinary excretion (biliary)	Serum, liver
Fluorine 18–sodium fluoride [^{18}F]NaF	Surface bone matrix	Bone metastasis (malignant or benignant) bone abnormalities, cardiac calcification process	Renal	Bone

5.7.2 ^{68}Ga-Labelled Radiopharmaceuticals

^{68}Ga is an excellent positron emitter with a half-life of 68 min. Its role represents an important milestone in functional and metabolic imaging. Recent studies have shown that radiolabelled compounds with ^{68}Ga provide better imaging quality than those with ^{111}In and ^{18}F tracers.

One significant advantage is the rapid labelling process done just before diagnostic examinations, with minimal activity loss due to the use of a generator installed directly in the radiopharmacy.

To use ^{68}Ga as a radiopharmaceutical, the compound must be resistant to hydrolysis and more stable than the Ga(III)-transferrin complex. Thus, the gallium complex must remain stable in the presence of transferrin (a plasma protein) [16, 17].

Various radiopharmaceuticals have been developed by conjugating ^{68}Ga with proteins, peptides, or small biological molecules (Table 5.4).

5.7.3 Other PET Radiopharmaceuticals

Many radiolabelled compounds in PET/CT imaging are now used in clinical practice, different from the most common ^{18}F or ^{68}Ga. However, due to their very short half-lives, most of these compounds require an on-site cyclotron for direct administration immediately after the radiolabelling process. These radiopharmaceuticals have very specific metabolic pathways and biodistribution, permitting a focused visualization of the target area (Table 5.5) [18].

Table 5.4 Characteristics of the most common radiopharmaceuticals labelled with ^{68}Ga

Radiopharmaceutical	Target/target category	Function	Excretion via	Normal biodistribution
[68Ga]PSMA-I&T [68Ga]PSMA-617 [68Ga]PSMA-11	Prostate-specific membrane antigen	Tumor with increased PSMA expression	Renal	Salivary gland, lacrimal gland, liver, spleen, kidney, bladder, small intestine
[68Ga]DOTA-TOC [68Ga]Ga-DOTA-NOC [68Ga]Ga-NODAGA-JR11 [68Ga]Ga-DOTA-TATE	Somatostatin receptor 2	Neuroendocrine tumors	Renal	Neuroendocrine gland, liver, spleen, intestine, kidney, bladder
[68Ga]Ga-FAPI-04 [68Ga]Ga-FAPI-21 [68Ga]Ga-FAPI-46	Fibroblast activation protein α fibroblast-activation-protein inhibitors	Solid malignancies	Renal	Kidneys, bladder

Table 5.5 Characteristics of the other most common radiopharmaceuticals in use

Radiopharmaceutical	Target/target category	Function	Excretion via	High uptake
L-[methyl-11C] Methionine	L-type amino acid transporter system and Na$^+$-dependent system	Brain gliomas and metastases	Renal	Blood, liver, spleen, kidney, bladder
N-[11C]-methyl-flumazenil	Binds to the benzodiazepine sites of GABAA receptors	Neuronal damages, epilepsy, stroke-induced penumbral, infarction and AD	Renal	Blood, liver, spleen, kidney, bladder
[11C-methoxyl] raclopride	Dopamine D$_1$ receptor	Neurological imaging	Renal	Blood, bladder
[^{11}C]Acetate	TCA cycle, fatty acid synthetase	Myocardical oxydative process, renal, pancreatic and prostate cancer	Renal	Blood, bladder
[^{11}C]Choline	Choline kinase	Prostate tumor, brain tumor, lung cancer, oesophagal cancer	Renal	Kidney, liver, pancreas, small intestine, salivary gland
[^{13}N]Ammonia	Glutamine synthetase	Assessing regional blood flow in tissue, coronary artery disease, hepatic encephalopathy	Renal	Myocardium, brain, liver, kidneys, skeletal muscle
[^{15}O]CO	Oxygen metabolism	Oxygen consumption in the brain and blood volume	Lung	Lung, brain, heart, blood
[^{15}O] H$_2$O	Follow the metabolism of water in blood flow	Cerebral blood flow Myocardial perfusion	Renal	Blood flow
[^{82}Rb] Rubidium chloride	Potassium-mimicking behavior	Cardiac flow	Renal	Heart

5.8 Applications of Artificial Intelligence in PET Imaging

Artificial intelligence (AI) has made remarkable progress in recent years, and its use is increasingly widespread even in the medical field.

The introduction of AI and PET imaging to clinical applications presents significant potential for improving image quality, dose reduction, diagnostic accuracy, and predictive analytics, indicating a promising future for AI-assisted nuclear medicine.

Specific AI subsets, such as machine learning (ML) and deep learning (DL), are playing an increasing role in PET/CT imaging in terms of image enhancement and clinical applications.

Image enhancement:

- *Photon detection:* Neural networks are used for precise photon position detection, improving DOI decoding and TOF PET imaging, which enhances spatial resolution and timing accuracy.
- *Data correction:* AI models generate accurate attenuation maps from non-AC PET data and enhance scatter distribution predictions, improving overall image quality. In particular, AI-based attenuation correction is crucial for PET-only or PET/MR scanners that lack CT images, providing accurate quantitative imaging without the need for additional CT scans.
- *Image reconstruction:* AI, especially DL algorithms, optimizes PET/CT image reconstruction processes. These advanced techniques

can refine reconstruction algorithms, leading to clearer and more precise images.

- *Low-dose imaging:* AI enables low-dose imaging, crucial for reducing radiation exposure to patients. Techniques like GANs (Generative Adversarial Networks) and DL algorithms allow for the generation of high-quality images even with reduced radiopharmaceutical doses, maintaining image interpretability and diagnostic accuracy [10, 11].

Clinical applications:

- *Tumor delineation and detection:* AI assists in accurately segmenting tumors and delineating metabolic tumor volumes, reducing delineation time for nuclear medicine and interobserver variability. Consequently, this points to potential improvements in the speed and consistency of treatment planning and increased biomarker stability
- *Pathological phenotype classification and radiogenomics*: AI models correlate imaging features with pathological and genetic data, aiding in the classification of tumor phenotypes and understanding of genetic mutations.
- *Therapeutic response and prognosis prediction*: AI improves the prediction of therapeutic responses and patient prognosis, supporting personalized treatment planning. AI-based models have been applied in evaluating responses to chemoradiotherapy and targeted therapies.

AI has the potential to revolutionize PET imaging by improving image quality, and reducing radiation exposure, leading to improved predictive performance [12].

5.9 Radiation Dosimetry and Protection in PET

The radiation dose to staff in a PET/CT facility can be optimized by adhering to fundamental radiological protection practices. These include maintaining a safe distance from the radiation source or patient, minimizing the time spent performing operations, and using appropriate shielding whenever feasible.

An essential tool in reducing staff exposure is the implementation of automatic dispensing and infusion systems. These systems minimize the need for manual administration of radiopharmaceuticals, eliminating direct contact and reducing the risk of exposure to extremities.

Technological advancements in PET/CT scanners have further contributed to reducing worker exposure. With improved detector and system designs, digital PET/CT allows for the detection of small lesions with lower administered activity, resulting in reduced dose exposure for both patients and staff. Efforts to minimize exposure for patients and technologists adhere to the ALARA (as low as reasonably achievable) principle, without compromising exam quality or patient care.

Whole-body monitoring should be conducted, and a Hp(10) measurement from a dosimeter worn on the upper body will provide an approximate indication of the dose to the eye lens. Equivalent dose monitoring is typically performed using an extremity dosimeter, which should be positioned as close as possible to the most exposed part of the skin. Monitoring extremity doses with ring dosimeters is recommended. Routine hygienic measures, such as wearing gloves and protective clothing, help limit skin contamination. However, contamination can still occur in cases of accidental spills or cross-contamination.

Distance from the patient should be maximized when escorting and positioning the patient. Unless the patient needs special assistance, it has been recommended that, when setting up a scan, staff should be encouraged to stand at the end of the bed or to the side of the gantry.

New tools based on artificial intelligence techniques have recently been developed that allow automatic patient positioning, reducing the need for operators to enter the PET/CT imaging room and thus decreasing their exposure [19].

References

1. Khalil MM. Positron emission tomography (PET): physics and instrumentation. In: Khalil MM, editor. Basic sciences of nuclear medicine. Cham: Springer; 2021.
2. Schmitz RE, Alessio AM, Kinahan PE. The physics of PET-CT scanners. PET PET-CT. Published online 2019, p. 1–16.
3. Mariani G, Erba PA, Volterrani D. Fondamenti di medicina nucleare. Berlin: Springer; 2011.
4. Volterrani D, Erba PA, Carrió I, Strauss HW, Mariani G. Nuclear medicine textbook: methodology and clinical application. Cham: Springer; 2019.
5. Jones T, Townsend D. History and future technical innovation in positron emission tomography. J Med Imaging. 2017;4(1):011013.
6. Bailey DL, Humm JL, Todd-Pokropek A, van Aswegen A. Nuclear medicine physics. A handbook for teachers and students. Vienna: International Atomic Energy Agency; 2014.
7. Powsner RA, Palmer MR, Powsner ER. Essentials of nuclear medicine physics, instrumentation, and radiation biology. 4th ed. Hoboken: Wiley Blackwell; 2022.
8. Saha GB. Basics of PET imaging: physics, chemistry, and regulations. 3rd ed. New York: Springer; 2016.
9. Reader AJ, Pan B. AI for PET image reconstruction. Br J Radiol. 2023;96(1150):20230292.
10. Gong K, Kim K, Cui J, Wu D, Li Q. The evolution of image reconstruction in PET: from filtered back-projection to artificial intelligence. PET Clin. 2021;16(4):533–42.
11. Dai J, Wang H, Xu Y, Chen X, Tian R. Clinical application of AI-based PET images in oncological patients. Semin Cancer Biol. 2023;91:124–42.
12. Matsubara K, Ibaraki M, Nemoto M, Watabe H, Kimura Y. A review on AI in PET imaging. Ann Nucl Med. 2022;36(2):133–43.
13. EFOMP's guideline: quality control in PET-CT and PET/RM. Version 02.03.2022.
14. International Atomic Energy Agency. PET-CT atlas on quality control and image artefacts, IAEA human health series No. 27. Vienna: IAEA; 2014.
15. Crişan G, Moldovean-Cioroianu NS, Timaru DG, Andrieş G, Căinap C, Chiş V. Radiopharmaceuticals for PET and SPECT imaging: a literature review over the last decade. Int J Mol Sci. 2022;23(9):5023.
16. Lau J, Rousseau E, Kwon D, Lin KS, Bénard F, Chen X. Insight into the development of PET radiopharmaceuticals for oncology. Cancer. 2020;12:1312.
17. Huang YY. An overview of PET radiopharmaceuticals in clinical use: regulatory, quality and pharmacopeia monographs of the United States and Europe. In: Nuclear medicine physics. London: IntechOpen; 2019.
18. Shahhosseini S. PET radiopharmaceuticals. Iran J Pharm Res. 2011;10(1):1–2.
19. Dannoon SF, Alenezi S, Alnafisi N, Almutairi S, Dashti F, Osman MM, Elgazzar A. Reducing radiation exposure from PET patients. J Nucl Med Technol. 2022;50(3):263–8.

Foundations of PET/MR

6

Sami Jeljeli, Gary Cook, Alexander Hammers,
Amedeo Chiribiri, Harriet Rogers,
Shawna Kinsella, Georgios Krokos,
and Radhouene Neji

6.1 Introduction

Despite the idea of combining positron emission tomography (PET) with MRI (magnetic resonance imaging) being proposed approximately 40 years ago [1], it took another 25 years for the first PET/MR system to be introduced in the clinical and research setting due to the engineering challenges that had to be overcome in combining the two modalities. An early intuitive approach [2] was to keep the two systems separate either by moving the bed from one bore to the other (sequential approach) or by moving the whole bed from the PET/CT to the MR scanner (trimodal approach). However, the scientific community was interested in the ground-breaking possibilities a simultaneous scan would unlock from a clinical perspective, such as complementary information by simultaneously imaging physiological function using a large pool of tracers in PET with functional and anatomical MRI, and from a technical perspective, such as the possibility to use MRI for motion correction on PET images [3] and to potentially improve PET spa-

S. Jeljeli (✉) · G. Cook · S. Kinsella
King's College London and Guy's and St Thomas' PET Centre and Department of Cancer Imaging, School of Biomedical Engineering and Imaging Sciences, King's College London, London, UK
e-mail: sami.jeljeli@kcl.ac.uk; gary.cook@kcl.ac.uk; shawna.kinsella@kcl.ac.uk

A. Hammers
King's College London and Guy's and St Thomas' PET Centre, Research Department of Biomedical Computing, and Research Department of Early Life Imaging, School of Biomedical Engineering, London, UK
e-mail: alexander.hammers@kcl.ac.uk

A. Chiribiri
Research Department of Cardiovascular Imaging and Research Department of Imaging Physics and Engineering, King's College London, Heart and Lung Critical Care Clinical Group, Guys and St Thomas' NHS Foundation Trust, London, UK
e-mail: amedeo.chiribiri@kcl.ac.uk

H. Rogers
MRI Physics Section, Medical Physics and Clinical Engineering, Guy's and St Thomas' NHS Foundation Trust, London, UK
e-mail: harriet.rogers@kcl.ac.uk

G. Krokos
King's College London and Guy's and St Thomas' PET Centre, Faculty of Life Sciences and Medicine, School of Biomedical Engineering and Imaging Sciences, London, UK
e-mail: georgios.krokos@kcl.ac.uk

R. Neji
Research Department of Imaging Physics and Engineering, School of Biomedical Engineering and Imaging Sciences, King's College London, London, UK
e-mail: radhouene.neji@kcl.ac.uk

© The Author(s), under exclusive license to Springer Nature Switzerland AG 2025
L. Camoni, L. Mansi (eds.), *Nuclear Medicine Hybrid Imaging for Radiographers & Technologists*,
https://doi.org/10.1007/978-3-031-86228-1_6

tial resolution by exploiting the decrease in positron range due to the magnetic field [4]. Moreover, the logistical benefits, and subsequently the higher patient throughput, and smaller footprint along with the decrease in patient dose quickly led to making the simultaneous design synonymous with 'PET/MR'. Consequently, according to [5], as of 2023, only one tri-modal PET/CT/MR was still in use out of a total 43 scanners worldwide, with the rest being the two currently available systems for simultaneous scanning.

Therefore, this chapter will focus on simultaneous PET/MR scanners. A short overview of the clinical applications conducted on PET/MR scanners is provided, and the fundamental principles of the scanner along with its technical characteristics are described. Finally, an educational overview of the steps and responsibilities involved is outlined, particularly focusing on the critical role of the PET/MR Radiographer/Technologist, using the King's College London and Guy's and St Thomas' PET Centre as an example. The first PET/MR scanner in the UK was installed at the University College London Hospitals (UCLH).

6.2 Clinical Applications

6.2.1 Oncology

Since its inception, PET/MR has gained significant grounds towards the diagnosis and treatment planning of various oncological diseases. Efficacy has been shown, for example, in malignant pleural mesothelioma [6], Hodgkin and non-Hodgkin lymphoma [7], prostate cancer [8], and breast cancer [9]. Its ability to deliver excellent soft tissue contrast and physiological function (e.g. blood flow, tissue diffusion) of MRI combined with the detailed metabolic and molecular information of PET allows for enhanced tumour delineation, staging, and therapy response assessment. It has been shown that PET/MR can perform at least as well as PET/CT in the majority of cancer imaging applications [10], but clinical translation has been impeded by slower scan

acquisition and economic viability. For instance, in cases of head and neck cancers, PET/MR combined with diffusion-weighted imaging (DWI) can differentiate between post-therapeutic changes and residual or recurrent disease more effectively than either PET/CT or MRI alone, but more multicentre trials are required to further assess the value of PET/MR in this clinical context [11]. Advantages are especially apparent in managing prostate cancer, where PET/MR contributes to more targeted biopsy strategies and optimized treatment plans with the potential to enhance patient outcomes [11]. In general, the stronger clinical applications are in cancers that require PET imaging and are often also imaged with MRI rather than CT, e.g. prostate cancer, brain tumours, gynaecological cancers.

6.2.2 Cardiology

One of the most common applications of PET/MR in cardiology is the evaluation of coronary artery disease (CAD). This is due to the ability of PET imaging to quantitatively assess myocardial perfusion and detect ischemic changes using radioactive tracers such as [^{13}N]ammonia among other tracers. This technique helps in identifying areas of reduced blood flow and determining the extent of myocardial viability, particularly useful in patients post-myocardial infarction for predicting recovery post-revascularization [12].

Supplementing PET/MR offers high-resolution images of cardiac structure and functional parameters. It is excellent at depicting areas of scar tissue through late gadolinium enhancement, providing valuable information on myocardial viability and tissue characterization [13]. When combined, PET/MR leverages PET's quantitative capabilities with MRI's detailed anatomical visualization and inherently excellent spatial resolution, significantly improving the diagnostic accuracy for CAD and other cardiac conditions. Simultaneously acquiring the two scans offers additional advantages, such as enhanced scanning efficiency, motion correction, and partial volume correction. The radiation exposure is lower compared to hybrid PET/computed tomography scanning, which is especially beneficial for younger patients who might require multiple scans [14].

Additionally, PET/MR is pivotal in diagnosing and managing inflammatory and infiltrative cardiac diseases such as myocarditis and sarcoidosis. The ability of PET to highlight metabolic activity using [^{18}F]FDG and gadolinium-enhanced MRI to delineate structural abnormalities allows for precise localization and assessment of disease activity [15]. Additionally, this hybrid modality is beneficial in evaluating cardiac tumours and systemic conditions affecting the heart, providing a comprehensive overview of both anatomical and metabolic changes [16].

6.2.3 Neurology

In neurology, PET is used mainly in neurodegenerative diseases such as Alzheimer's and Parkinson's disease; in epilepsy for the presurgical evaluation; and in the management of brain tumours. In all of these cases, PET/MR provides additional useful information from MRI, and the simultaneous acquisition is particularly useful in neuro-oncology where the patient status may quickly change between separate PET/CT and MRI acquisitions.

In the diagnosis and management of neurodegenerative diseases such as Alzheimer's and Parkinson's disease, PET/MR with [^{18}F]FDG PET provides metabolic information that helps in the early detection of these conditions, while MRI offers high contrast and spatial resolution images of the brain which can be used to detect changes in the hippocampi and/or brain atrophies. Selective radiopharmaceuticals are also used, e.g. [^{18}F]F-Dopa for demonstrating degeneration of the dopaminergic system, and amyloid or tau tracers for demonstrating deposition of those proteins in Alzheimer's disease, even before the patient develops symptoms or before functional ([^{18}F]FDG) or structural (MRI) changes become visible.

PET/MR is a valuable one-stop shop imaging tool in epilepsy for identifying seizure foci for surgical planning where [^{18}F]FDG PET is ideally interpreted together with the structural MRI. There is now evidence that simultaneous PET/MR has an advantage over post hoc co-registered PET/CT and MRI [17].

In neuro-oncology, PET/MR enhances the diagnosis and treatment of brain tumours by integrating metabolic and anatomical data. PET imaging, especially with amino acid tracers like [^{18}F]FET ([^{18}F]fluoro-ethyl-tyrosine), is superior in distinguishing tumour recurrence from radiation necrosis and in detecting low-grade gliomas that may not be visible on MRI alone. There has been sufficient evidence [16]. This capability is critical for accurate treatment planning and monitoring therapeutic responses.

PET/MR also shows promise in studying the microenvironment of brain tumours, which can help in developing personalized treatment strategies. For example, it aids in assessing tumour perfusion, hypoxia, and metabolic activity, providing a comprehensive understanding of tumour biology [18]. This information is important for planning targeted therapies and evaluating their effectiveness.

6.3 Fundamentals and Instrumentation of PET/MR

6.3.1 Basic MRI Principles of PET/MR

The fundamentals of MRI within a PET/MR scanner are no different to those within a standard MRI-only scanner. The following provides an overview of the basic principles of MRI.

An MRI scanner is composed of various coils (loops of wire). A typical scanner will consist of the main magnet (which produces the strong static magnetic field, B_0), gradient coils, and RF (radiofrequency) coils. It is possible to generate an image through a combination of the static magnetic field, gradient magnetic fields, and RF pulses, using the abundance of hydrogen particles in the human body.

The human body is primarily composed of water, which in turn is composed of hydrogen atoms. Each hydrogen nucleus consists of a single positively charged proton which spins around its axis. This spinning charge generates a small magnetic field, known as a magnetic moment. When a proton is placed in the large static external magnetic field (B_0), it tries to align itself with the direction of this field. However, due to the principles of quantum mechanics, the proton cannot align perfectly and instead spins or precesses, around the direction of the magnetic field. The precessional frequency is proportional to the external magnetic field; therefore, a higher external magnetic field produces a higher frequency. This relationship is given by the Larmor equation:

$$\omega = \gamma \bullet B_0$$

ω precession/Larmor frequency, γ the gyromagnetic ratio (a constant = 42.57 MHz T^{-1} for hydrogen nuclei), B_0 the external magnetic field.

These protons can be oriented in any direction, resulting in a nearly spherical distribution; however, there is a tendency to align with the external magnetic field (B_0). When this magnetic field is applied by placing an object inside the scanner, it causes the proton distribution to precess around this fixed axis. Given the vast number of protons in the human body, the spins can be represented as a vector of the average magnetic moments instead of each individual proton. This net magnetization, M_0, aligns with B_0. However, M_0 is much smaller than B_0 and so when it is parallel to B_0, as has just been described, it cannot be measured. To measure M_0, an RF pulse is applied which flips M_0 90° into the transverse plane. This RF pulse is applied at the Larmor frequency. After the RF pulse is turned off, the spins gradually return to equilibrium in a process called relaxation. This process has two main components: the dephasing of spins in the transverse plane (transverse relaxation) and the realignment of the net magnetization along the z-axis (longitudinal relaxation).

The dephasing of the spins in the transverse plane occurs not only due to inhomogeneities in the main static magnetic field, but also due to the interactions between the spins (spin-spin relaxation). This can be quantified by the transverse relaxation time or T_2.

Longitudinal relaxation occurs when the protons interact with the surrounding tissue resulting in a loss of energy (spin-lattice relaxation). This process is quantified by the longitudinal relaxation time, T_1. Transverse (spin–spin) relaxation, quantified by T_2, is independent and proceeds more rapidly than T_1 dephasing.

In addition to the main external magnetic field (B_0) and the applied RF pulse, magnetic gradients are also needed. When placed in the static magnetic field, the protons will be experiencing approximately the same magnetic field and can all be excited by the same frequency RF pulse (applied at the Larmor frequency). However, we need to be able to interpret where the received MRI signal is coming from. For this, we need to localize the signal by applying additional magnetic field gradients. Gradients are simply additional magnetic fields that have linear variations to alter the strength of the external magnetic field. When these gradients are applied, the protons are experiencing slightly different magnetic field strengths and thus have different precessional frequencies. It is the application of these gradients in combination with the RF pulse that allows for the localization of the signal.

Furthermore, various alterations can be made to the duration and strength of the applied pulses and gradients to give us different MRI sequences. Each sequence provides images with different contrast; for example, on a T_1-weighted image CSF will appear dark, whereas on a T_2-weighted image CSF will appear bright. Each clinical indication can require multiple contrasts relevant to the specific pathology, and so several MRI sequences are needed for each MRI exam.

6.3.2 Basic PET Principles of PET/MR

The fundamental principles for PET scanning in PET/MR are the same for PET/CT or PET-only cameras which have been described in other chapters of this book. In brief though, PET applications take advantage of positron rich isotopes which undergo β^+ decay where a proton (p) is converted into a neutron (n) with the concurrent emission of a positron (β^+) and a neutrino (ν).

$$p = n + \beta^+ + \nu$$

Since the neutron is one electron mass heavier than the proton, the parent isotope needs to have a transition energy higher than two electron masses (2×511 keV) for the above reaction to take place. Any excess energy is given to the positron which will then travel through matter, gradually losing energy through interactions with the surrounding particles until it annihilates with an electron of the medium to two photons, each carrying an energy of 511 keV and travelling in almost opposite directions. The path travelled by the positron before it annihilates is called positron range and introduces blurring to the PET images due to the uncertainty of the point of annihilation.

However, according to MRI physics, we know that when a magnetic field is applied to a charged particle, this will follow a spiralling trajectory along the direction of the magnetic field as shown in Fig. 6.1. Consequently, the distance travelled by the positron will be decreased along the x–y direction with increasing magnetic field, potentially reducing the blurring in the images due to positron range. Monte Carlo simulations have also been employed to confirm this behaviour corroborating the potential benefits in PET spatial resolution by the introduction of a PET/MR scanner [4]. This benefit was especially expected to be demonstrated in the increasing clinical applications using highly energetic radioisotopes such as rubidium-82, gallium-68, oxygen-15, and others.

The other main differences in the acquisition of PET data compared to a conventional PET/CT scanner are related to the compatibility of various components between PET and MRI scanners that exhibited certain challenges in the design of the hybrid scanner. In addition, one of the main requirements in PET image reconstruction is some a priori knowledge of the attenuating medium which would be usually given by the CT images or emission data. All those challenges and how they were addressed are further outlined in the following sections on technical foundations.

6.3.3 Technical Challenges of Integrated PET/MR

6.3.3.1 Effect of the Magnetic Field on PET

The integration of the PET with the MRI components was far from a straightforward process and unearthed significant challenges from an engineering perspective. Most of the issues were related to the metallic components of the PET detectors and particularly in the photomultiplier tubes (PMTs). More specifically, PMTs are very

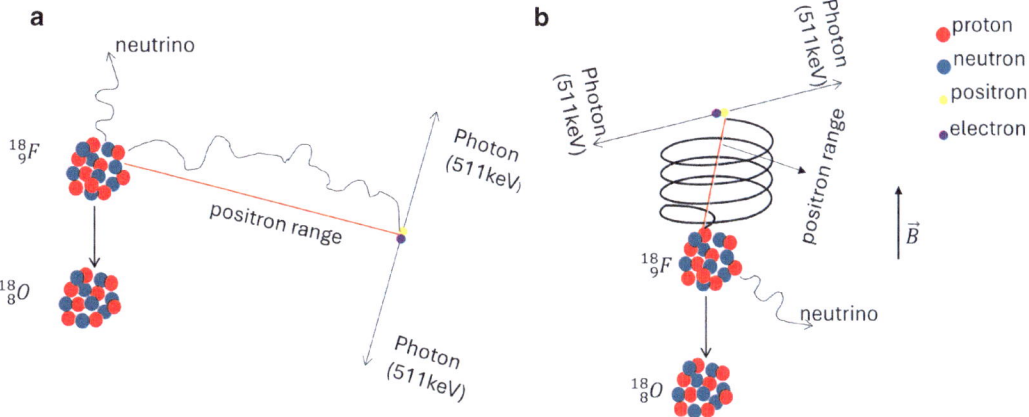

Fig. 6.1 Beta decay of fluorine-18 (F-18) to oxygen-18 (O-18) when (**a**) no magnetic field is present and (**b**) under the influence of a magnetic field

sensitive to magnetic fields (even the earth's magnetic field could affect their performance) as they could bend the trajectory of the electrons and as a result decrease their collection efficiency. To prevent such issues, a magnetic shield case made of metallic components could be used. However, this causes bi-directional problems with the MRI performance and function being affected by the presence of those PET components and vice versa [19, 20]. Moreover, the bulky design of the PMTs as indicated in Fig. 6.2 was quite impractical for this task as it made the design of a simultaneous system even more challenging.

6.3.4 Field Inhomogeneity

The isocentre of the MRI bore should have a highly homogeneous magnetic field where the protons (within the patient being imaged) are experiencing approximately the same precessional frequency. When other materials are placed within the scanner's field of view (FOV), the homogeneity is distorted which, in turn, results in image quality issues such as signal degradation, shading, image distortion, and other artifacts. Most modern PET scanners use lutetium or lutetium-yttrium oxyorthosilicate scintillator (LSO or LYSO) or bismuth germanate (BGO) crystals which have similar magnetic susceptibility to human tissue and cause minimal distortion which can be corrected by shimming (a process

used to improve magnetic field homogeneity). However, the metallic parts of the PMTs can cause greater distortion.

6.3.5 Radiofrequency Interference

The PET electronics can cause electromagnetic interference. Taking into account how low the radiofrequency signal received by the coils is in MRI, one can easily imagine that even the slightest interference could result in distorted MRI images [3, 19, 20]. This electromagnetic interference can also affect PET electronics and lead to a drop of the count rate. An easy approach to this problem is to use lightproof non-ferromagnetic RF shielding such as copper to enclose the PET components.

As per Faraday's law, a changing magnetic field generates electrical currents. Due to how an MRI scanner operates, with rapidly changing magnetic field gradients, these currents (known as eddy currents) are produced when imaging is performed. Eddy currents can cause degradation in gradient switching and shifts in the main magnetic field, therefore once again causing image artifacts such as mis-registration and blurring. Higher field strengths and fast imaging sequences (and those where there is rapid gradient switching) produce the greatest eddy current problems. In this context, eddy currents could increase the temperature in PET electronics while the copper shielding required to enclose PET components can in turn induce eddy currents on its surface.

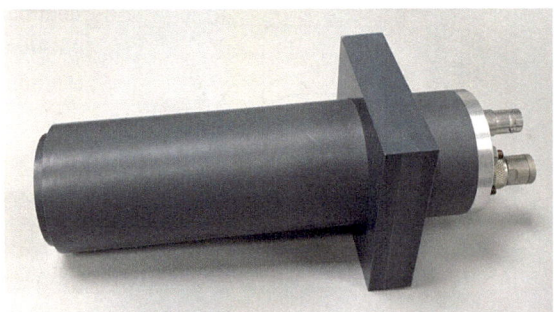
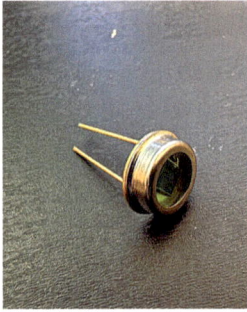
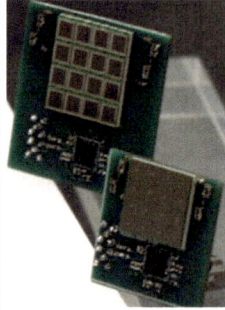

Fig. 6.2 Photos of a PMT (centre), an APD (left) and a SiPM (right, Wikimedia Commons/CC-BY-SA-3.0) detector [21]. The images have been magnified for better visualization, but the height of a PMT is approximately 15 cm while the diameter of an APD is approximately 0.5 cm and the SIPM array is approximately 4 cm wide and comprised of single APDs with dimensions of <0.01 cm each

6.3.6 Solutions for Designing a Simultaneous PET/MR

Evidently, an alternative to the PMTs within a simultaneous PET/MR system needed to be found. An intuitive approach was to place the PMTs far away from the scanner. As such, one of the earliest solutions to the problem was to use long optical fibers that connected the PMTs (which were placed far from the magnetic field) with the scintillation crystals and direct the light across [22]. Although this technique was easier to set up in a smaller system such as preclinical scanners, it would have been a much more complex task to set up in a clinical PET/MR facility, with many long cables that were connected to PMTs far from the scanner itself creating a much larger footprint. Moreover, since the photons had to travel a long distance in the fiber cables, they were experiencing additional attenuation while it was challenging to perfectly align the crystals with the PMT tubes to ensure direct detection of photons. Due to these effects, the systems experienced some light loss and decreased timing and energy resolution compared to a system with coupled scintillation crystals-PMTs.

A more practical alternative to the previous solution was the use of solid-state photodetectors such as avalanche photodiodes (APD). These are much more compact, can be directly connected to the crystals, and are insensitive to magnetic fields making them a perfect candidate for PET/MR systems. The incident photon results in an avalanche of electrons that builds an internal gain and has the advantage of achieving more than three times higher the quantum efficiency (ability to convert photons into electrons) compared to PMTs. On the other hand, the stochastic process of the avalanche phenomenon in APDs leads to increased noise that can subsequently affect the signal-to-noise ratio of the PET images. Therefore, the gain applied for operating the system is usually relatively small compared to PMTs. In addition, the generation of the electrical signal from the avalanche process is slower compared to PMTs which does not allow for time-of-flight (TOF) capabilities. The first scanner to take advantage of this technology was launched in 2010 and was the first PET/MR system commercially available for clinical use. Interference of the magnetic field to the PET components and vice versa was minimal [23].

The next stop in further improving the performance of the PET/MR systems was the use of silicon photomultipliers (SiPMs) instead of conventional APDs. Despite the difference in name, it needs to be noted that this is not a completely different technology. SiPMs are essentially an array of small cells of APDs operating in Geiger-mode. This means that the diode can be operated slightly above the breakdown voltage threshold (the voltage at which the semiconductor begins to fail) which can be prevented using a quench circuit. At such high voltage, even a single electron can result in a strong avalanche. The small cells act independently with the summed output from all cells being proportional to the deposited energy in the scintillation crystal. At the same time, light sharing between cells is eliminated leading to better spatial resolution. Moreover, digital SiPMs exhibit better timing resolution allowing for TOF capabilities. This technology was used in PET/MR that achieved a smaller than 400 ps timing resolution allowing for TOF capabilities. An illustration of the various detectors can be seen in Fig. 6.2 while a cross-sectional view of the scanner components within the bore of a PET/MR scanner which allows simultaneous scanning can be seen in Fig. 6.3.

6.3.7 Additional Practical Problems

The integration of the PET components within the MRI coils also resulted in a smaller bore diameter of 60 cm. Even though this is approximately just 10 cm smaller compared to existing PET/CT and MRI systems, it made positioning of patients with arms up more difficult, and as a result, all patients on the PET/MR are scanned with arms down. Due to the limited FOV of the MRI, this leads to 'truncation artefacts' in the arms and consequently inaccurate attenuation correction for the PET data. Various approaches have been employed in order to address this issue including the prediction of the attenuation correction map during recon-

Fig. 6.3 Illustration of the various components enclosed within a PET/MR bore

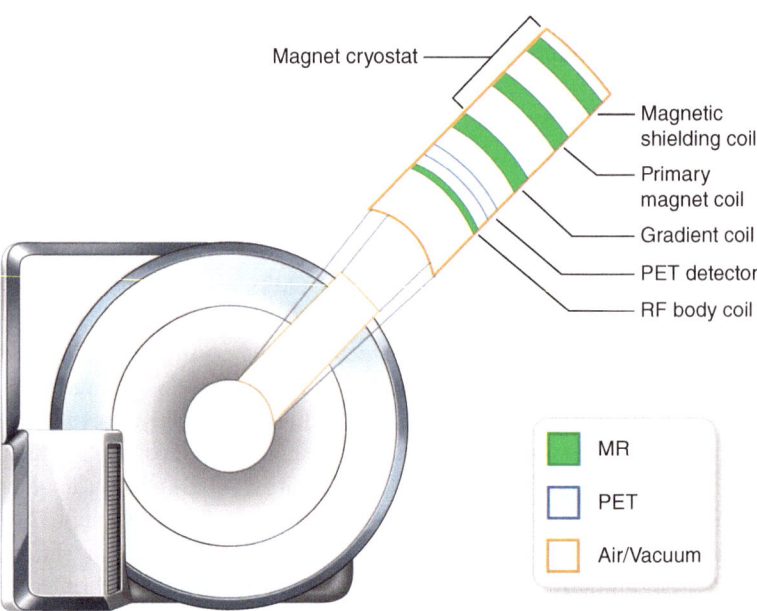

Magnet cryostat

Magnetic shielding coil

Primary magnet coil

Gradient coil

PET detector

RF body coil

MR

PET

Air/Vacuum

struction (more details in the next section) and the more commonly used 'B0 homogenization using gradient enhancement' (HUGE), a sequence technique which results in an extended FOV. In addition, the smaller bore has resulted in more patients experiencing claustrophobia [24]. For brain scans, this can be mitigated with the use of a mirror on the head coil. For body scans, the head could be scanned first and then the patient could be repositioned feet-first after the first bed position. Most importantly, PET/MR staff need to be appropriately trained to make sure the patient is relaxed and as comfortable as possible and they are prepared about what the examination involves, this can be achieved through frequently using the intercom.

Another practical issue that is indirectly related to the design and the inherent properties of the PET/MR is the accurate scheduling and scanning of patients which is mainly relevant in a busy clinical environment. Delays in a PET department are not usually easily tolerated as the production and delivery of the radiopharmaceutical is scheduled for a certain time and the patients need to arrive promptly to their appointment so that all scheduled patients receive the appropriate dose for their examination. A delay, for example,

in scanning the first patient, would have a knock-on effect on all subsequent appointments which could result in appointment cancellation for the last patients as the radiotracer might have decayed below the permissible dose for performing a diagnostic PET examination. The positioning of the patient for an oncology scan on the PET/MR is less straightforward compared to the PET/CT due to the use of multiple coils, use of headphones and/or earplugs (acoustic noise reduction) and ensuring that the patient is lying comfortably without arms crossed (to prevent closed loops and tissue burns), a process which could also lead to delays in the subsequent patient scans and increased staff dose.

Therefore, the radiographers need to be adequately trained on PET and MRI properties, to be able to confidently position patients securely, and carefully plan accordingly for each day's appointments.

6.3.8 The Issue of Attenuation Correction

One of the main hurdles for absolute quantification on PET images when performing PET/MR is attenuation correction. As MRI signal is related to proton density and not photon attenuation (as is the case for CT on PET/CTs or emission scans on PET-only scanners), the density of the materials within the PET's FOV is difficult to determine. This also applies to the attenuation of the photons due to MRI coils and hardware which lie within the PET's FOV. To address such issues, casing from low attenuating materials such as polyethylene is generally used. Nonetheless, biases of approximately 20% have still been observed in high attenuating areas of the coils such as the locks [25]. A workaround to this problem is to use integrated hardware attenuation maps, i.e. pre-defined CT-based attenuation maps of the patient's bed and head coils which are available in the scanner's software. These are then superimposed to the patient's attenuation map during image reconstruction. This method has been found to significantly reduce bias, although inclusion of flexible surface coils is still a challenge as it is difficult to predict their exact location on the patient. Manufacturers have yet to include a method to deal with these flexible surface coils or the use of additional hardware such as headphones and flatbeds for radiotherapy planning. However, research has proposed various approaches, such as the use of oil capsules on the patient and the coil [26] or a depth camera to track the actual position of the coil during scanning [27].

Another challenge is to develop a method that could convert MRI signal to attenuation coefficient values for 511 keV photons for the patients. A number of approaches have been proposed in the literature which can be largely categorized as (a) MR-based, (b) emission-based, (c) atlas-based, and (d) machine learning-based methods [28].

6.3.8.1 MR-Based Methods

These methods aim to exploit the information from the MRI images in order to create attenuation coefficient maps for PET. These are also called segmentation approaches, as the task usually relates to identifying different classes of tissue and applying a uniform attenuation coefficient for each class. The most commonly used approach is the Dixon method which was originally suggested almost 40 years ago [29]. This method uses two slightly different echo times resulting in two images: one with the water and fat molecules precessing in-phase and one out-of-phase. Using simple algebra, fat-only and water-only images can then be generated which can then be combined to generate an image of two classes (fat and water) as shown in Fig. 6.4. This method still led to bias due to bone not being included in the final map. A more recent version of this method uses a bone atlas that is registered to the final attenuation correction map leading to improved quantification. An alternative method to visualize bone is to use very short echo times to receive signal from regions with very short T_2^* (T_2 imaging which incorporates field inhomogeneities) in what is known as ultra-short time echo (UTE) or zero-time echo (ZTE). A comparison of all methods can be seen in Fig. 6.5. The advantage of MR-based methods is that they are readily available on the scanner, easy to use, and for most regions provide relatively low bias and are sufficient for qualitative purposes. However, it has still been reported that these approaches (particularly UTE and the bone atlas in the Dixon method) are not always reproducible, as classification of human physiology into a very limited number of classes with uniform values might not be the most accurate approach. Moreover, motion between MRI and PET can lead to additional artifacts in the reconstructed images, while motion during the MRI image can lead to artifacts on the images that are inevitably propagated on the PET images. Various methods such as breath-holding and radial sampling of the k-space have been proposed, and in most cases have successfully addressed motion artifacts [30].

6.3.8.2 Emission-Based Methods

The main principle of these methods is to use the emission PET data along with the radioactivity distribution to jointly estimate the attenuation correction map, during iterative image reconstruction. The most popular method is the maximum-likelihood reconstruction of attenuation and activity algorithm (MLAA) [31]. In order to better estimate the attenuating medium,

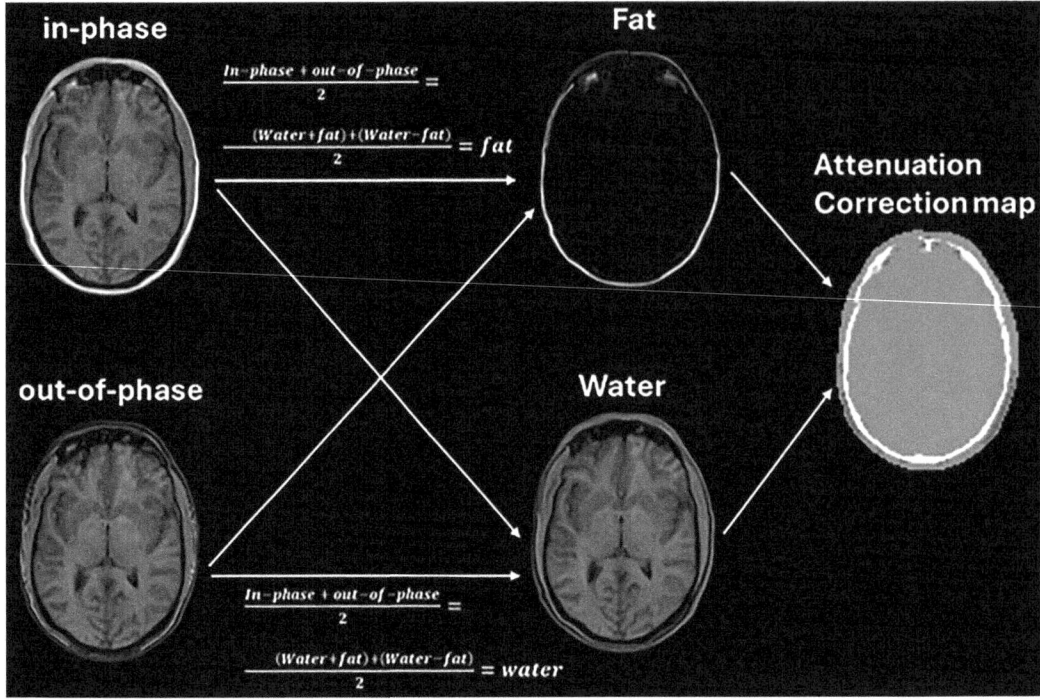

Fig. 6.4 Visual representation of the Dixon sequence principle for a head scan. A bone atlas has been applied on the final attenuation correction map in this case

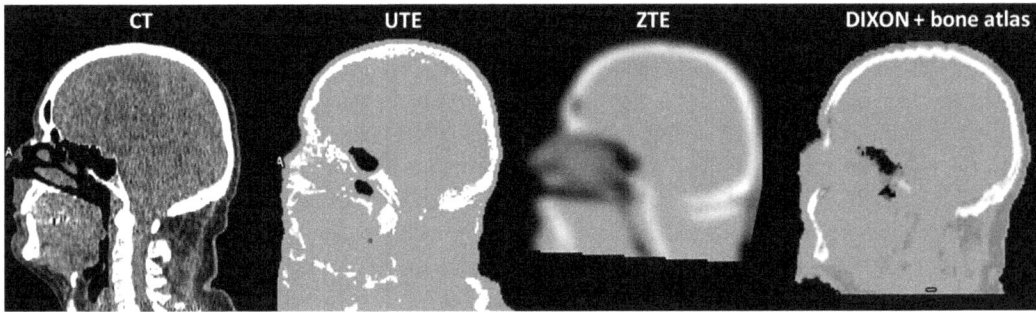

Fig. 6.5 MR-based provided methods for the brain along with the corresponding CT image in brain [28]

TOF (time of flight) images are usually better suited for this purpose while non-TOF images could result in artefacts and high noise in the images [28]. Another problem that has been reported is that the attenuation coefficient values can only be estimated up to an additive constant. A few workarounds have been proposed that usually involve the use of tissue priors for accurate estimation. On the other hand, this method does not rely on an anatomical image which makes it highly attractive for both PET/CT and PET/MR applications, and it has been used on the first PET/MR system to address the truncation artefacts due to the limited FOV as described earlier. Nonetheless, the more recent approach using HUGE has provided more accurate results. Finally, this method takes longer than the MR-based methods to be implemented as the reconstruction process is much slower.

6.3.8.3 Atlas-Based Methods

This simple and intuitive approach makes use of large databases of either CT images or paired CT and MRI images. The database is then applied on the MRI image of the patient (target) using a range of methods with the simplest approach being direct registration of the database to the target image and selecting the CT (pseudo-CT since the actual CT was never acquired) that better matches the target image or even trying to estimate the pseudo-CT by segmenting the target image into small patches and estimating the best prediction for each patch. Currently, at least one commercially available PET-MR system implement such an approach for the brain that uses a CT-only database and applies it on the target image. Depending on the atlas method, accuracy on the reconstructed PET images varies although many methods have shown promising results for the brain [32]. Two of the main limitations of the atlas methods though are the time needed to be implemented which can be of the order of 30 min to several hours, and the fact that it is more difficult to be implemented in non-rigid areas such as lungs and bowel.

6.3.8.4 Machine Learning Methods

The rapid advancements in graphic processing units and the accessibility of data from online repositories have given rise over the last few years to machine learning and more specifically to deep learning methods. These methods also make use of databases of paired MRI and CT, non-attenuation corrected and attenuation corrected PET images, non-attenuation corrected and CT images, etc. to be able to predict one from the other [28]. This is done by using neural networks that can find and utilize a large number of features most of which are not visible by the human eye and can be used to predict one image from the other. Most studies make use of a U-net architecture, named after its shape which has a contracting (encoding) path in which the image is encoded into features and an expanding path (decoding) in which the features are used to predict the image. Most deep learning approaches have provided very promising results with high accuracy and can generate the predicted image very rapidly making this approach extremely popular. Nonetheless, accuracy and generalizability of those methods heavily rely on the diversity and the magnitude of the database used to train the network [28]. A recent technique to expand the training dataset is the application of federated learning where various centres can train their own network and then provide the trained model to a central server where the results are aggregated. With this method, no patient data are shared avoiding potential data confidentiality issues while large numbers of patients are used to train highly generalizable models [33]. All those attributes are expected to make deep learning approaches more widely used in the future.

6.3.9 Quality Assurance on the PET/MR

In principle, the PET scanner of a PET/MR system should undergo the same procedures for acceptance testing and quality assurance as the PET/CT scanners according to the latest NEMA procedures (at the time of writing those would be NEMA NU 2-2018) [34]. These include measuring the scanner's spatial resolution, sensitivity, scatter fraction, count losses and randoms, accuracy, image quality, and time-of-flight resolution and alignment between PET and MRI. To assess the scanner's sensitivity, aluminium 'sleeves' are used with varying diameters which are successively added to a line source and is extrapolated to zero attenuating material. Since aluminium is a nonferrous material, these measurements can be performed on PET/MR scanners without issues. All other measurements other than the image quality are also not affected by the presence of the MRI scanner. Previous reports on performance measurements of two commercially available PET-MR systems [23, 35] have indicated that the PET component performs equally well as other state-of-the-art PET/CT systems.

As far as the image quality is concerned, the challenge is again the attenuation correction of the NEMA IEC PET body phantom. As described earlier, there are certain challenges when trying to image materials like bone or plastic due to their short transverse relaxation times. Moreover, the procedure for filling the phantom includes dissolving ^{18}F in water to fill the background and spheres of the phantom. The low conductivity of water though usually leads to artefacts in the attenuation correction map as shown in Fig. 6.6c. To tackle this issue, a CT-based attenuation correction map can be used, the conductivity of water can be increased (e.g. by adding salt in the solution) or a different liquid with higher conductivity and higher relative permittivity can be used for filling the phantom such as triethylene glycol [36]. In our experience, simply using tap water with approximately 1% concentration of salt has proven the easiest and most practical approach for accurately determining the border of the phantom as shown in Fig. 6.6. Still though, since plastic borders cannot be imaged, the AC map will be a binary image of just water and air. Using

a CT-based attenuation correction, it has been previously shown that the PET/MR scanners perform similarly to the PET/CTs and could potentially participate in multi-centre trials along with the PET/CT scanners (Fig. 6.7).

Moreover, both the European Federation of Organisations for Medical Physics (EFOMP) and the European Association of Nuclear Medicine (EANM) have recently published detailed procedures for quality control in PET/MR systems [37, 38]. Again, the PET-related QC processes are identical to the QC processes performed on a conventional PET/CT scanner and include inspection of image uniformity using a uniform cylinder (Ge-68 or F-18), inspection of sinogram data, alignment of PET and MRI, QC of peripheral equipment such as weighing scales and dose calibrators, etc.

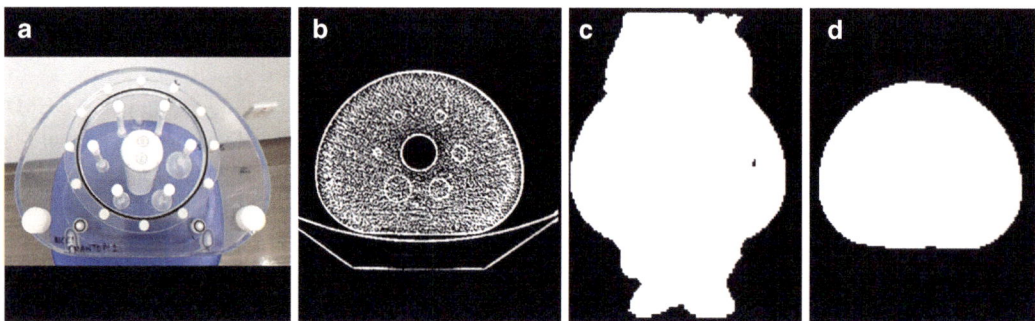

Fig. 6.6 (**a**) Photo of the NEMA IEC PET body phantom, (**b**) CT scan of the phantom, and (**c**) attenuation correction map as generated from the Dixon sequence on the PET/MR when filling the phantom with water and (**d**) water with salt. Due to water's low conductivity the atten-

uation map in (**c**) suffers from artefacts and it is improved by increasing its conductivity with the inclusion of water in (**d**). Since the attenuation map can only image water and fat, those are binary images displaying air and water

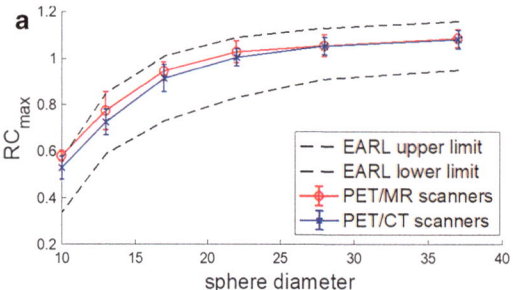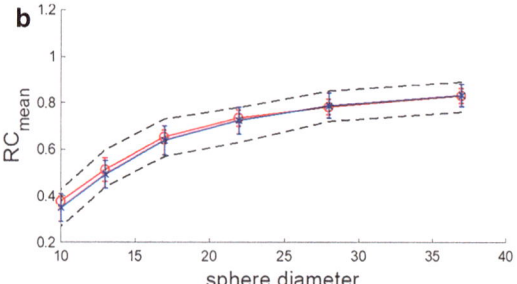

Fig. 6.7 Recovery coefficient curves for the (**a**) maximum and (**b**) mean value within the spheres in the NEMA IEC body phantom. Red curves are averaged over 8 PET/MR scanners and blue curves are averaged over 25

PET/CT scanners accredited for participation in multicentre trials. Error bars represent the standard deviation across the sites and dashed black curves the EARL limits

For the MRI component, various QC procedures should also be in place. An initial acceptance test includes various image quality tests using a range of phantoms (for example, MagNET phantoms) to assess SNR, signal uniformity, spatial resolution, geometric linearity and distortion, slice width and position, and ghosting. The results of these imaging tests are compared to MagNET type test data and use tolerances suggested by IPEM report 112 [39]. Additionally, regular coil QC should also be performed on each coil. Regular inspection of coils is needed to ensure there is not a drop in signal-to-noise ratio and that all coils are performing adequately. At our site, these coils checks are performed weekly. Further checks such as recording and monitoring liquid helium levels, and temperature should also be con-ducted. Besides, of the recommended checks described before, the scientific community is still interested in specific checks directly related to the simultaneous use of the PET/MR systems. Additional checks performed in our department to investigate count rate performance of PET when sequences of high specific absorption rate (SAR), and when echo planar imaging (EPI) is performed which requires high gradient switching, revealed no effect on the PET performance (Fig. 6.8). Moreover, even if a different solution to water is used, phantom walls are not visible in MRI. Therefore, various attempts have also been employed to concurrently assess PET and attenuation correction performance such as phantoms made of polymer or even including animal cadavers [40, 41].

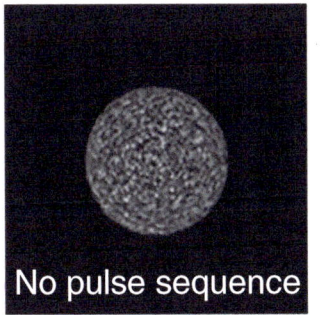 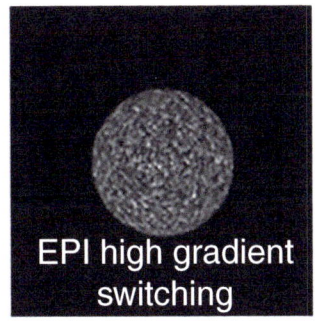 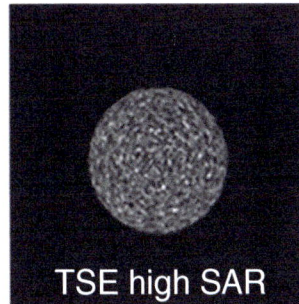

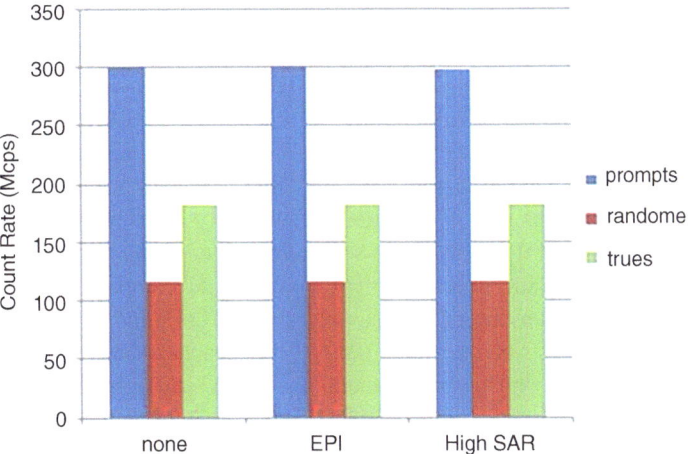

Fig. 6.8 Count rate performance of PET scanner under no pulse sequence and during simultaneous scanning when performing an EPI and a turbo spin echo (TSE) image. Image kindly provided by Dr Jane Mackewn

6.4 Best Practices for Radiographers

PET training is essential for understanding PET imaging principles, handling and administering radioactive tracers, and assessing image quality and data validity. A key component in PET training is having a sound knowledge and understanding of PET physics. This includes the various stages of PET data formation, from tracer injection and accumulation in target tissue, tracer decay by positron emission, annihilation, coincidence detection, and subsequent image reconstruction.

Of equal importance is the understanding of radiation safety protocols to protect patients and staff is fundamental. PET/MR radiographers must be well-versed in handling radioactive materials safely, minimizing exposure to themselves and to the patients. Of equal importance is the radiographer's ability to effectively manage cases of inadvertent radiation incidents. This is done in accordance with the departmental standard operating procedure (SOP) and includes the following steps: immediately informing the department's radiation protection supervisor and PET Physicist, isolating the contaminated area if the radiation incident involves contamination of equipment and space within the PET/MR unit, allowing sufficient time for the contamination readings to reach a zero level indicating that it is now safe for other users to enter and use the PET/MR working area. If, however, the radiation incident involves accidental extravasation of the radiopharmaceutical agent, the radiographer must inform the PET physicist on duty in order to determine the dose of tracer that has been injected into the circulating system versus the dose of tracer that extravasated. This step is essential in order to determine whether it is feasible to scan the patient or re-cannulate and inject them with an additional dose to compensate for the amount of tracer that extravasated. In summary, PET radiopharmaceuticals are powerful tools in medical diagnostics. However, careful consideration of radiation exposure is essential to balance the benefits with the potential risks associated with their use. These include carcinogenesis due to repeated exposure over a patient's lifetime and acute effects like radiation sickness resulting from short-term exposure to high radiation doses. Another essential part of PET training is the accurate calculation of radioactive tracer dosage, and this must be done according to ARSAC notes of guidance. This ensures that the patient receives the correct amount of tracer, optimizing image quality and diagnostic accuracy while ensuring safety [42].

Following dose calculation, the radiopharmaceutical must be injected according to very strict protocols which ensure the patient's safety and data validity. Skills for handling various radioactive tracers used in different studies are developed through hands-on experience. This includes knowing the specific properties and safety requirements of each tracer as well as an understanding of their physiological function that relates to how organs and tissues are working at the cellular and molecular levels. PET imaging is uniquely suited for this because it can visualize metabolic processes, receptor activity, blood flow, and other functional aspects. Additionally, managing the timing and coordination of tracer administration with MRI sequences is crucial. PET/MR radiographers must understand how different tracers interact with the body and their optimum uptake time based on their biodistribution. Also, the tracer injection delay is dependent on whether the radiopharmaceutical kinetics have been established or not. If the answer is yes, then a fixed delay between the tracer injection and start of the PET is employed. This fixed delay is dependent on the physiological and chemical properties of the tracer. If not, the tracer is injected on the scanning table at the start of the PET acquisition in order to capture the early kinetics as well as the late part of the time activity curve [42]. In order to maintain the skills and competencies necessary for handling and injecting radioactive tracers safely, PET/MR radiographers and technologists are regularly assigned shifts in the PET/CT department where they operate in exactly the same capacity as PET/CT technologists. This rotation also helps ensure that the PET/MR staff stay updated with the latest protocols and changes in PET/CT.

Once the data has been acquired, it must be carefully evaluated by the scanning radiographer. This includes identifying software errors on the uMAPS acquired alongside the PET. Artifacts on the latter may cause image degradation and false positives on the PET data, thereby affecting the validity of the data acquired. Other commonly encountered artifacts include halo effect resulting from increased activity in the bladder when using GA68 PSMA for prostate imaging. After investigation, this was found out to be due to scatter correction around the bladder (as illustrated in Fig. 6.9). In this case, a specific combination of extended FOV (HUGE) and scatter correction option is essential to reduce or eliminate this artifact.

Considering the complexity of PET/MR scanners, scanning radiographers must be proficient in using the machine's controls, troubleshooting common issues, and performing regular quality checks to ensure the integrity of the acquired data. Of equal importance is the requirement to label every piece of hardware or equipment that is brought in the PET/MR environment in order to eliminate the risk of patient or staff injury or death. Equipment classification includes three categories described as Conditional, Safe, and Unsafe. Conditional equipment can be brought into the magnet room but must be kept at a safe distance from the bore of the magnet depending on the properties of the conditional device itself. Safe equipment can be taken anywhere in the magnet room, even inside the bore, while unsafe equipment must be kept out of the magnet room entirely.

PET/MR research often involves the use of special pieces of equipment essential for the various aspects of the study. These include stopwatches, arterial blood sampling module, tracer injection trolley, leaded tracer-syringe holder, infusion pump, etc. It is often essential to make some adjustments some of which logistic in order to carry out all the tasks required. One example is to draw arterial blood during the PET/MR scan, placing them on a paper tray, open the hatch situated inside the magnet room and placing the tray there. Once the hatch is closed, it is opened by a second member of staff from the technical room who will take the blood samples to the blood lab for analysis. Another example is to place the

a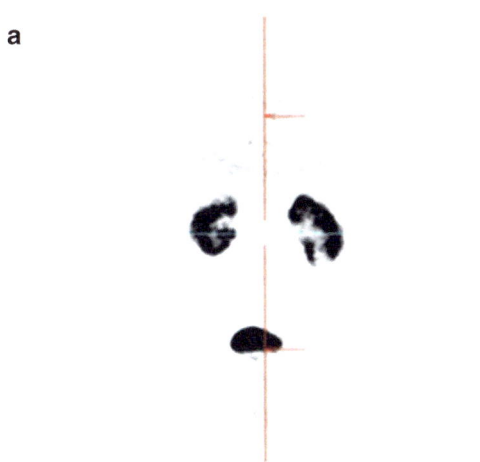

MRAC_HUGE_OFF_SCATTER_CORR_RELATIVE

b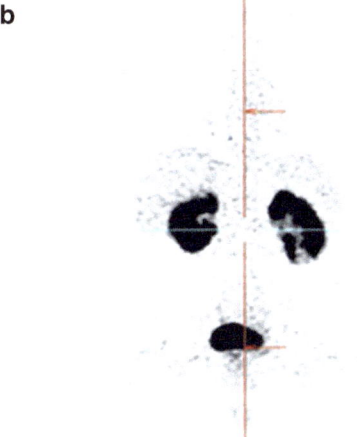

MRAC_HUGE_ON_SCATTER_CORR_ABSOLUTE

Fig. 6.9 Patient undergoing [⁶⁸Ga]Ga-PSMA-11 PET/MR examination displaying (**a**) HALO artifact around the bladder and kidneys with relative scatter correction. (**b**) Elimination of the artifact when absolute scatter correction was applied. In addition to PET training, a sound knowledge of advanced MRI techniques is required for optimizing image quality and adapting scanning parameters when necessary. Practical examples include adjusting specific parameters to minimize image artifacts, reduce breath-hold durations, and enhance cardiac gating, all of which contribute to the overall quality of the MRI data

pump used for blood sampling inside an MRI conditional metal cage in order to reduce interference from the MRI scanner. This cage, however, needs to be kept at a certain distance from the scanner bore and is therefore tethered to the wall using an MRI-safe strong cord.

Ensuring no non-MR Conditional equipment is brought into the magnet room to prevent projectile hazards. This involves thorough checks and training. It is also important to have the patients changed into scrubs in order to eliminate the risk of introducing metal objects into the scanning environment and to avoid clothing-related artifacts.

A special emphasis is placed on Cardiac PET/MR scanning due to its technical complexity. In order to be independently proficient in PET/MR, a rotation through the Cardiac MRI department is essential in order to equip the PET/MR radiographer with the required skills for carrying out complex cardiac PET/MR studies. This is due to the complexity and demanding nature from a technical perspective of cardiac MRI in comparison to other MRI disciplines. This rotation is ongoing to maintain a high level of scanning expertise. For cardiac PET/MR scans, additional steps must be taken to ensure the quality of the data acquired is high. To capture clear images of the moving heart, an MRI-compatible ECG is attached to the patient (Fig. 6.10).

This device allows gating of the patient's cardiac cycle during the scan, enabling the acquisition of data at consistent time points of the cardiac cycle. This helps in reduce motion artifacts caused by the beating heart. Proper training for PET/MR radiographers on correct ECG placement is essential for optimal image quality, safety, and scan efficiency. The patient's skin must be cleansed of any lotion or oils, and any hair must be removed for proper electrode placement. MRI-safe electrodes must be used, with special care taken to position the ECG module to avoid any loops or contact with the patient's skin.

Following ECG placement, it is important to allow adequate time for the ECG module to learn the patient's cardiac cycle (8–10 heartbeats) outside the bore of the magnet, without disruption from coil placement or breath coaching with the patient. If this step is skipped, it could lead to triggering errors during the scan. Additionally, a peripheral pulse unit (PPU) is placed as an alternative for gating should the ECG encounter any issues. A respiratory bellow is also used to monitor patient's compliance with any required breathing instructions.

6.4.1 Integrated PET/MR Training

Integrated PET/MR training necessitates through knowledge of both pre-scan procedures and the regulatory frameworks that govern the use of radioactive tracers, which are key to ensuring both patient safety and compliance with legal standards. In fact, although PET/MR involves lower radiation doses than PET/CT due to the absence of X-ray radiation, the use of radioactive tracers necessitates the same regulatory approvals as PET/CT. The Ionising Radiation (Medical Exposure) Regulation (IR(ME)R) addresses the rules around radiation exposure of individuals as part of medical and biomedical research. Additionally, radiopharmaceutical administration as part of a research project can only take place once approved by the Administration of Radioactive Substances Advisory Committee [42]. Also, before a PET/MR research study can commence, ethics approval must be in place. The Patient Information Sheets (PISs) need to be appropriately written while being comprehensive and simple enough for the public to fully understand the study and its potential risks and benefits. Close collaboration with the local research coordinator and the principal investigator from the early stages of the study is essential to ensure all the above. On the day of scanning, the PET/MR Radiographer coordinates with research teams to gather the necessary documents which mainly include an electronic request vetted by a Consultant PET Clinician to ensure the study's appropriateness and safety, a consent form obtained from the research team and signed by the patient, ensuring they understand the procedure and agree to participate, as well as an MRI questionnaire completed and double-checked with the patient to ensure no contraindications,

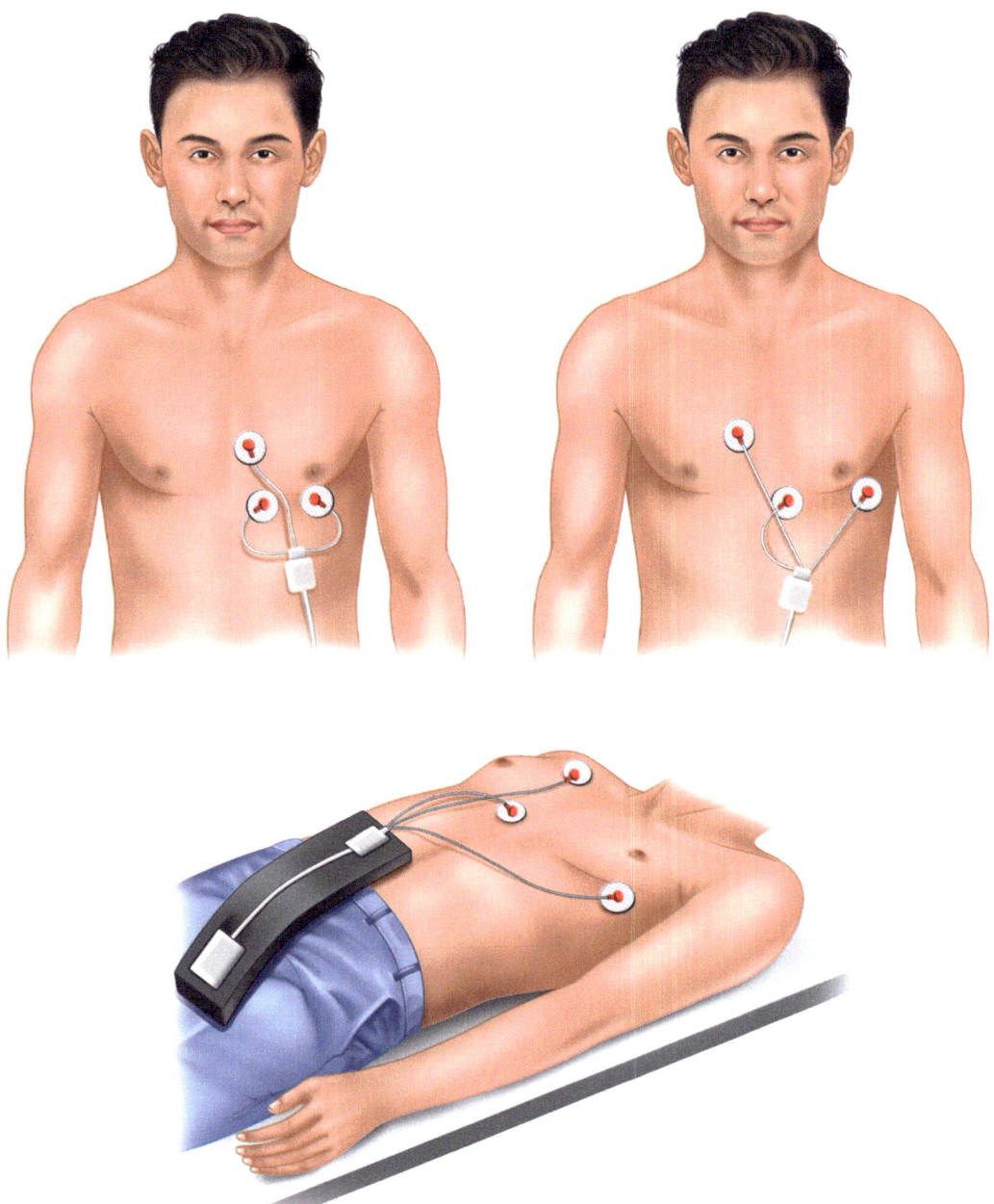

Fig. 6.10 Positioning the ECG electrodes (left, centre) and the PERU (right)

such as certain implants like pacemakers or intracardiac defibrillators, are present.

Before proceeding with the tracer injection and scan, additional checks are required to assess the patient's renal function and disease, allergies to GBCA, pregnancy status, and medical history in general. The scanning radiographer/technologist reviews the patient's renal profile by evaluating the eGFR value to ensure the safe administration of gadolinium-based contrast agents (GBCAs). Patients with impaired renal function may be at risk for nephrogenic systemic fibrosis (NSF), a serious condition characterized by the thickening and hardening of the skin, connective tissues, and sometimes internal organs. Additionally, patients must be screened for severe allergies to GBCA and kidney disease. GBCAs are primarily excreted through the kidneys, and for patients with severe kidney disease (GFR <30 mL/min/1.73 m^2), there is a risk of NSF [43]. Moreover, extra checks are required for female patients of childbearing age. This is because radioactive tracers and gadolinium-based contrast agents (GBCAs) are usually avoided during pregnancy and are often excluded from PET/MR research studies. The pregnancy status is established at the stage of prepping the patient once they arrive for their scan appointment and a pregnancy test is performed if they cannot confidently exclude being pregnant.

Of equal importance is the pre-PET questionnaire which is used to gather information on the patient's medical history and current medications as some of these may affect tracer bio-distribution thereby affecting the validity of the PET/MR data acquired. The questionnaire also captures information about specific treatment plans such as chemotherapy and radiotherapy. This information is crucial in order to assess treatment response using PET data. This procedure also holds true for patients having their clinical scans as standard of care.

Once all the checks have been completed, the next step is to explain to the patient exactly what to expect from participating in the PET/MR study. This is because patient compliance is crucial for the success of a study involving a PET/MR scanner, especially considering its smaller bore size compared to other modern MRI scanners. Whole-body scanning necessitates the use of multiple coils to ensure adequate coverage from the vertex to the mid-thigh. This set-up can sometimes induce claustrophobia in patients, requiring additional measures to make them comfortable. Maintaining constant communication throughout the scan is essential to alleviate their anxiety, particularly given the typical duration of PET/MR research scans, which ranges from 60 to 90 min. Another important factor to consider is explaining the noise gener-

ated by the various pulse sequences used, the potential for increased temperature in the area being scanned, possible itching on the nose, and peripheral nerve stimulation. By providing detailed information and reassurance, patients are more likely to remain calm and compliant throughout the procedure. In addition to earplugs and/or headphones being provided to reduce the acoustic noise, an emergency buzzer is also provided. This can be used if the patient needs to communicate with the radiographer should they feel anxious and wish to stop the scan. Once the patient is presented with all the information about the scan, they are given the opportunity to ask any questions should they need more information. The patient is also informed about the use of the radioactive tracer and gadolinium-based contrast, ensuring they understand the purpose of these two agents and any possible sensation they may experience during or immediately after the injection process.

6.4.2 Post-Scan Procedures and Data Management

Upon scan completion, certain procedures are carried out in order to ensure patient safety and integrity of the data acquired.

Firstly, the patient is advised to increase fluid intake to expedite the removal of the radiopharmaceutical. This helps lower radiation exposure to the gonads and bladder by promoting faster tracer elimination from the body [42]. Secondly, equipment contamination check is required to exclude any contamination resulting from the radiopharmaceutical injection. Due to the restrictions imposed by the strong magnetic field of the scanner, equipment monitoring must be done by swabbing the equipment and scanning table and then checking for any readings using a portable Berthold contamination device placed outside the magnet room. Thirdly, the patient is invited to complete a satisfaction questionnaire as providing feedback is crucial for improving future research and clinical experiences. Patient feedback helps identify areas for improvement and enhances the overall quality of care.

Once this is all done, the acquired and reconstructed data (MRI raw data, PET raw data, PET and MRI reconstructed images) must be stored in a secure and organized manner in accordance with the local GDPR regulations. Proper data management ensures data integrity and accessibility for future analysis.

6.4.3 PET/MR Research Radiographer Prerequisites

A flexible approach is vital in the research environment to accommodate the specific needs of different patient cohorts and the availability of radioactive tracers. Flexibility also ensures that studies can proceed smoothly despite varying patient conditions and tracer availability. Moreover, the PET/MR Radiographer must be able to anticipate potential issues and troubleshoot effectively, prioritize patient need, assess their conditions thoroughly, and adapt the scanning conditions in order to maximize patient compliance depending on their tolerance level and communicate insights and feasibility findings to the Principal Investigator.

6.5 Future Directions and Conclusion

The role of the PET/MR Radiographer is multifaceted and critical to the success of PET/MR studies. From training and patient preparation to executing the scan and handling post-scan procedures, the radiographer ensures the highest standards of safety, accuracy, and patient care are met. By following this guide, PET/MR Radiographers can effectively conduct PET/MR studies, contributing to advancements in medical research and patient care. Their expertise and dedication are instrumental in the successful implementation of PET/MR technology, providing valuable insights into various medical conditions and improving patient outcomes.

References

1. Iida H, Kanno I, Miura S, Murakami M, Takahashi K, Uemura K. A simulation study of a method to reduce positron annihilation spread distributions using a strong magnetic field in positron emission tomography. IEEE Trans Nucl Sci. 1986;33(1):597–600.
2. Musafargani S, Ghosh KK, Mishra S, Mahalakshmi P, Padmanabhan P, Gulyas B. PET/MRI: a frontier in era of complementary hybrid imaging. Eur J Hybrid Imaging. 2018;2(1):12.
3. Vandenberghe S, Marsden PK. PET-MRI: a review of challenges and solutions in the development of integrated multimodality imaging. Phys Med Biol. 2015;60(4):R115–54.
4. Huang SY, Savic D, Yang J, Shrestha U, Seo Y. The effect of magnetic field on positron range and spatial resolution in an integrated whole-body time-of-flight PET/MRI system. IEEE Nucl Sci Symp Conf Rec. 2014;2014:1006.
5. Prakken NHJ, Besson FL, Borra RJH, Buther F, Buechel RR, Catana C, et al. PET/MRI in practice: a clinical centre survey endorsed by the European Association of Nuclear Medicine (EANM) and the EANM Forschungs GmbH (EARL). Eur J Nucl Med Mol Imaging. 2023;50(10):2927–34.
6. Tian T, Xie H, Huang M. Epithelial malignant pleural mesothelioma mimics lymphoma on 18 F-FDG PET/MRI: a case report. Clin Nucl Med. 2024;49(4):359–60.
7. Morakote W, Baratto L, Ramasamy SK, Adams LC, Liang T, Sarrami AH, et al. Comparison of diffusion-weighted MRI and [(18)F]FDG PET/MRI for treatment monitoring in pediatric Hodgkin and non-Hodgkin lymphoma. Eur Radiol. 2024;34(1):643–53.
8. Duan H, Song H, Davidzon GA, Moradi F, Liang T, Loening A, et al. Prospective comparison of (68) Ga-NeoB and (68)Ga-PSMA-R2 PET/MRI in patients with biochemically recurrent prostate cancer. J Nucl Med. 2024;65(6):897–903.
9. Chau OW, Islam A, Lock M, Yu E, Dinniwell R, Yaremko B, et al. PET/MRI assessment of acute cardiac inflammation 1 month after left-sided breast cancer radiation therapy. J Nucl Med Technol. 2023;51(2):133–9.
10. Spick C, Herrmann K, Czernin J. 18F-FDG PET/ CT and PET/MRI perform equally well in cancer: evidence from studies on more than 2,300 patients. J Nucl Med. 2016;57(3):420–30.
11. Mukherjee S, Fischbein NJ, Baugnon KL, Policeni BA, Raghavan P. Contemporary imaging and reporting strategies for head and neck cancer: MRI, FDG PET/MRI, NI-RADS, and carcinoma of unknown primary-AJR Expert Panel Narrative Review. AJR Am J Roentgenol. 2023;220(2):160–72.

12. Ratib O, Nkoulou R. Potential applications of PET/MR imaging in cardiology. J Nucl Med. 2014;55(2):40–6.

13. Hartiala J, Knuuti J. Imaging of the heart by MRI and PET. Ann Med. 1995;27(1):35–45.

14. Robson PM, Dey D, Newby DE, Berman D, Li D, Fayad ZA, et al. MR/PET imaging of the cardiovascular system. JACC Cardiovasc Imaging. 2017;10(10):1165–79.

15. Rischpler C, Nekolla SG, Kunze KP, Schwaiger M. PET/MRI of the heart. Semin Nucl Med. 2015;45(3):234–47.

16. Ruddy TD, Al-Mallah M, Arrighi JA, Bois JP, Bluemke DA, Di Carli MF, et al. SNMMI/ACR/ASNC/SCMR joint credentialing statement for cardiac PET/MRI: endorsed by the American Heart Association. J Nucl Med. 2023;64(1):149–52.

17. Flaus A, Mellerio C, Rodrigo S, Brulon V, Lebon V, Chassoux F. (18)F-FDG PET/MR in focal epilepsy: a new step for improving the detection of epileptogenic lesions. Epilepsy Res. 2021;178:106819.

18. Holzgreve A, Albert NL, Galldiks N, Suchorska B. Use of PET imaging in neuro-oncological surgery. Cancer. 2021;13(9):2093.

19. Catana C. Principles of simultaneous PET/MR imaging. Magn Reson Imaging Clin N Am. 2017;25(2):231–43.

20. Muzic RF, DiFilippo FP. Positron emission tomography-magnetic resonance imaging: technical review. Semin Roentgenol. 2014;49(3):242–54.

21. Deng Z, Li A. A novel visible light communication system prototype based on SiPM receiver. arXiv preprint arXiv:190900641. 2019.

22. Mackewn JE, Strul D, Hallett W, Halsted P, Page R, Keevil S, et al. Design and development of an MR-compatible PET scanner for imaging small animals. IEEE Trans Nucl Sci. 2005;52(5):1376–80.

23. Delso G, Furst S, Jakoby B, Ladebeck R, Ganter C, Nekolla SG, et al. Performance measurements of the Siemens mMR integrated whole-body PET/MR scanner. J Nucl Med. 2011;52(12):1914–22.

24. Shortman RI, Neriman D, Hoath J, Millner L, Endozo R, Azzopardi G, et al. A comparison of the psychological burden of PET/MRI and PET/CT scans and association to initial state anxiety and previous imaging experiences. Br J Radiol. 2015;88(1052):20150121.

25. Eldib M, Bini J, Calcagno C, Robson PM, Mani V, Fayad ZA. Attenuation correction for flexible magnetic resonance coils in combined magnetic resonance/positron emission tomography imaging. Investig Radiol. 2014;49(2):63–9.

26. Kartmann R, Paulus DH, Braun H, Aklan B, Ziegler S, Navalpakkam BK, et al. Integrated PET/MR imaging: automatic attenuation correction of flexible RF coils. Med Phys. 2013;40(8):082301.

27. Frohwein LJ, Hess M, Schlicher D, Bolwin K, Buther F, Jiang X, et al. PET attenuation correction for flexible MRI surface coils in hybrid PET/MRI using a 3D depth camera. Phys Med Biol. 2018;63(2):025033.

28. Krokos G, MacKewn J, Dunn J, Marsden P. A review of PET attenuation correction methods for PET-MR. EJNMMI Phys. 2023;10(1):52.

29. Dixon WT. Simple proton spectroscopic imaging. Radiology. 1984;153(1):189–94.

30. Lamare F, Bousse A, Thielemans K, Liu C, Merlin T, Fayad H, et al. PET respiratory motion correction: quo vadis? Phys Med Biol. 2022;67:3.

31. Glatting G, Wuchenauer M, Reske SN. Simultaneous iterative reconstruction for emission and attenuation images in positron emission tomography. Med Phys. 2000;27(9):2065–71.

32. Ladefoged CN, Law I, Anazodo U, St Lawrence K, Izquierdo-Garcia D, Catana C, et al. A multi-centre evaluation of eleven clinically feasible brain PET/MRI attenuation correction techniques using a large cohort of patients. NeuroImage. 2017;147:346–59.

33. Shiri I, Vafaei Sadr A, Akhavan A, Salimi Y, Sanaat A, Amini M, et al. Decentralized collaborative multi-institutional PET attenuation and scatter correction using federated deep learning. Eur J Nucl Med Mol Imaging. 2023;50(4):1034–50.

34. Nema N. NU 2-2018-performance measurements of positron emission tomographs. Rosslyn: National Electrical Manufacturers Association; 2018.

35. Demir M, Toklu T, Abuqbeitah M, Cetin H, Sezgin HS, Yeyin N, et al. Evaluation of PET scanner performance in PET/MR and PET/CT systems: NEMA tests. Mol Imaging Radionucl Ther. 2018;27(1):10–8.

36. Ziegler S, Braun H, Ritt P, Hocke C, Kuwert T, Quick HH. Systematic evaluation of phantom fluids for simultaneous PET/MR hybrid imaging. J Nucl Med. 2013;54(8):1464–71.

37. Matheoud R, Boellaard R, Pike L, Ptacek J, Reynes-Llompart G, Soret M, et al. EFOMP's protocol quality controls in PET/CT and PET/MR. Phys Med. 2023;105:102506.

38. Koole M, Armstrong I, Krizsan AK, Stromvall A, Visvikis D, Sattler B, et al. EANM guidelines for PET-CT and PET-MR routine quality control. Z Med Phys. 2023;33(1):103–13.

39. McRobbie D SS. IPEM Report 112 (2017). Quality control and artefacts in magnetic resonance imaging. 2017. Report No.: 112.

40. Rausch I, Valladares A, Sundar LKS, Beyer T, Hacker M, Meyerspeer M, et al. Standard MRI-based attenuation correction for PET/MRI phantoms: a novel concept using MRI-visible polymer. EJNMMI Phys. 2021;8(1):18.

41. Lennie E, Tsoumpas C, Sourbron S. Multimodal phantoms for clinical PET/MRI. EJNMMI Phys. 2021;8(1):62.

42. Notes for guidance on the clinical administration of radiopharmaceuticals and use of sealed radioactive sources. Administration of Radioactive Substances Advisory Committee; 2024.

43. Fraum TJ, Ludwig DR, Bashir MR, Fowler KJ. Gadolinium-based contrast agents: a comprehensive risk assessment. J Magn Reson Imaging. 2017;46(2):338–53.

Advances in Hybrid Imaging: SPECT/CT

7

Valentina Ferri and Francesca Bisello

7.1 Introduction

This chapter provides an overview of the latest hybrid imaging systems, focusing on advancements in SPECT/CT technology. It discusses the principles, components, and capabilities that distinguish these systems from older models. The drive behind these innovations is the demand for faster, more precise, and personalized imaging tools to map and quantify complex physiological processes affecting patients. As medicine becomes more personalized, the need for integrated, sophisticated tools grows. Innovation trends focus on improving image quality, system performance, integration, and patient comfort. To assess the impact of these advancements, it is essential to first understand the benchmarks of traditional SPECT/CT systems and the steps toward improvement.

V. Ferri (✉)
Division of Nuclear Medicine and Molecular Imaging, Department of Radiology, Stanford University Medical Center, Stanford, CA, USA
e-mail: vferri@stanford.edu

F. Bisello
Division of Medical Physics, IRCCS Azienda Ospedaliero-Universitaria Policlinico S.Orsola-Malpighi, Bologna, Italy
e-mail: francesca.bisello@aosp.bo.it

7.2 SPECT/CT

Single-photon emission computed tomography (SPECT) is used to image the radiotracers characterized by a single-photon emission. Traditional SPECT devices are based on the gamma camera principle by Hal Anger [1] and produce three-dimensional images. The essential components of a SPECT camera are collimators, scintillation crystals (mainly sodium iodide doped with thallium, NaI(Tl)), which are read out by photomultipliers, and subsequent electronics. These components constitute the detectors. One or multiple detectors are mounted on the gantry, which enables the movements of the detector heads. Their dimensions are typically 40 × 40 cm or smaller and commonly 9.5 mm thick (in order to optimize the stopping power for the 140 keV photons of technetium-99m, the most used radionuclide). Dual detector-head cameras are the standard in clinical practice, due to their balance between photon sensitivity and costs, single or triple detector head cameras are less common. The SPECT/CT system also includes a bed for patient positioning and workstations (computers) for the acquisition, reconstruction, and postprocessing of the imaging data.

Since the introduction of commercial SPECT/CT in the late 1990s, the field has seen rapid expansion and development, establishing the role of SPECT/CT as a clinical routine imaging tool. SPECT/CT provides better contrast than planar imaging (two-dimensional) and an opportunity to quantify in vivo activity distribution. The difficulties in interpreting SPECT signals are very much improved with CT localization. Still, traditional SPECT studies continue to be more time-consuming than planar studies, and several factors affect the quality of the resulting images (e.g., poor resolution, low sensitivity, noise, and partial volume effect) and the ability to perform absolute quantification (e.g., attenuation, scatter, motion, and poor resolution).

The last development efforts of SPECT/CT focus on multiple components of the system, both hardware and software. In fact, at this present stage of technological development, minor changes could also lead to considerable improvements. These advances in terms of detector hardware, system design, and software improvement, which will be soon discussed, ultimately aim to increase both spatial resolution and sensitivity of the scanners (together with software upgrades necessary to handle increased data stream and processing needs) to obtain improved image quality and decreased overall acquisition time (or reduction of the dose to the patients).

Those improvements pave the way to a greater number of clinical applications and ultimately new imaging paradigms, including fast SPECT/CT whole-body scans, dual isotope imaging, three-dimensional dynamic scans, and, finally, going toward reliable and clinically relevant semiquantitative and/or quantitative images.

In the following paragraphs, the CZT (cadmium zinc telluride)-based detectors and the multidetector SPECT/CT systems will be discussed.

7.3 CZT Detectors

CZT (cadmium zinc telluride—sometimes also referred to as CdZnTe) detectors directly convert incoming gamma rays into electrical signals (Fig. 7.1). When a gamma ray interacts within the CZT crystal, an electron-hole pair is generated. These pairs create an electrical signal that is measured by the detector, which allows the gamma ray's energy to be determined with precision. This direct conversion process results in higher energy resolution compared to traditional detectors, based on indirect conversion methods such as converting gamma rays into visible light first using a scintillation material (like Na(I)) and then converting it into electrical signals for analysis. While indirect conversion methods are still widely used and have their own advantages, direct conversion techniques like those utilized in CZT detectors tend to offer better energy resolution and spatial resolution, making them a preferred choice for clinical needs (Fig. 7.2)

As an example, if a 140 keV photon interacts within the CZT detector, approximately 30,000 electrons are produced, which is about 20 times more than the yield of a traditional Anger camera based on NaI(Tl) crystal [4]. The most relevant consequences of this difference are that the resulting energy resolution is improved by a factor of 2 and the sensitivity is improved by a factor of 4–7 [5, 6]. However, it is important to remember that these enhancements cannot be attributed to CZT detectors alone, but are also due to additional improvements, including dedicated collimation systems and pixelated (digital) detectors [7].

The first clinical introduction of CZT semiconductor detectors happened in the late 2000s when dedicated SPECT-only cameras for myocardial imaging entered the market: their improved energy resolution and higher sensitivity made them important players in the space of nuclear cardiology. These cameras are characterized by a compact design, which features separate multielement detectors, each with a specialized collimator, centered on a common region that encompasses the heart. Cardiac perfusion studies could be acquired in one-third [8] of the time required by a conventional SPECT without compromising on the image quality. The high count-rate capability allowed by the CZT element also enables dynamic acquisitions. The first of two general-purpose CZT dual head SPECT/CT devices was introduced for clinical commercial use in 2017.

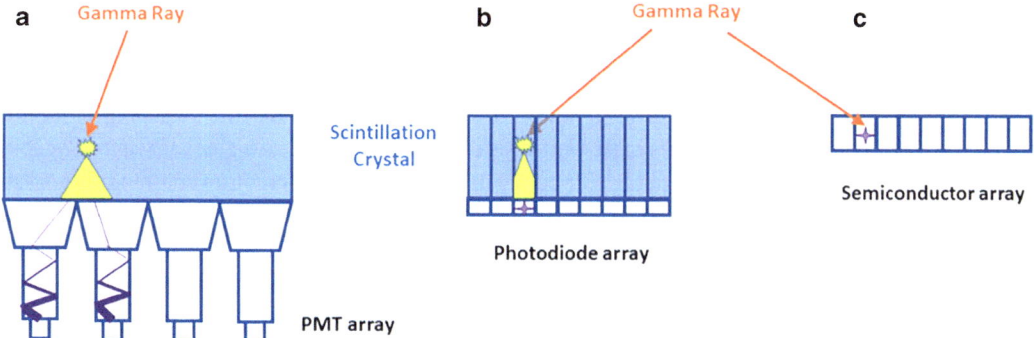

Fig. 7.1 SPECT detectors. (**a**) Monolithic scintillation crystal backed by a photomultiplier (PMT) array. The gamma ray (orange) is converted into a shower of light photons (yellow), which are converted into an electronic signal (purple). (**b**) Pixelated scintillation crystals backed by a photodiode array. The light from the gamma ray interaction is funneled to a solid-state photodiode array, which converts the light into an electronic signal. (**c**) Pixelated semiconductor detector (CZT): The gamma ray is converted directly into an electronic signal. Reproduced and adapted with permission from Dorbala, S., Ananthasubramaniam, K., Armstrong, I.S. et al. Single Photon Emission Computed Tomography (SPECT) Myocardial Perfusion Imaging Guidelines: Instrumentation, Acquisition, Processing, and Interpretation. J. Nucl. Cardiol. 25, 1784–1846 (2018) [2] published under a Creative Commons Attribution 4.0 International License

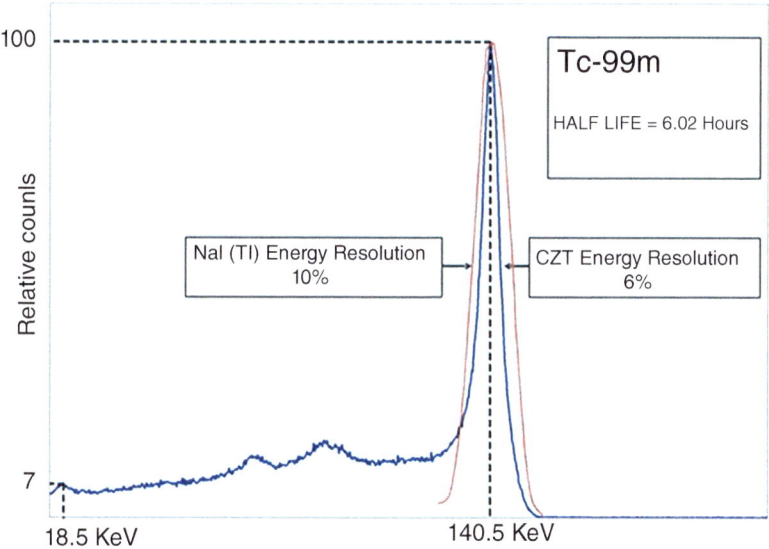

Fig. 7.2 Energy resolution on CZT cameras. Reproduced and adapted with permission from Agostini, D., Marie, PY., Ben-Haim, S. et al. Performance of cardiac cadmium-zinc-telluride gamma camera imaging in coronary artery disease: a review from the cardiovascular committee of the European Association of Nuclear Medicine (EANM). Eur J Nucl Med Mol Imaging 43, 2423–2432 (2016) [3] published under a Creative Commons Attribution 4.0 International License

7.4 Multidetector SPECT/CT Systems

The idea of CZT-based multidetector design has recently (2019) been translated from single-organ imaging systems to whole-body general-purpose systems by the same vendors that first introduced CZT cameras in the nuclear cardiology space (see previous paragraph). The SPECT portion of the system is characterized by multiple pixelated CZT detectors configured as retractile columns disposed in a radial configuration. The SPECT is coupled with a state-of-art CT, to produce, at present, the most advanced SPECT/CT camera design for clinical use (Fig. 7.3).

The advantage of these classes of systems, at present (2024) produced by two manufacturers and commercially available for clinical use, lies in the ability of the detectors to approach the patient's surface at a 360-degree angle, maximizing the count collection by minimizing the distance to the radiation source (the patient). This combination given by this innovative design together with the CZT-based detector performances results in increased energy resolution and sensitivity, thus enhancing the overall performance of the imaging system and paving the way to new clinical applications.

7.4.1 Acquisition and Collimation Geometries

This class of systems presents a ring-shaped gantry (80 cm bore diameter), equipped with 12 independent detectors. Each detector consists of a CZT module capable of radial (in/out) and rotational (sweep) motion. Each detector has a differ-

ent sweep range up to 105° and 180°, depending on the system considered.

The multiple projections are thus acquired during the rotation and the sweeping motion of the detector columns, in a novel scanning geometry (Fig. 7.4). Different sweep modes are supported: step-and-shoot sweep mode and continuous sweep mode. Once multiple views are acquired by the 12 detectors, a single SPECT Bed Position is formed. On each detected event, even at high count rates, the uniformity, real-time energy, and isotope decay corrections are performed.

These systems are designed to acquire consecutive multiple bed positions followed by multiple CT scans, to produce up to eight hybrid SPECT/CT FOVs. For example, in one of the systems considered, the whole-body SPECT scan range is 195 cm, while the hybrid SPECT/CT and CT standalone scan range is up to 185 cm for axial scan or 180 cm for helical scans.

The collimators on both systems are parallel-hole type, made of tungsten and aligned with the CZT pixels on the detectors. The collimator is fixed and does not require to be changed in the current version of these cameras.

The optimal proximity of each detector to the patient surface is achieved by different methods: in one system through an optical scouting, enabled by sensors that detect and map the patient's 3D outline, while the other system uses a capacitance board mounted on each detector [6]. Both approaches ultimately guide the movement of each detector column to the final position, which can sit just a few millimeters away from the patient's surface.

These cameras are equipped with the latest generation computed tomography (CT) devices.

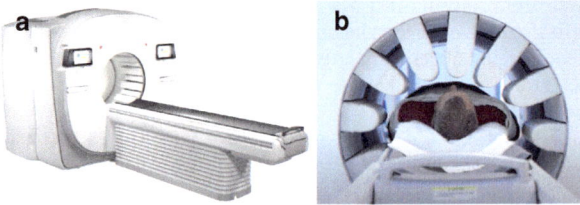

Fig. 7.3 (**a**) Whole-body multidetector SPECT/CT system. (**b**) Detail of a patient acquisition. Detector columns move independently toward close proximity to the patient surface. Image courtesy of GE HealthCare

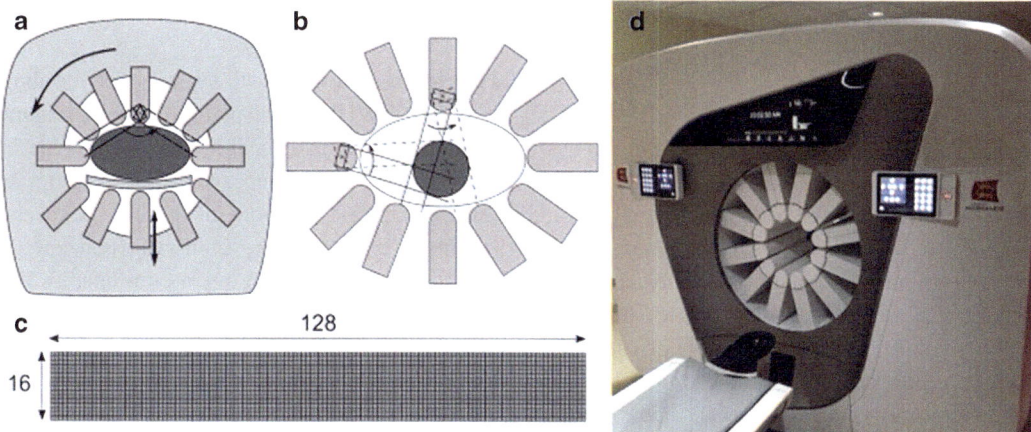

Fig. 7.4 (**a**) General camera architecture showing the different movements of the 12 detectors, (**b**) schematic principle of the focus mode showing the reduced swipe motion of detectors to a predefined region of interest shown in dark gray, (**c**) design of the detection column consisting of an array of 16 × 128 pixel units and (**d**) picture of the system. Published under a Creative Commons Attribution 4.0 International License, from "360° CZT gamma cameras for nuclear medicine and molecular imaging, Nuclear Medicine and Molecular Imaging, Elsevier, 2022" by Laetitia Imbert, Achraf Bahloul, Antoine Verger, Pierre-Yves Marie

CT detectors are available in rows of 16 or 32 and 16 or 64, respectively.

7.4.2 Detector Design

The two systems feature seven and eight CZT modules, respectively. The axial field of view (longitudinal coverage) is 28 cm and 32 cm, respectively. The surface area of the square face of each CZT pixel is 2.46 × 2.46 mm² for both cameras, with pixel thicknesses of 7.25 mm for one system and 5 mm for the other.

The thicker CZT detectors (7.25 mm) can image a wide range of isotopes, with photons' energies of up to 270 keV (i.e., low and medium energies), such as those from the higher energy peaks of lutetium-177 (208 keV) and indium-111 (245 keV).

For the thinner CZT detectors (5 mm), the same isotopes need instead to be acquired on their lower energy peaks, such as 113 keV for lutetium-177 and 171 keV for indium-111. This system is therefore capable of imaging energies from 40 to 200 keV.

At present, neither of the systems can image iodine-131 accurately as the energy peak is out of range (364 keV).

7.4.3 Reconstruction Algorithms and Image Quality

Both systems offer dedicated algorithms for image reconstruction due to their novel acquisition and collimation geometries. Those algorithms are still based on iterative reconstruction (OSEM—ordered subset expectation maximization) with corrections for attenuation, scatter, and resolution recovery.

In addition, each vendor developed proprietary algorithms to fully exploit the system capability and design. For example, one vendor implemented a Bayesian penalized-likelihood reconstruction algorithm (BSREM) [9], which improves image quality and quantification by minimizing the noise level on reconstructed tomographic images. Such an approach was previously introduced and validated for PET imaging. Specific postprocessing aiming to improve spatial resolution is also available for bone scans and it is based on CT information.

The other vendor implemented an algorithm first introduced in CZT-based cameras for nuclear cardiology to improve image sharpness. Additionally, partial volume effect (PVE) correction is available for bone imaging, and it is made possible by incorporating information from the CT scan.

7.4.4 SPECT Quantification

These systems' advanced technology coupled with novel approaches to image reconstruction enables reliable quantitative analysis of the images (i.e., images can be expressed in units of activity instead of traditional units of counts). In fact, the option to correct for additional degrading factors typical of SPECT imaging (i.e., beyond the traditional attenuation and scatter), such as resolution recovery, noise regularization, and partial volume effect (PVE), not only improves overall image quality but also improves SPECT quantification.

The option to produce PET-like images expressed in SUV, or other quantitative metrics, allows to add information to visual assessment only, like in the case of traditional imaging.

The process of image quantification involves the acquisition of specific phantoms for activity calibration (uniform activity distribution) and PVE correction (inserts such as spheres or other geometries with different volumes). PVE correction is used to recover the measured activity concentration in clinical images, improving the accuracy of quantification. Moreover, dedicated image reconstruction parameters may be necessary if the purpose of the imaging is quantitation instead of visualization only [9, 10]. Quantification accuracy and performances (Fig. 7.5) has been evaluated for both systems as it was measured as the difference between the SPECT-based and the radionuclide calibrator-based activity on dedicated phantoms.

Current research is focusing on determining how to best use quantitative SPECT SUV data, which still needs harmonization and community efforts to be validated. Recent studies show promising results, in particular its importance in interpreting bone SPECT images and in the prediction of therapy response in lutetium-177 post therapy imaging [11].

7.4.5 System Performances

Energy Resolution Both systems deliver about a 5–6% FWHM (full width half maximum) energy resolution on technetium-99m scans (at 140 keV). The system capable of imaging the main lutetium-177 photo peak (208 keV) also reaches a 5% energy resolution at that energy. This outstanding energy resolution enables differentiation between simultaneously acquired isotopes with smaller differences in peak energies. In traditional systems, energy resolution at 140 keV is commonly around 9–10%.

Spatial Resolution The tomographic spatial resolution (SPECT resolution) of this class of systems is a major element in achieving the overall image quality, beyond the CZT technology, the pixel size, and the reconstruction.

Both systems feature similar central, radial, and tangential resolution with technetium-99m: about 3.4–4.3 mm, 3.5–4 mm, and 3–3.4 mm, respectively [6, 12, 13]. A range of values were presented to reflect different results from different authors.

For comparison, traditional clinical SPECT systems can achieve spatial resolutions around 10–12 mm in routine clinical settings, while high-performance systems, particularly those optimized for cardiac or neurological imaging, can achieve resolutions closer to 7–8 mm (Fig. 7.6). Small animal imaging systems using pinhole or multipinhole collimators can achieve resolutions as fine as 1–2 mm.

System Volume Sensitivity For one system, it was measured acquiring a cylindrical phantom filled with an homogenous radioactive solution, which led to 542.4 kcount s^{-1}/(MBq ml^{-1}) for technetium-99m and 152.1 kcount s^{-1}/(MBq ml^{-1}) for lutetium-177 (two photopeaks summed) [12, 13]. For the other system, the tomographic sensitivity was measured with a point source in air, and it was estimated at 236 counts $s^{-1}\cdot MBq^{-1}$. Using focus mode, it increased to 1159 counts

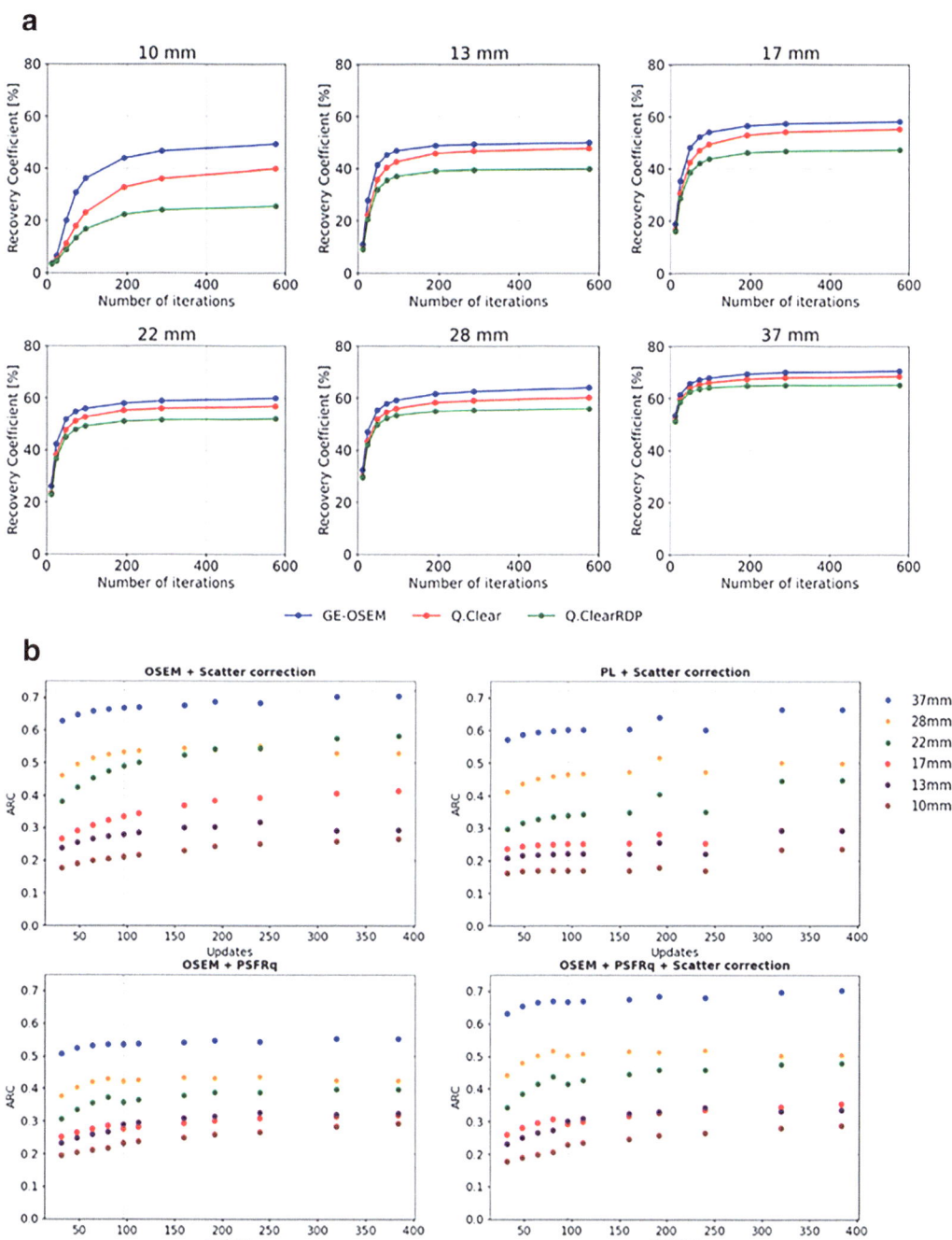

Fig. 7.5 Characterization of quantitative performances for the two systems using lutetium-177-based NEMA IEC phantom with spherical inserts (10–37 mm diameters). (**a**) Recovery coefficients (%) as a function of the number of iterations for three different reconstruction algorithms. Published under a Creative Commons Attribution 4.0 International License from Danieli, R., Stella, M., Leube, J. et al. Quantitative ^{177}Lu SPECT/CT imaging for personalized dosimetry using a ring-shaped CZT-based camera. EJNMMI Phys 10, 64 (2023) [9]. https://doi.org/10.1186/ s40658-023-00586-z—https://creativecommons.org/ licenses/by/4.0/. (**b**) Activity concentration recovery coefficient for different volumes of spheres as a function of the number of updates, for four different reconstruction approaches. Published under a Creative Commons Attribution 4.0 International License, from "360° CZT gamma cameras for nuclear medicine and molecular imaging, Nuclear Medicine and Molecular Imaging, Elsevier, 2022" by Laetitia Imbert, Achraf Bahloul, Antoine Verger, Pierre-Yves Marie

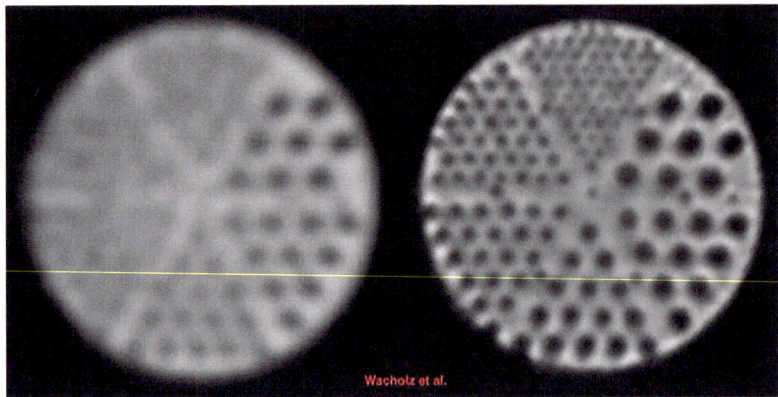

Fig. 7.6 Comparison of images of the cold rod section of the Jaszczak phantom obtained on a multidetector system (right) with comparable images obtained on a conventional dual-detector SPECT/CT system (left—circa 2018). On the right side, all cold rods can be visualized (4.8–12.7 mm diameters). Image courtesy of O'Connor, Michael K., Ph.D

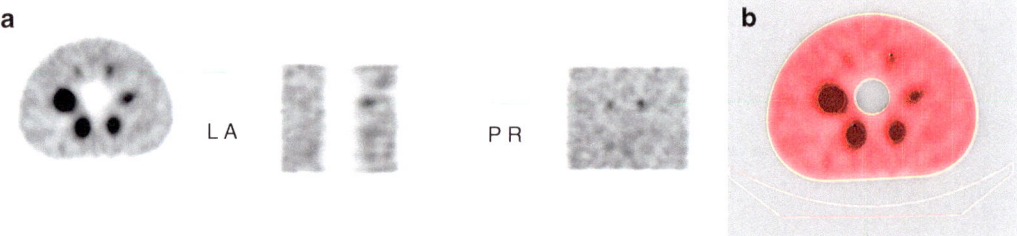

Fig. 7.7 NEMA IEC Phantom with spherical inserts (10–37 mm diameters), filled with lutetium-177. Spheres to background concentration: 8:1. Both lutetium photopeaks contribute to the image (113 and 208 keV). The smallest sphere is visible. (**a**) Axial, coronal, and sagittal views of the SPECT only image. (**b**) SPECT and CT fusion

$s^{-1}\cdot MBq^{-1}$, which was 1.6 times and 8 times greater than the sensitivity measured on the scintillation camera (144 counts $s^{-1}\cdot MBq^{-1}$) [14].

Image Quality Image quality is typically evaluated by acquiring standard SPECT phantoms like the NEMA IEC (Image Quality Phantom with spherical inserts). Both systems demonstrated the detectability of the smallest 10 mm diameter sphere (range: 10–37 mm) when technetium-99m was imaged. For the system able to image the lutetium-177 main peak at 208 keV, that same 10 mm diameter sphere is also visible (Fig. 7.7).

7.5 Clinical Applications

Focal SPECT Recording Both systems feature a focus mode acquisition, a modality that targets specific regions of interest, like small organs, or small regions like the thyroid, parathyroid, brain, heart, and kidneys. This mode exploits the swiveling motion of the detectors to collect more counts through increased angular sampling and increased time spent acquiring projections of the target region. Focus mode works similarly to dedicated organ-specific cameras previously mentioned, but for these whole-body general purpose SPECT/CT systems, a low-dose CT scan can be added to correct for photon attenuation, making it particularly useful in myocardial perfusion imaging to reduce artifacts and improve diagnostic accuracy. High-quality attenuation-corrected images have been obtained in patients with obesity using short acquisition times and low-dose protocols [6]. Additionally, CT scans enable absolute quantification of results expressed in SUVs values, which has shown promise in diagnosing cardiac conditions using technetium-99m-PYP SPECT imaging [15].

Whole-Body Bone SPECT Imaging The improved sensitivity of these systems allows to reach high-quality whole-body imaging within acquisition times of less than 20 min. This scan duration is comparable to that of traditional whole-body planar bone scintigraphy but with the significant advantage of achieving full 3D whole-body acquisition in a single scan, eliminating the need for additional SPECT sessions. Acquisition times can be adjusted based on the body region, with longer times for the abdomen and thorax (3–4 min) and shorter times for the head and legs (2–3 min). The SPECT image can be coupled with a low-dose whole-body CT scan to correct for attenuation and partial volume effects [16].

Lung SPECT Imaging The high sensitivity of multidetector CZT cameras enables effective dual isotope ventilation and perfusion scans [17] with high image quality and shorter acquisition times. Overall, although in the study there was no difference in terms of final diagnosis compared to the conventional SPECT/CT camera, a better delineation of pulmonary embolism was achieved [18].

7.5.1 Advanced Clinical Applications

Dual Isotope Imaging The higher energy resolution of CZT detectors on multidetector CZT cameras allows for the simultaneous recording of two different isotopes. This capability, previously demonstrated with dedicated cardiac CZT cameras, can be extended to these general purpose cameras. This enables dual isotope studies for cardiac applications, for example, thallium-201/technetium-99m dual acquisition for stress/rest myocardial perfusion imaging, thallium-201/iodine-123, or technetium-99m/^{123}I for myocardial perfusion and sympathetic innervation or technetium-99m/iodine-123 for myocardial perfusion and fatty acid tracer metabolism.

Additionally, while still needing further validation, the technetium-99m/iodine-123 dual acquisition could be useful for noncardiac appli-

cations, such as parathyroid SPECT imaging [19] and analyzing brain uptake of technetium-99m-HMPAO and iodine-123-ioflupane.

Dynamic 3D SPECT Imaging Compared to the traditional SPECT imaging, this class of systems enables the transition from 2D dynamic planar scans to 3D dynamic SPECT scans. 3D dynamic scans were first introduced in clinical practice with dedicated cardiac CZT SPECT cameras. Its translation in the context of multidetector CZT SPECT systems allows the cardiac protocol to measure myocardial flow and flow reserve to be used with these cameras. Additionally, these cameras can image the vascular phase of bone scintigraphy, enabling a comprehensive three-phase analysis (perfusion, blood pool, metabolism) with the benefit of achieving 3D recording and CT imaging. This improves the localization of bone and relative soft tissue lesions in all those phases.

Lutetium-177-based radiopharmaceutical therapies became very prominent in the past years for treating neuroendocrine tumors and prostate cancer. The therapy is administered in multiple cycles through subsequent radiopharmaceutical injections.

Routine quantification of lutetium-177 distribution across the whole body and dosimetric applications could be beneficial to personalize the therapy or for predicting therapy response on an individual basis [20]. Such optimization is possible through 3D post-therapy imaging, which has been often hampered by the long acquisition times (about 20 min per bed position) and lack of standardization in clinical protocols. Multidetector SPECT cameras address these challenges by offering high energy resolution and high-count sensitivity images in a fraction of time [20], enabling rapid whole-body recordings with adequate image quality, even in low count rate scenarios.

For example, two peaks acquisition at 3 min per bed position is possible both for reading and quantitation purposes. The camera acquires vertex to mid-thighs post-therapy SPECT/CT scans with four to five bed positions at 3 min/bed and a total scan time of 12–15 min [20]. Short scanning time like this is an important factor in helping improve patient comfort and enabling the patient to remain still during the entire exam. Additionally, post-therapy imaging can be performed for all patients receiving the treatment, instead of just a few selected cases.

Lister The List Mode data can be collected and used to retrospectively reframe the acquired scan with different parameters. Therefore the Lister enables research applications and/or can be employed to optimize the image acquisition per each patient.

7.6 Quality Controls and Acceptance Testing

Daily quality controls (DQCs) are performed on both systems with a cobalt-57 line source mounted on a jig arm, designed to suspend the source in air in the center of the field of view (Fig. 7.8). Information on detector uniformity, detector registration, energy resolution, and system sensitivity are obtained through focused scanning of such sources.

Acceptance testing of these systems is unique since many traditional NEMA tests [21] cannot be applied to this novel design, since there is no acquisition in planar mode and collimators cannot be removed. However, different publications are available with the first performance evaluation of these systems [10, 13, 14]. Also, the latest technical publication by NEMA [22] includes a

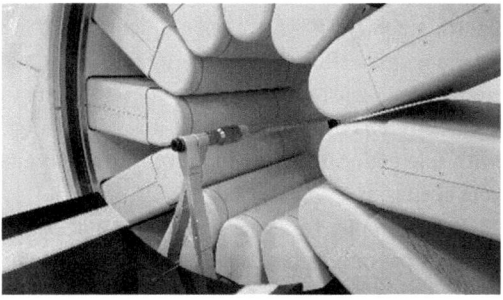

Fig. 7.8 Photograph of cobalt-57 line source mounted on a jig arm for daily QCs

section describing tests specific to gamma camera whole-body scanning systems.

References

1. Decuyper M, Maebe J, Van Holen R, et al. Artificial intelligence with deep learning in nuclear medicine and radiology. EJNMMI Phys. 2021;8(1):81.
2. Dorbala S, Ananthasubramaniam K, Armstrong IS, et al. Single photon emission computed tomography (SPECT) myocardial perfusion imaging guidelines: instrumentation, acquisition, processing, and interpretation. J Nucl Cardiol. 2018;25(5):1784–846.
3. Agostini D, Marie P-Y, Ben-Haim S, et al. Performance of cardiac cadmium-zinc-telluride gamma camera imaging in coronary artery disease: a review from the cardiovascular committee of the European Association of Nuclear Medicine (EANM). Eur J Nucl Med Mol Imaging. 2016;43(13):2423–32.
4. Anger HO. Scintillation camera. Rev Sci Instrum. 1958;29:27–33.
5. Hyafil F, Gimelli A, Slart RHJA, et al. EANM procedural guidelines for myocardial perfusion scintigraphy using cardiac-centered gamma cameras. Eur J Hybrid Imaging. 2019;3(1):11.
6. Imbert L, Bahloul A, Verger A, Marie P-Y. 360° CZT gamma cameras for nuclear medicine and molecular imaging. In: Nuclear medicine and molecular imaging. Amsterdam: Elsevier; 2022. p. 390–9.
7. Ritt P. Recent developments in SPECT/CT. Semin Nucl Med. 2022;52(3):276–85.
8. Hutton B, Occhipinti M, Thie J, et al. Origins of SPECT. Eur J Nucl Med Mol Imaging. 2014;41(Suppl 1):S3–S16.
9. Danieli R, Stella M, Leube J, et al. Quantitative 177Lu SPECT/CT imaging for personalized dosimetry using a ring-shaped CZT-based camera. EJNMMI Phys. 2023;10(1):64.
10. Vergnaud L, Badel JN, Giraudet AL, et al. Performance study of a 360° CZT camera for monitoring 177Lu-PSMA treatment. EJNMMI Phys. 2023;10(1):58.
11. Song H, Leonio MI, Ferri V, et al. Same-day post-therapy imaging with a new generation whole-body digital SPECT/CT in assessing treatment response to [177Lu]Lu-PSMA-617 in metastatic castration-resistant prostate cancer. J Nucl Med. 2021;62(Suppl 1):1125.
12. Le Rouzic G, Zananiri R. First performance measurements of a new multi-detector CZT-based SPECT/CT system: GE StarGuide. J Nucl Med. 2021;62(Suppl 1):1125.
13. Ferri V, Zananiri R, Iagaru A. Performance evaluation of a novel multi-detector CZT-based SPECT/CT system using Tc99m and Lu177. J Nucl Med. 2022;63(Suppl 2):2440.

14. Desmonts C, Bouthiba MA, Enilorac B, et al. Evaluation of a new multipurpose whole-body CzT-based camera: comparison with a dual-head Anger camera and first clinical images. EJNMMI Phys. 2020;7(1):18.

15. Dorbala S, Park MA, Cuddy S, et al. Absolute quantitation of cardiac 99mTc-pyrophosphate using cadmium-zinc-telluride-based SPECT/CT. J Nucl Med. 2021;62(5):716–22.

16. Yamane T, Kondo A, Takahashi M, et al. Ultrafast bone scintigraphy scan for detecting bone metastasis using a CZT whole-body gamma camera. Eur J Nucl Med Mol Imaging. 2019;46(8):1672–7.

17. Bajc M, Schümichen C, Grüning T, et al. EANM guideline for ventilation/perfusion single-photon emission computed tomography (SPECT) for diagnosis of pulmonary embolism and beyond. Eur J Nucl Med Mol Imaging. 2019;46(12):2429–51.

18. Bailly M, Kosovezer H, Le Rouzic G, et al. Dual-isotope lung SPECT using 3D-ring CZT StarGuide SPECT/CT: first clinical results and head-to-head comparison with a conventional camera. J Nucl Med. 2021;62(Suppl 1):1128.

19. Bailly M, Le Rouzic G, Zananiri R, et al. Dual-isotope procedures using 3D-ring CZT StarGuide SPECT/CT: first clinical results from parathyroid acquisitions and head-to-head comparison with a conventional camera. J Nucl Med. 2021;62(Suppl 1):1127.

20. Song H, Ferri V, Duan H, Aparici CM, Davidzon G, Franc BL, Moradi F, Nguyen J, Shah J, Iagaru A. SPECT at the speed of PET: a feasibility study of CZT-based whole-body SPECT/CT in the post ^{177}Lu-DOTATATE and ^{177}Lu-PSMA617 setting. Eur J Nucl Med Mol Imaging. 2023;50(8):2250–7.

21. National Electrical Manufacturers Association. NEMA standards publication NU 1-2018 performance measurements of gamma cameras. Rosslyn: National Electrical Manufacturers Association; 2018.

22. National Electrical Manufacturers Association. Performance measurements of gamma cameras NEMA NU 1 - 2023. Rosslyn: National Electrical Manufacturers Association; 2023.

Advances in Hybrid Imaging: PET/CT

8

Francesca Bisello and Valentina Ferri

8.1 Introduction

The following chapter aims to offer an overview of the latest generation of hybrid imaging systems. The technological advancements in the newest Positron emission tomography/computed tomography (PET/CT) systems will be discussed along with the principles, components, and capabilities that set them apart from earlier models.

The vision that guides the newest technological improvements is based on the need for increasingly personalized, fast, and precise imaging tools, able to study, map, and quantify the considerable number of physiological processes that impact a patient's life. The growing complexity linked to a more personalized medicine calls for more sophisticated and integrated tools. The trends in innovation aim to keep improving the standards in image quality, system performance and system integration, and, most importantly, patient experience and comfort.

To understand the impact of all these recent technological developments, it is important to first clarify the benchmarks for traditional PET/CT systems and understand the steps toward the technological improvement.

8.2 PET/CT as an Integration of Functional and Anatomical Imaging for Diagnosis and Therapy: Steps Toward a Full Total Body Acquisitions

Positron emission tomography/computed tomography (PET/CT) combines two powerful imaging techniques into a single system, providing both functional and anatomical information. PET uses radioactive tracers—molecules labeled with positron-emitting isotopes like fluorine-18—which are injected into the body to target specific biological processes. The PET scanner detects the gamma rays emitted when the positrons interact with electrons in the body, creating detailed images of metabolic and molecular activity. CT, on the other hand, produces high-resolution X-ray images, allowing for precise anatomical localization of PET-detected changes. The integration of PET and CT allows clinicians to visualize both how tissues function and their structure, making it an invaluable tool in the diagnosis and management of various diseases [1, 2].

Today, positron emission tomography (PET) systems are widely available in medical centers

F. Bisello
Division of Medical Physics, IRCCS Azienda Ospedaliero-Universitaria Policlinico S.Orsola – Malpighi, Stanford, CA, USA
e-mail: francesca.bisello@aosp.bo.it

V. Ferri (✉)
Stanford University Medical Center, Division of Nuclear medicine and Molecular Imaging, Department of Radiology, Bologna, Italy
e-mail: francescavferri@stanford.edu

L. Camoni, L. Mansi (eds.), *Nuclear Medicine Hybrid Imaging for Radiographers & Technologists*,
https://doi.org/10.1007/978-3-031-86228-1_8

across the globe, and they have become indispensable tools in both diagnostic and therapeutic settings. PET's ability to provide detailed molecular and metabolic information makes it essential for early disease detection, precise diagnosis, and accurate staging of conditions like cancer, neurological disorders, and cardiovascular diseases.

In addition to its diagnostic power, PET plays a critical role in therapy management. It helps clinicians evaluate treatment efficacy, monitor changes in tumors or diseased tissues, and adjust therapies based on real-time data.

The following section will discuss the latest developments in PET imaging, such as total body PET/CT, which holds promise to bring a significant change of paradigm in the field, in terms of both technology and clinical and research applications.

8.2.1 From Analog to Digital PET/CT Systems

The evolution from analog to digital systems (Fig. 8.1) has been a pivotal advancement in the development of modern PET/CT technology,

particularly in enabling the realization of full-body PET/CT scanners. Early PET systems relied on analog components such as photomultiplier tubes (PMTs), which were effective but limited in their sensitivity, spatial resolution, and timing accuracy. These limitations restricted the performance of PET/CT systems, especially in applications requiring comprehensive whole-body imaging, which demands significantly higher sensitivity and the ability to manage large amounts of data [1].

One of the most crucial developments in this transition has been the introduction of silicon photomultipliers (SiPMs) [3], which replaced traditional analog PMTs with fully digital detection systems. SiPMs offer far superior performance in terms of timing resolution and photon detection efficiency.

This has allowed for the advancement of time-of-flight (TOF) PET technology [4], which improves the signal-to-noise ratio by precisely measuring the time difference between gamma photons reaching the detectors. With TOF, PET/CT scanners are now able to produce clearer and more accurate images, even with lower doses of radioactive tracers, making it ideal for applica-

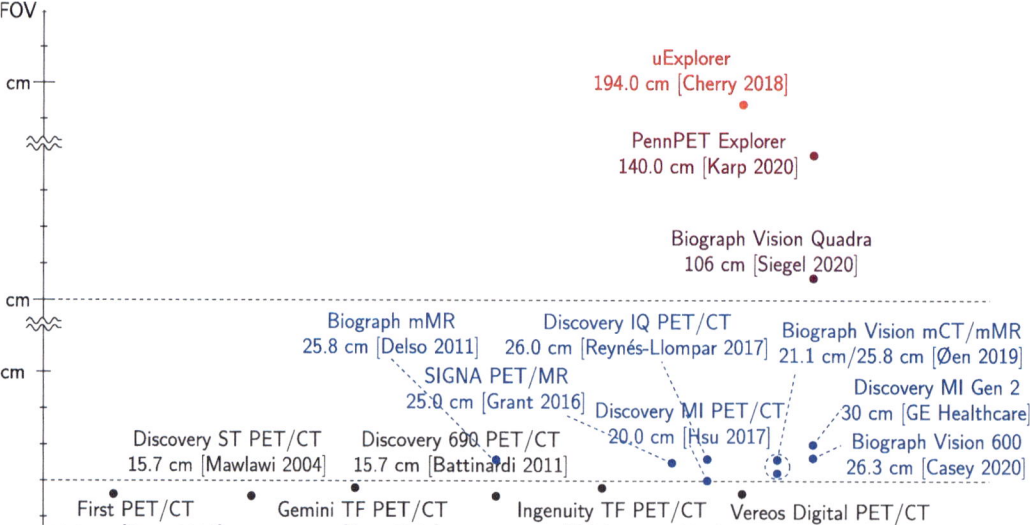

Fig. 8.1 Evolution of aFOV of research and commercial PET/CT or PET/MR systems. Reproduced and adapted with permission from Nadig, V., Herrmann, K., Mottaghy, F.M. et al. Hybrid total-body pet scanners—current status and future perspectives. Eur J Nucl Med Mol Imaging 49, 445–459 (2022). https://doi.org/10.1007/s00259-021-05536-4 published under a Creative Commons CC BY license

tions like whole-body imaging, where high-resolution detail across larger fields of view is essential [5].

Moreover, digital systems have enabled the scalability of detector arrays, which is critical for total-body imaging. Full-body PET/CT scanners, such as the uEXPLORER and Biograph Vision Quadra, require detectors that can cover the entire human body in a single scan, capturing data from organs and tissues simultaneously. The increased channel count and improved data processing capabilities made possible by digital systems have been fundamental in achieving the extended axial fields of view (aFOV) that these scanners offer [3, 6]. Analog systems, in contrast, were limited in their ability to scale up to this degree, making full-body imaging impractical.

The shift to digital systems has also had a significant impact on image reconstruction and analysis techniques. The higher-quality data generated by digital detectors can be fed into advanced iterative reconstruction algorithms, which create more precise images. Additionally, recent developments in machine learning (ML) and deep learning (DL) have introduced greater automation and accuracy in image analysis, helping clinicians interpret the complex datasets produced by full-body PET/CT scans [7, 8].

These methods are particularly useful for dynamic imaging, where tracer kinetics need to be monitored in real-time across multiple organs.

The transition from analog to digital systems is thus not just an incremental improvement but a necessary leap forward that has unlocked new possibilities for PET/CT technology. With the enhanced resolution, timing accuracy, scalability, and data handling made possible by digital systems, the development of full-body PET/CT has moved from a conceptual goal to a clinical reality.

8.2.2 From Whole-Body Scan to Total Body PET/CT: Technical Challenges and New Routine

8.2.2.1 Evolution of Axial Field of View

The axial field of view (aFOV) of standard PET/CT scanners is limited, requiring patient bed translations with slightly overlapping aFOV positions to capture images of the whole torso or body ("from head to thighs"). These translations can lead to quantification errors due to varying noise levels in different regions with different tracer uptake, issues with alignment, motion artifacts, and variations in data acquisition time, ultimately affecting the quality and accuracy of the resulting images. As PET systems have improved, in coincidence timing resolution (CRT) and acquired time-of-flight (TOF) information, this process is becoming more efficient. The trend toward larger aFOVs, now exceeding 20 cm in most modern multimodal PET systems, has contributed to significantly shortening acquisition times for a whole-body PET/CT examination [3].

The latest PET/CT scanners, released in the late 2010s, offering an expanded axial field of view (aFOV) up to 1–2 m and allowing for whole-body imaging in less than 60 s, provide real-time insights into physiological and pathological processes and simultaneous imaging of multiple organs (Fig. 8.2).

These systems, such as the Biograph Vision Quadra (by Siemens Healthineers) and Uexplorer (by United Imaging), are designed to capture a full-body image in a single acquisition, reducing the time needed for multibed imaging and minimizing patient discomfort, thanks to their enhanced sensitivity. Higher sensitivity means the system can identify smaller amounts of radiotracer or detect changes in tracer distribution more effectively. Such an increase enables the detection of smaller lesions and improves signal-

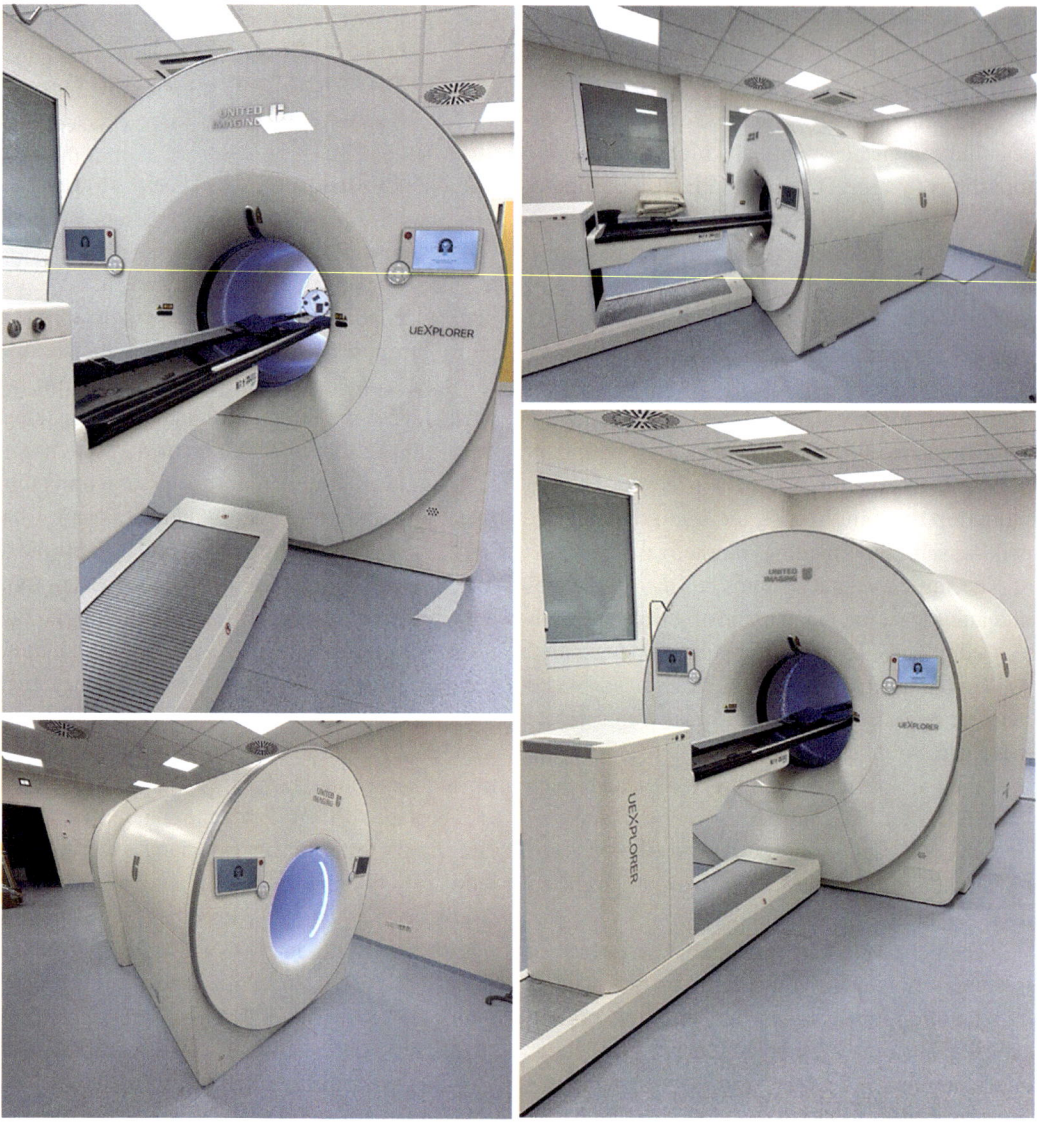

Fig. 8.2 Photographs of the total body PET/CT (uEX-PLORER by United Imaging Healthcare) installed in the Nuclear Medicine Division of IRCCS Azienda Ospedaliero Universitaria di Bologna, Italy—Policlinico di Sant'Orsola. By courtesy of Prof. Stefano Fanti

to-noise (SNR) ratios, which is critical for accurate diagnostics. Other systems are based on a modular design, where additional modules can be added to the standard one to extend the resulting axial FOV (Omni Legend by GE HealthCare).

The transition to full-body PET/CT systems is marked by advancements that push the boundaries of imaging technology. Full-body PET/CT encompasses not only the capacity for total-body imaging but also integrates dynamic imaging capabilities, allowing clinicians to observe complex physiological processes in real time. This is particularly useful in evaluating the kinetics of radiotracers as they move through different tissues and organs. Such capabilities are vital for comprehensive assessments in oncology, cardiology, and other medical fields, as they provide insights into disease progression, response to therapy, and overall patient health.

The gain in sensitivity is achieved by the fact that the geometric coverage is increased over the full patient body, which is completely surrounded by detector material. Simulations and the first comparative studies suggest that expanding a PET scanner from a standard 20-cm aFOV to a 200-cm aFOV results in roughly a 40-fold increase in effective sensitivity when the whole body is imaged, as indicated by the noise-equivalent counting rate measurement. In the case of brain imaging or the heart, in which the whole area is included in the aFOV even in traditional ~20 cm aFOV scanners, the sensitivity can still be increased by four- to fivefold, thanks to the increased number of detectors surrounding the areas.

Achieving true whole-body coverage in PET/CT imaging represents a significant technical challenge. While advancements in technology have led to the development of total-body and full-body PET/CT systems, several hurdles have been addressed to optimize performance and maximize clinical utility.

8.2.2.2 Detector Sensitivity and Design

Sensitivity refers to the ability of the PET system to detect positron annihilation events (i.e., the two 511 keV photons emitted in opposite directions). Higher sensitivity means more accurate and reliable images can be produced with fewer radiotracers, reducing patient dose and shortening scan times. Whole-body PET systems feature larger and more densely packed detector arrays, increasing the solid angle covered by the detectors, which in turn increases the number of detected annihilation events and improves sensitivity.

For comparison, transitioning from traditional PET/CT systems (15–25 cm aFOV) to extended FOV systems (1–2 m aFOV) involves a transition in "point" peak sensitivity of 4–6% to a 12–24% (increase of 3–5 times) and a "body" imaging sensitivity of 7–21 cps/kBq to a 200–500 cps/kBq (increase of 30–50 times). This ultimately leads to decrease of acquisition time for a whole-body image from roughly 20–0.5 min (decrease of 20–40 times).

Modern whole-body PET systems utilize higher-performance scintillation crystals like lutetium oxyorthosilicate (LSO) or lutetium-yttrium oxyorthosilicate (LYSO), which have higher stopping power for 511 keV photons, faster scintillation decay times, and higher light output compared to earlier materials like BGO. This leads to better photon detection efficiency and timing resolution in combination with SiPM and TOF technology discussed before.

This expansion required addressing challenges in geometrical efficiency and ensuring the detection of photon pairs with high precision. Whole-body systems needed to optimize detector materials and configurations to maximize photon capture without introducing additional noise or artifacts. Innovations such as hexagonal detector arrays (reducing dead space), depth of interaction (DOI) detection (correcting for parallax errors), and layered detectors (capturing photons across multiple layers) have improved sensitivity. Additionally, arc-shaped geometries [9, 10] better match the body's shape, optimizing photon detection from all angles. These advances ensure high sensitivity, better image quality, and shorter scan times in whole-body PET imaging.

8.2.2.3 Image Reconstruction Algorithms

Another significant technical challenge lies in the development of advanced image reconstruction algorithms that can effectively handle the vast amount of data generated by true whole-body scans. Current reconstruction techniques, while effective, struggle with the complexity of simultaneously capturing information from numerous organs and tissues, leading to potential issues with noise and resolution. Iterative reconstruction methods have improved image quality, but optimizing these algorithms for true whole-body coverage remains an area of active research. The incorporation of machine learning and artificial intelligence into reconstruction processes may offer solutions, yet these technologies are still evolving.

8.2.2.4 Motion Artifacts and Patient Management

Patient motion during imaging presents another challenge for achieving true whole-body coverage in PET/CT. Even slight movements can lead to artifacts that compromise the quality of the images obtained. This is particularly relevant for long scanning procedures, which can be uncomfortable for patients. Strategies to mitigate motion artifacts, such as breath-hold techniques or respiratory gating, can help, but they add complexity to the imaging process. Future systems must incorporate user-friendly features that minimize patient discomfort while ensuring optimal image quality.

8.2.2.5 Data Processing and Integration

The processing and integration of data from true whole-body PET/CT scans pose significant challenges in terms of the large volumes of data generated, which require efficient storage, processing, and interpretation systems. Integrating data from multiple sources, including PET and CT, necessitates sophisticated software that can manage and analyze the information seamlessly. Developing robust data management systems is vital to facilitate clinical workflows and ensure timely and accurate diagnostics.

8.2.3 State of the Art and Systems Performance

The development of total-body PET/CT systems marks a significant advancement in the field of nuclear medicine and molecular imaging, offering enhanced imaging capabilities compared to traditional systems. As outlined in Table 8.1 [11], several research and commercial total-body PET/CT scanners have emerged, including the Biograph Vision Quadra (by Siemens Healthineers), Uexplorer (by United Imaging Healthcare), and PennPET Explorer. Each of these systems is designed for clinical applications and features an extended aFOV, which allows for comprehensive imaging of the entire human body.

A critical aspect of these systems is their impressive axial coverage. The Uexplorer boasts the largest aFOV at 194 cm, enabling simultaneous imaging of the entire body and thereby reducing scan times while improving patient comfort. In contrast, the Biograph Vision Quadra has an aFOV of 106 cm, while the PennPET offers a more moderate coverage of 64 cm, with plans for an eventual expansion to 140 cm. This extended coverage is essential for achieving true whole-body imaging.

Table 8.1 Overview on existing of total-body PET scanning systems

System	Biograph Vision Quadra	Uexplorer	PennPET explorer
Company/facility	Siemens Healthineers	UC Davis and United Imaging Healthcare	UPenn, KAGE Medical, and Philips
Purpose	Clinical (human)	Clinical (human)	Clinical (human)
Bore diameter (cm)	78	76	NA
aFOV (cm)	106	194	64 (140 planned)
tFOV (cm)	NA	68.6	57.6
Photosensors	Analog SiPMs	Analog SiPMs (SensL)	Digital SiPMs (PDPC)
Scintillators	LSO (20 mm)	LYSO (18.1 mm)	LYSO (19 mm)
CTR (ps)	219	430	250
dE/E (%)	10.1	11.7	12
Spatial res. (mm)	3.4	2.9	4
Sensitivity (kcps/MBq)	174	174	55
NECR/Mcps (kBq/cc)	<2.5 (26)	<1.855 (9.6)	>0.001 (30)

Sensitivity is another vital performance metric highlighted in Table 8.1. Both the Uexplorer and Biograph Vision Quadra achieve a sensitivity of 174 kcps/MBq, indicating their ability to detect low levels of radioactivity efficiently. The PennPET, while exhibiting a lower sensitivity of 55 kcps/MBq, still contributes to the overall advancements in imaging technology.

Spatial resolution, crucial for accurate lesion detection, ranges from 2.9 mm to 4.0 mm across these systems, with the Uexplorer demonstrating superior performance at 2.9 mm. This enhanced spatial resolution facilitates the identification of smaller lesions, which is particularly important in oncology.

Additionally, the CTR (Coincidence Timing Resolution) plays a significant role in the accuracy of image reconstruction. The Biograph Vision Quadra achieves a CTR of 219 ps, whereas the Uexplorer and the PennPET have CTRs of 430 ps and 250 ps, respectively. Lower CTR values indicate better timing resolution, which is essential for optimizing time-of-flight (TOF) imaging capabilities, further enhancing the precision of diagnostics.

Another interesting commercial system in the extended axial field of view space is the Omni Legend by GE HealthCare, which features a modular design where multiple modules can be added to a standard aFOV (16 cm). At present, Omni Legend is characterized by a 32-cm axial field of view which can be expanded in the future to 64 cm, or 128 cm, and employs digital bismuth germanate (BGO) crystals, designed to improve spatial resolution and sensitivity while containing costs. Performance evaluations according to NEMA NU 2-2018 standards reach a full width at half maximum of less than 4.0 mm at 1.0 cm off-center and a sensitivity of 1478 cps/MBq/cm (or up to 46 cps/kBq across a 32 cm aFOV), ranking it among the highest sensitivity levels for current PET/CT systems. This is attributed to its long aFOV and thick (30 mm) BGO crystals. The energy resolution is measured at 9.8%, with an optimized energy window of 435–580 keV, facilitating effective scatter management. The reconstruction framework uses an image-processing algorithm based on artificial intelligence that can

mimic image quality obtained with a TOF-based system. These advancements in spatial resolution and sensitivity, together with "Precision Deep Learning" algorithms to support reconstruction, contribute to improved image quality and lesion detection, although further research is necessary to evaluate the system's efficacy across diverse clinical examinations [12].

8.2.4 Clinical and Research Applications of Total Body PET (TB-PET)

Total-body PET/CT systems represent a significant leap forward in medical imaging, offering comprehensive coverage and enhanced sensitivity for a wide array of applications. These systems are increasingly being integrated into routine clinical practice, providing valuable insights in various medical fields, including oncology, cardiology, neurology, and infectious disease management enabling accurate disease assessment and detection of small lesions missed by traditional imaging.

Intrinsically, they have the potential to be highly effective in reducing patient radiation exposure allowing lower injected activity.

8.2.4.1 Applications in Clinical Practice
General Healthcare Applications TB-PET promises improved image quality, reduced radiation doses, and faster scanning times—potentially completing examinations in 15–30 s, thus increasing patient throughput. While the high initial costs may limit widespread adoption, the demand in high-volume hospitals could drive early investment. The ongoing development and optimization of TB-PET technology may eventually enhance affordability and expand its clinical applications. The ongoing development and optimization of TB-PET technology will likely make these systems more affordable in the future. Advances in detector materials, electronics, and software optimization, combined with economies of scale as production increases, may reduce costs and make the technology more accessible to a broader range of healthcare facilities. This will

not only expand the clinical applications of TB-PET, from cancer diagnosis to infection imaging and metabolic studies but also make high-sensitivity, low-dose imaging available to more patients worldwide.

Dose Reduction Protocols Another major benefit is the potential for reduced radiation doses. Traditional PET/CT scans require a relatively high dose of radiotracer due to the need for longer scan times and lower sensitivity. In contrast, TB-PET systems, with their increased sensitivity and efficiency, can achieve the same diagnostic results with significantly lower amounts of radiotracer. For example, some studies suggest that radiation doses in TB-PET can be reduced by up to 40–70% without compromising image quality [13]. In some cases, ultra-low-dose PET techniques using up to 1/20th of the standard dose have been achieved, enabling longitudinal imaging with reduced exposure to radiation, which is particularly beneficial for vulnerable populations [14].

Oncology TB-PET significantly enhances the detection of small, low-density tumor deposits (micrometastases) that traditional imaging methods struggle to identify. Current techniques like MRI and ^{18}F-FDG PET/CT can detect tumors as small as ~5 mm^3, but TB-PET offers the potential for noninvasive detection of even smaller deposits. This capability could improve cancer staging, inform treatment decisions, and enable better assessment of therapy responses. Although small micrometastases might not be visualized individually due to spatial resolution limitations, dynamic imaging combined with quantitative modeling could allow detection within larger tissue regions. By leveraging kinetic models and compartmental analysis, such systems can capture microkinetic parameters like the tracer delivery rate, K1, and fractional blood volume (vb), which are crucial for understanding the tumor's microenvironment. These developments provide a more detailed characterization of tumor biology, even when the micrometastases themselves remain undetected as distinct visual entities. The integration of high temporal resolution with TB-PET allows precise mapping of fast tracer kinetics and differentiates the various phases of tracer distribution in tissues. For example, the system can monitor the influx and retention of tracers like ^{18}F-FDG, which provides insights into tumor perfusion and metabolic activity, indirectly signaling the presence of micrometastases [14]. The exploration of novel imaging biomarkers is anticipated to further enhance TB-PET's effectiveness in oncology and could extend to the detection of infectious diseases and inflammation.

Cardiology Cardiology has benefited from PET/CT imaging for many years, particularly in assessing myocardial perfusion and viability. However, the advent of total-body PET/CT systems offers notable enhancements in this field. Traditional PET/CT scanners are effective for cardiovascular imaging, but they are limited by their smaller field of view and lower sensitivity, which require longer scan times and higher doses of radiotracer. Whole-body coverage and increased sensitivity allow for simultaneous imaging of the heart and peripheral tissues, enabling comprehensive assessments that are not possible with traditional systems. For instance, dynamic imaging of tracer kinetics across the entire body offers new insights into systemic factors influencing cardiac function, such as blood flow and metabolism throughout the vasculature. The system's ability to produce high-resolution, whole-body images in a single pass allows for more accurate evaluation of coronary artery disease, myocardial viability, and perfusion without the need for multiple scans. Additionally, the high temporal resolution of TB-PET enables more precise measurement of fast-moving cardiac dynamics and better differentiation of myocardial blood flow patterns. This is particularly useful in detecting early changes in coronary artery disease or in complex cases where perfusion and viability need to be assessed simultaneously with high accuracy. Moreover, the potential for reduced radiation doses and faster scan times improves patient comfort and safety, particularly for those requiring frequent follow-up scans, such as patients with chronic cardiovascular conditions [14, 15].

Neurological Imaging While traditional PET systems can perform dynamic imaging in a specific region (e.g., the brain), TB-PET/CT allows for whole-body dynamic imaging. This is important because certain neurological conditions, such as epilepsy or brain tumors, might have systemic manifestations that traditional scanners would miss [16]. For example, TB-PET can track how a radiotracer like ^{18}F-FDG is metabolized not just in the brain but throughout the vascular and metabolic systems, offering a broader understanding of how neurological diseases affect the body. TB-PET systems are designed with faster temporal resolution, meaning they can capture changes in the brain's metabolic or functional activity with higher accuracy over time. This becomes particularly useful in conditions like epilepsy, where the ability to capture fast-moving metabolic changes (such as during seizure onset) is crucial for accurate diagnosis and surgical planning. Additionally, total-body systems allow for more advanced motion correction algorithms, reducing the impact of patient movement on image quality [17]. This is especially important for patients with movement disorders (e.g., Parkinson's disease) who may find it hard to remain still [18]. The dose reduction possibility is beneficial also in this field for neurological patients who require frequent follow-up scans, such as those with chronic neurodegenerative diseases (like Alzheimer's or multiple sclerosis) or (more relevant) children with epilepsy [19]. Lower radiation doses reduce the long-term risks of repeated imaging while maintaining diagnostic quality.

Infectious Disease Management Total-body PET/CT can be used to detect and localize infections, such as abscesses or osteomyelitis. The comprehensive imaging capabilities allow for effective evaluation of the entire body, facilitating prompt and accurate diagnosis. For example, studies indicate that PET scans demonstrate high sensitivity (90%) and specificity (85%) in identifying osteomyelitis, impacting clinical management decisions in about 67% of cases. The ability to visualize infections that may not be confined to one region of the body enhances the overall assessment and treatment planning for patients [20].

8.2.4.2 Research Applications

Drug Development TB-PET holds promise for early pharmaceutical development by enabling high-sensitivity investigations during early clinical trials. It allows for detailed studies of drug biodistribution and pharmacokinetics, even at microdoses, and can assess the effects of potential toxic compounds.

Novel Imaging Biomarkers The growing interest in novel biomarkers and multiparametric imaging techniques also holds promise. Dual-tracer imaging and the enhanced sensitivity of TB-PET create opportunities for more robust identification of cancer spread and response to treatment. As a result, the continued development of these techniques is anticipated to make TB-PET systems even more effective for early detection and monitoring of cancer progression. These advancements are highlighted by studies which demonstrate the potential for high-quality total-body kinetic modeling to provide insights into complex biological processes at a micro-level, supporting the potential for more effective oncology imaging with TB-PET systems [21].

Cell Tracking and Function This imaging technology can aid in the development of stem cell and cancer immunotherapies by tracking labeled cells over extended periods. It also allows for imaging of therapeutic cell functionality, enhancing our understanding of these therapies.

Maternal-Fetal and Pediatric Studies TB-PET's ultra-sensitive imaging capabilities can facilitate research in maternal-fetal medicine, enabling noninvasive assessments of placental transport and fetal health with minimal radiation exposure. It also opens avenues for pediatric research, particularly in understanding developmental disorders.

Multisystem Disease TB-PET's ability to conduct whole-body imaging could enhance the understanding of complex conditions involving multiple organ systems, such as metabolic syndrome, neurodegenerative diseases, and mental health disorders.

8.2.5 Daily Use and Best Practices for Technicians

Incorporating total-body PET/CT systems into clinical practice presents unique operational challenges and opportunities for staff involved in patient examinations. These systems may require adjustments in scheduling due to their faster scanning capabilities, allowing for increased patient throughput while also necessitating more complex dynamic imaging protocols which require examination duration up to 60 min.

Moreover, the implementation of total-body PET/CT systems in clinical settings introduces a diverse range of applications that require multiple imaging protocols tailored to specific clinical needs. These protocols can vary significantly based on the intended use—whether for oncology, cardiology, or neurology—thus necessitating a high level of teamwork and communication among various professionals.

Physicists play a crucial role in ensuring the technical accuracy and safety of imaging protocols. They are responsible for optimizing scanner performance, implementing quality assurance measures, and providing training on new technologies. Technicians are vital for the practical aspects of imaging, including patient preparation, operating the equipment, and managing data acquisition. Physicians, particularly radiologists and specialists in the relevant fields, must interpret the imaging results and integrate them into patient care decisions.

Effective communication and collaboration among these teams are essential for achieving optimal patient outcomes. As the complexity of total-body PET/CT imaging increases, the need for a multidisciplinary approach becomes even more pronounced. Research supports this notion, indicating that integrated care teams enhance diagnostic accuracy, improve patient management, and lead to better health outcomes.

The ongoing development and clinical implementation of total-body systems indicate a need for tailored operational protocols that address the complexities and demands of these advanced imaging modalities, and it's expected that dedicated guidelines will be developed, focusing on specific operational and safety considerations unique to these systems. In the meantime, utilizing existing protocols and fostering an environment of continuous improvement among the imaging staff will be essential.

8.2.6 Quality Controls and Acceptance Testing

The advancement of total-body PET/CT technology necessitates the investigation in the establishment of new standards and the development of specialized tests beyond the state of art recommendation NEMA Standards Publication NU 2-2018, Performance Measurements of Positron Emission Tomographs (PETS) to accurately validate the performance of these systems, as evaluated in the study by Spencer et al. [22], where ad hoc tests have been development for the acceptance of uEXPLORERs long axial field of view (aFOV) of 194 cm.

Moreover, this expanded aFOV also brings challenges and intense validation activity in ensuring consistent performance across various imaging protocols [13] and SUV quantifications and harmonization. The topic of standardized uptake value (SUV) quantification and the harmonization of new total-body PET/CT systems is crucial for ensuring consistency and accuracy in imaging results across different platforms.

A study highlighted the need for standardized protocols in SUV quantification, particularly for total-body PET scans, which can significantly impact clinical outcomes. Variability in SUV measurements can arise due to differences in PET/CT scanners, reconstruction algorithms, and patient preparation methods (Song et al. 2023). Therefore, the implementation of consistent guidelines and techniques is essential to mitigate these variations and enable reliable comparisons in multicenter studies.

References

1. Gonzalez-Montoro A, Ullah MN, Levin CS. Advances in Detector Instrumentation for PET. J Nucl Med. 2022;63(8):1138–44. https://doi.org/10.2967/jnumed.121.262509.

2. IAEA. Radiation protection during PET/CT. 2024. https://www.iaea.org/resources/rpop/health-professionals/nuclear-medicine/pet-ct. Accessed 6 October 2024.

3. Nadig V, Herrmann K, Mottaghy FM, Schulz V. Hybrid total-body pet scanners-current status and future perspectives. Eur J Nucl Med Mol Imaging. 2022;49(2):445–59. https://doi.org/10.1007/s00259-021-05536-4.

4. Lecoq P, Gundacker S. SiPM applications in positron emission tomography: toward ultimate PET time-of-flight resolution. Eur Phys J Plus. 2021;136(3):292. https://doi.org/10.1140/epjp/s13360-021-01183-8.

5. Surti S, et al. Impact of time-of-flight PET on whole-body oncologic studies: a human observer lesion detection and localization study. J Nucl Med. 2011;52(5):712–9. https://doi.org/10.2967/jnumed.110.086678.

6. Vandenberghe S, Moskal P, Karp JS. State of the art in total body PET. EJNMMI Phys. 2020;7(1):35. https://doi.org/10.1186/s40658-020-00290-2.

7. Hosch R, et al. Artificial intelligence guided enhancement of digital PET: scans as fast as CT? Eur J Nucl Med Mol Imaging. 2022;49(13):4503–15. https://doi.org/10.1007/s00259-022-05901-x.

8. Hashimoto F, Onishi Y, Ote K, Tashima H, Reader AJ, Yamaya T. Deep learning-based PET image denoising and reconstruction: a review. Radiol Phys Technol. 2024;17(1):24–46. https://doi.org/10.1007/s12194-024-00780-3.

9. Badawi RD, et al. First human imaging studies with the EXPLORER total-body PET scanner. J Nucl Med. 2019;60(3):299–303. https://doi.org/10.2967/jnumed.119.226498.

10. Cherry SR, Jones T, Karp JS, Qi J, Moses WW, Badawi RD. Total-body PET: maximizing sensitivity to create new opportunities for clinical research and patient care. J Nucl Med. 2018;59(1):3–12. https://doi.org/10.2967/jnumed.116.184028.

11. Katal S, Eibschutz LS, Saboury B, Gholamrezanezhad A, Alavi A. Advantages and applications of total-body PET scanning. Diagnostics. 2022;12(2):426. https://doi.org/10.3390/diagnostics12020426.

12. Dadgar M, Verstraete A, Maebe J, et al. Assessing the deep learning based image quality enhancements for the BGO based GE omni legend PET/CT. EJNMMI Phys. 2024;11:86. https://doi.org/10.1186/s40658-024-00688-2).

13. Huang Y, et al. Optimal clinical protocols for total-body ^{18}F-FDG PET/CT examination under different activity administration plans. EJNMMI Phys. 2023;10(1):14. https://doi.org/10.1186/s40658-023-00533-y.

14. Shiyam Sundar LK, Gutschmayer S, Maenle M, Beyer T. Extracting value from total-body PET/CT image data - the emerging role of artificial intelligence. Cancer Imaging. 2024;24(1):51. https://doi.org/10.1186/s40644-024-00684-w.

15. Wang Y, Li E, Cherry SR, Wang G. Total-body PET kinetic modeling and potential opportunities using deep learning. PET Clin. 2021;16(4):613–25. https://doi.org/10.1016/j.cpet.2021.06.009.

16. Sun Y, Cheng Z, Qiu J, Lu W. Performance and application of the total-body PET/CT scanner: a literature review. EJNMMI Res. 2024b;14(1):38. https://doi.org/10.1186/s13550-023-01059-1.

17. Wang J, et al. Motion-correction strategies for enhancing whole-body PET imaging. Front Nucl Med. 2024;4:1257880. https://doi.org/10.3389/fnume.2024.1257880.

18. Sun X, et al. 11C-CFT PET brain imaging in Parkinson's disease using a total-body PET/CT scanner. EJNMMI Phys. 2024a;11(1):40. https://doi.org/10.1186/s40658-024-00640-4.

19. Gennari AG, et al. Long-term trends in total administered radiation dose from brain [18F]FDG-PET in children with drug-resistant epilepsy. Eur J Nucl Med Mol Imaging. 2024;52(2):574–85. https://doi.org/10.1007/s00259-024-06902-8.

20. Uy N, Tavakoli-Tabasi S, Tamara L, Musher D. The clinical utility of PET scans for evaluation of osteomyelitis: do results actually impact management? Open Forum Infect Dis. 2015;2:1512. https://doi.org/10.1093/ofid/ofv133.1065.

21. Gu F, Wu Q. Quantitation of dynamic total-body PET imaging: recent developments and future perspectives. Eur J Nucl Med Mol Imaging. 2023;50(12):3538–57. https://doi.org/10.1007/s00259-023-06299-w.

22. Spencer BA, McBride K, Hunt H, Jones T, Cherry SR, Badawi RD. Practical considerations for total-body PET acquisition and imaging. In: Witney TH, Shuhendler AJ, editors. Positron emission tomography: methods and protocols. New York: Springer; 2024. p. 371–89. https://doi.org/10.1007/978-1-0716-3499-8_21.

23. Song Y, Meng X, Cao Z, Zhao W, Zhang Y, Guo R, Zhou X, Yang Z, Li N. Harmonization of standard uptake values across different positron emission tomography/computed tomography systems and different reconstruction algorithms: validation in oncology patients. EJNMMI Phys. 2023;10(1):19. https://doi.org/10.1186/s40658-023-00540-z. PMID: 36920590; PMCID: PMC10017904.

Quality Control For Single-Photon Emission Computed Tomography (SPECT/CT) in Nuclear Medicine

9

Federica Savino and Vincenzo Rizzo

9.1 Introduction

Establishing a routine quality control (QC) program of instrumentation used within a nuclear medicine department, such as hybrid single-photon emission computed tomography (SPECT/CT) and positron emission tomography (PET/CT) scanners, represents a crucial effort to ensure the correct diagnostic performance and quantitative accuracy.

Routine QC testing starts after installation of the instrument, so after the acceptance tests, a periodic QC program is specifically required to test the constancy of the performance of the equipment throughout its lifetime. Several recommendations by national and international agencies exist for periodic SPECT/CT and PET/CT QC, such as from the European Association of Nuclear Medicine (EANM), International Atomic Energy Agency (IAEA), American Association of Physicists in Medicine (AAPM) and International Electrotechnical Commission (IEC). Also, National Electrical Manufacturers Association (NEMA) tests, which are intended to verify the performance of the PET and SPECT scanner at their installation and acceptance, could be used as routine tests. These recommendations

must be considered in the light of any national guidelines and legislation, which must be followed. An effective QC program is able to detect subtle changes in the performance of the PET or SPECT scanner, using simple, practical and reproducible procedures, and through the use of selected and measurable parameters directly linked to the quality of clinical images; in other words, it helps to detect problems before they can impact clinical studies in terms of safety, image quality, quantify accuracy, and patient radiation dose.

9.2 Acceptance and Reference Tests

After installation, and before it is put into clinical use, a nuclear medicine instrument must undergo thorough and careful acceptance testing, the aim being to verify that the instrument performs according to its specifications and its clinical purpose. Each instrument is supplied with a set of basic specifications, which have been produced by the manufacturer according to standard test procedures, which should be traceable to standard protocols, such as the NEMA and IEC performance standards. By following such standard protocols in the clinical setting, with support from the vendor for supplying phantoms and software where necessary, specifications can be verified and baseline performance data created.

F. Savino · V. Rizzo (✉)
Division of Nuclear Medicine, Azienda Ospedaliera
G. Moscati, Avellino, Italy
e-mail: Federica.savino@aornmoscati.it;
Vincenzo.rizzo@aornmoscati.it

These acceptance test results became the reference data for future QC tests, and some may be repeated periodically, such as at half-yearly or yearly intervals, or whenever a major service or component change has been carried out.

Once the instrument has been accepted for clinical use, its performance needs to be tested routinely with simple QC procedures that are sensitive to changes in performance. Tests must be performed by appropriately qualified and trained staff, and detailed local operating procedures should be written for this routine work. All test results must be recorded and monitored for variations, and appropriate actions taken when changes are observed. The QC tests are an important part of the routine work, and sufficient equipment time and staff time must be allocated for routine QC.

9.3 Routine Test Recommendations and Test Frequency

Recommendations for basic routine QC tests that should be scheduled and carried out for the main instruments of the nuclear medicine department are presented in the tables below. The tables give briefly the purpose of the test, suggested frequency, and a comment. These are not intended as national guidelines or national regulations, and the test frequencies given should be followed and adjusted according to observations of instrument stability and environmental stability (power supply, temperature, and humidity).

Test procedures can be found by reference to standard descriptions and national and international protocols mentioned above. It is recommended that each department create detailed written routine QC test procedures specific for each instrument in use.

9.4 Gamma Camera

In Table 9.1, the routine QC tests to be performed in a quality assurance program for a gamma camera are reported [1].

Usually, the radionuclides to be used for testing are the radionuclides that are used clinically. The most commonly used radionuclides are ^{99m}Tc, ^{57}Co, ^{123}I, ^{67}Ga, ^{131}I. The test phantoms most frequently used are a ^{57}Co sheet source, a quadrant-bar phantom, and a SPECT phantom.

The planar tests must be performed for each detector and collimator combination in a multiple detector system. The tests are categorized as being intrinsic or extrinsic. Intrinsic tests are performed without an installed collimator and are designed to measure the performance of the imaging detector only. Extrinsic tests include the collimator and detector combined.

Many of the performance measurements are made in reference to the gamma field-of-view size.

The convention adopting for defining the field size is used, namely:

- UFOV (useful field of view): the total area useful for gamma imaging whose dimension is defined by the manufacturer.
- CFOV (central field of view): the imaging area defined by scaling the linear dimension of the UFOV by 0.75.

Intrinsic measurements are performed with a point source that consists of a single near-spherical volume of 0.3 ml or less. When placed at a sufficient distance, the point source uniformly illuminates the detector UFOV. The activity that is used depends on the type of measurement and the source distance. Always refer to the gamma camera user's manual for manufacturer's recommendations for acceptable activities and count rates.

The line source is used for measuring spatial resolution and spatial linearity. For intrinsic measurements, the line source is fashioned with the use of a slit phantom defined by NEMA. For extrinsic measurements, the line source consists of a thin-walled plastic or glass tube into which a test radionuclide is placed. The inside diameter should be less than 1/4 times the expected spatial resolution. A line source with a minimum length of 100 mm is recommended. Capillary tubes of

Table 9.1 Routine QC test for gamma camera

Test	Purpose	Frequency	Comments
Physical inspection	To check collimator and detector head and to check any damage to the collimator	Daily	Inspect for mechanical and other defects that may compromise safety of patient or staff; if collimator damage is detected or suspected, immediately perform a high-count extrinsic uniformity test
Collimator touch pad and gantry emergency stop	To test that the touch pads and emergency stops are functioning	Daily	Both the collimator touch pads and gantry emergency stop must function if there is an unexpected collision with the patient or an obstacle during motion; the touch pads must be checked each time the collimators are changed
Energy window setting for ^{99m}Tc	To check and center the preset energy window on the ^{99m}Tc photopeak	Daily	The test is intended to check the correct ^{99m}Tc energy window
Energy window setting—other radionuclides to be used	To test that preset energy windows are properly centered for the energies of other clinically used radionuclides	Daily when used	Frequency of the test should be adapted to the particular camera and frequency of use of the radionuclides
Intrinsic/extrinsic uniformity and sensitivity for ^{99m}Tc (or ^{57}Co)—quantitative	To monitor the trend in uniformity with quantitative uniformity indices, and to check the sensitivity	Weekly/ monthly	Monitor uniformity indices: integral and differential uniformity in central and useful field of view from a high-count image; record cps/MBq to check sensitivity
Intrinsic uniformity for other radionuclides	To test the response of a spatially uniform flux of photons emitted by other clinically used radionuclides	Three-monthly	Uniformity of detector response for every radionuclide in use should be tested periodically; frequency of the test should be adjusted to the frequency of use of the radionuclide in question
Spatial resolution and linearity—visual	To detect distortion of spatial resolution and linearity	Six-monthly	Visual-quadrant bar or orthogonal hole pattern; intrinsic or extrinsic, depending on convenience; if an orthogonal hole pattern is used, the results can be quantified if special software is available
Multiple window spatial registration	To test that the images acquired at different photon energies superimpose when imaged simultaneously, in an additive or subtractive mode	Six-monthly/ yearly	Relevant for dual radionuclide studies or imaging of radionuclides with multiple energy windows (e.g., ^{67}Ga or ^{111}In)
Pixel size	To determine absolute pixel size	Six-monthly	Pixel size is especially important for quantitative imaging and multimodality matching and attenuation correction
Whole-body scan spatial resolution in air	To test spatial resolution both parallel and perpendicular to the direction of motion	Yearly	Line sources or point sources may be used, positioned at different positions along the length of the whole-body scan; attention should be paid to the spatial resolution at the start and end of the whole-body scan

(continued)

Table 9.1 (continued)

Test	Purpose	Frequency	Comments
COR alignment	To check that the mechanical and electronic CORs are aligned, i.e., COR offsets are within limits of acceptability, in X and Y directions	Weekly/monthly	The frequency of the test depends on detector COR stability and should be adjusted accordingly; the test should be done for all collimators used for SPECT studies, and for each multiple detector configuration used; ensure that procedure checks both X and Y directions
Tomographic spatial resolution in air	To check tomographic spatial resolution of the system in air, with no scatter	Six-monthly	To check that the tomographic spatial resolution is not degraded by data acquisition or the reconstruction process
Overall system performance	To test tomographic uniformity and contrast resolution, and attenuation correction if available	Six-monthly	A total performance phantom (e.g., Jaszczak) should be used; uniformity of reconstructed slices with a uniform activity (no sphere/rod inserts) and contrast resolution of slices with cold spheres or rods should be monitored; if software attenuation correction is available, it should be applied to the images

length of 100 mm or longer can be filled by capillary action.

For extrinsic performance measurements on a gamma camera with a collimator, a sheet source is necessary to uniformly illuminate the detector UFOV. In theory the sheet source would be a water-filled tank into which a test radionuclide is mixed. It is recommended, however, for practical reasons, that a sealed sheet source containing ^{57}Co be used. The optimal activity of the radionuclide depends on the radionuclide and collimator used, and may range from 80 to 600 MBq (~2 to 15 mCi) in order to produce a detector count rate between 10,000 and 40,000 cps.

9.4.1 Flood-Field Uniformity

The purpose of this test is to measure the sensitivity variation over the gamma camera UFOV by uniformly flooding the detector crystal with gamma radiation. The flood images are assessed both visually and quantitatively. Refer to the manufacturer procedure manual for recommendations of number of counts and count-rate. For quantitative analysis, are defined two measures

of nonuniformity: integral uniformity (IU) and differential uniformity (DU). The integral uniformity is based on the maximum and minimum pixel count in the image and can be expressed using the Eq. (9.1):

$$IU\% = \frac{Pixel_{Max} - Pixel_{Min}}{Pixel_{Max} + Pixel_{Min}} \times 100 \quad (9.1)$$

where max Pixel is considering the maximum pixel count and min Pixel considers the minimum pixel count within the image.

On the other hand, the differential uniformity is based on the maximum counts difference for any five consecutive pixels across all rows and columns of the image; mathematically can be expressed as:

$$DU\% = \frac{Pixel_{High} - Pixel_{Low}}{Pixel_{High} + Pixel_{Low}} \times 100 \quad (9.2)$$

where high Pixel refers to the maximum count difference for any five consecutive pixels (row or column) in the image and min Pixel refers to the minimum count difference for any five consecutive pixels (row or column) in the image.

Both parameters are evaluated within the Center Field of View (CFOV) and the Useful

Field of View (UFOV). The manufacturers are expected to provide the NEMA analysis software to calculate IU and DU [2].

9.4.1.1 Intrinsic Flood-Field Uniformity

This test measures the count density variation over the gamma camera UFOV without the influence of a collimator. This measurement is done with a point source without collimator. With the collimator removed, rotate the detector toward the point source, which had to be centrally located over the detector UFOV at a distance of at least five times the larger detector UFOV dimension.

9.4.1.2 Extrinsic Flood-Field Uniformity

This test checks the overall system uniformity, which includes checking for collimator defects. It should be noted that extrinsic floods with ^{57}Co are routinely used to assess the uniformity on a daily basis of both the collimator and detector and represent an efficient method for routine daily testing. Place the sheet source directly on the collimator with an air-gap of up to 15 cm, so that flood images for both detectors may be acquired simultaneously.

9.4.2 Spatial Resolution and Spatial Linearity

The spatial resolution is obtained by measuring the width of a line-spread-function (LSF) obtained by plotting a count density profile drawn orthogonally across a line source image. The spatial resolution is specified as the width of the LSF at half-height, better referred to as the full-width-at-half-maximum (FWHM). A second measurement taken at the full-width-at-tenth-maximum (FWTM) may also be specified. The results are expressed in mm. The FWTM provides a measure of image contrast losses that may occur from collimator septal penetration and scatter. Another and routine method for measuring spatial resolution is by imaging bar phantoms. The most common bar phantom is a quadrant bar phantom consisting of four different panels of parallel bars of decreasing size and spacing that covers the detector UFOV. The bar phantom should have a

bar width in the smallest quadrant that is approximately half of the expected intrinsic spatial resolution (the smallest commercially available bars are 2 mm). It is recommended that the bar phantom be purchased from the manufacturer that designed the gamma camera system. The objective for the bar phantom test is to identify the smallest quadrant of bars visible in the image. The FWHM of LSF is approximately 1.6 times the smallest visible bar size.

The spatial resolution test can be performed also using two capillaries (diameter <1 mm) filled with Tc-99m and placed on a support at 10 cm of the collimator (Fig. 9.1). One capillary is used to calculate the FWHM and FWTM. The second capillary is used to evaluate the pixel size.

Spatial linearity refers to the ability of a gamma camera to locate acquired events accurately, and it is measured by imaging line sources over the detector UFOV. For testing, a nonlinearity is measured and is expressed as a deviation in mm between the true and imaged line source locations. The most common cause of nonlinearity is associated with PMT calibrations. The non-

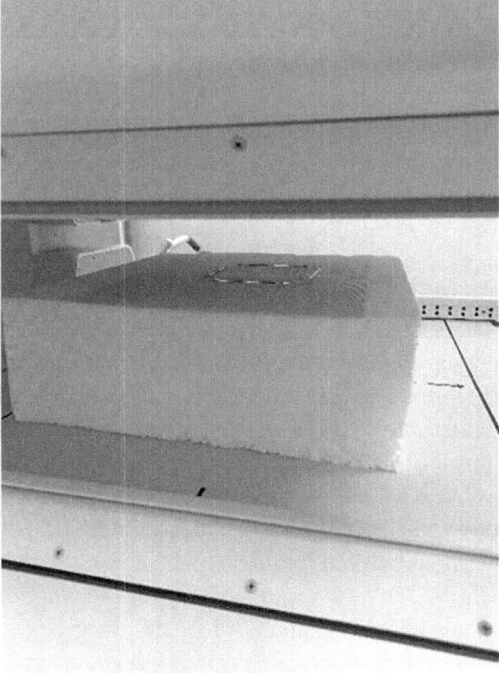

Fig. 9.1 Setup for spatial resolution test

linearity may be observed in line or bar pattern images, in which the bars appear to bend around the PMTs.

Both spatial resolution and linearity measurements involve imaging a line source and, therefore, may be obtained from the same image.

Also these tests are performed in intrinsic and extrinsic modality. Ordinarily, two patterns (horizontal and vertical) are used to separately measure spatial resolution in X and Y. It may be necessary to arrange for the gamma camera manufacturer to provide these phantoms.

They will be of the proper size to match the detector UFOV. Software for analysis may also be provided.

For intrinsic measurement, remove the collimator and install the slit phantom. The bar quadrant phantom should be in contact with the detector crystal. A point source is positioned at least 4 UFOV from and centered over the detector. For this measurement, the activity of the point source should be between 40–200 MBq (1–5 mCi). On a computer workstation, obtain LSFs by placing a wide profile (30 mm or as wide as the workstation software provides) orthogonally across each of the slit images.

The extrinsic test measures the overall spatial resolution of the gamma camera with an installed collimator. The measurement is made with a line source in air at a distance of 10 cm from the face of the collimator. Line sources are positioned parallel to and at a distance of 10 cm from the face of the collimator and perpendicular to the axis of measurement. Separate images should be acquired along the X and Y axis. The computer image matrix and camera zoom factor should be chosen so that the digital resolution perpendicular to the capillary tubes is less than 1/5 of the expected FWHM. On a computer workstation, obtain LSFs by placing a wide profile (30 mm or as wide as the workstation software provides) orthogonally across each of the slit images. Draw profiles at several locations spanning the detector UFOV. The peak of the LSF may be determined by applying a parabolic fit of the three largest count values of the LSF peak. Use linear interpolation to identify the half-maximum locations on either side of the LSF peak. For bar phantom images, visually identify the smallest perceptible bar size. It is necessary that at least one half of the length of the bars be observed in a portion of one quadrant for that quadrant to be considered visible [2].

9.4.3 Extrinsic Planar Sensitivity

The planar sensitivity of a gamma camera system is measured in units of counts per minute per unit activity, CPM/kBq (CPM/μCi), for radioactive sources placed within the detector's UFOV. The sensitivity is obtained by measuring the count rate from the radionuclide in a disk source of known activity under low attenuation and scatter conditions.

Position the sensitivity source centered over the gamma camera detector UFOV. The exact distance is not crucial, but it should be consistent for each measurement. A very low-attenuating source holder, such as a thin cardboard box, may be used to stand the source container off at the measurement distance from the collimator.

A distributed source of area smaller than the detector UFOV is used for measuring extrinsic sensitivity. The radionuclide shall be ^{99m}Tc. The test source had to be diluted into a layer of water of 2–3 mm depth in a 150 mm diameter flat plastic disk (e.g., a Petri dish) (Fig. 9.2). The activity used for the test radionuclide should range from

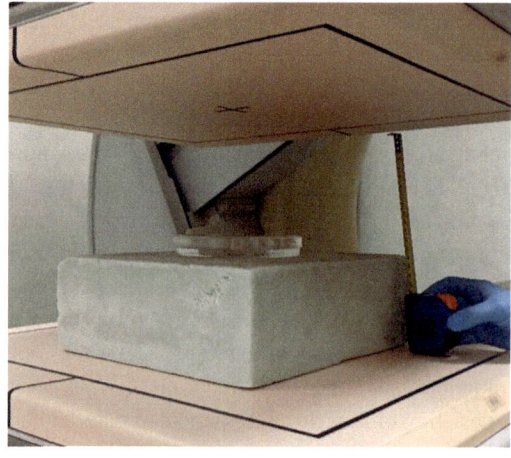

Fig. 9.2 Setup for sensitivity test

20–80 MBq (~0.5–2.0 mCi). It is critical that the exact activity in the test source be known. Residual activity in a source syringe or vessel used for transferring the source into a dish must be subtracted.

The acquisition time should be for at least 1 min. Repeat the acquisition for all detector, radionuclide, and collimator combinations selected to be measured. Record the time of the assay and the time of imaging. Calculate the system sensitivity for each detector, collimator, and radionuclide combination. Apply the appropriate background and decay corrections [2].

9.4.4 Energy Resolution

This test measures the energy resolution of the gamma camera detector by measuring the FWHM of an energy peak expressed as a percentage of the energy peak. The measurement of the 140 keV gamma energy of ^{99m}Tc is required. The energy resolution of other radionuclides may be measured. The energy spectrum is measured intrinsically using a point source such as the one prepared for uniformity imaging. Each detector is measured separately.

An intrinsic acquisition ensures that all PMTs are illuminated uniformly. Refer to the manufac-

turer's manual for instructions on how to acquire and store an energy spectrum. The manufacturer may have special software to perform this acquisition and to determine the FWHM of the spectral peak (Fig. 9.3). Use of this software is highly recommended [2].

9.4.5 Image Quality Phantom

The image quality SPECT phantom is a water-filled 20.4 cm diameter cylinder into which a test radionuclide is mixed. The phantom contains solid objects that displace the water in order to assess spatial resolution (rods) and contrast resolution of cold objects (spheres or cylinders) in a hot (radioactive) background (Fig. 9.4).

The phantom scan results are also very sensitive for identifying artifacts that may appear in the hot background as the result of improper gamma camera calibrations.

SPECT image quality is tested by evaluating phantom images for spatial resolution, contrast, and uniformity. The radionuclide shall be ^{99m}Tc. Other radionuclides may also be evaluated.

After the acquisition of the phantom, reconstruct the slices by FBP and with a Butterworth low-pass frequency filter using an order and cut-off frequency that would be used for clinical

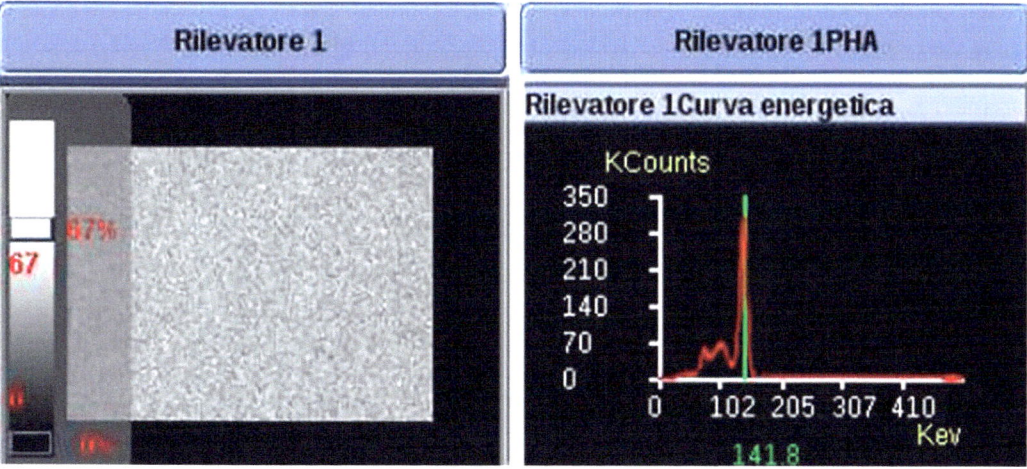

Fig. 9.3 Result of acquisition for energy resolution and uniformity tests

Fig. 9.4 A deluxe Jaszczak phantom model ECT/FL-DLX/P. (**a**) Components, (**b**) a cross-sectional schematic drawing of a Deluxe Jaszczak phantom showing the position and diameter of 148 rods in 6 sectors, (**c**) 6 spheres, and (**d**) the diameters for the objects are expressed in mm

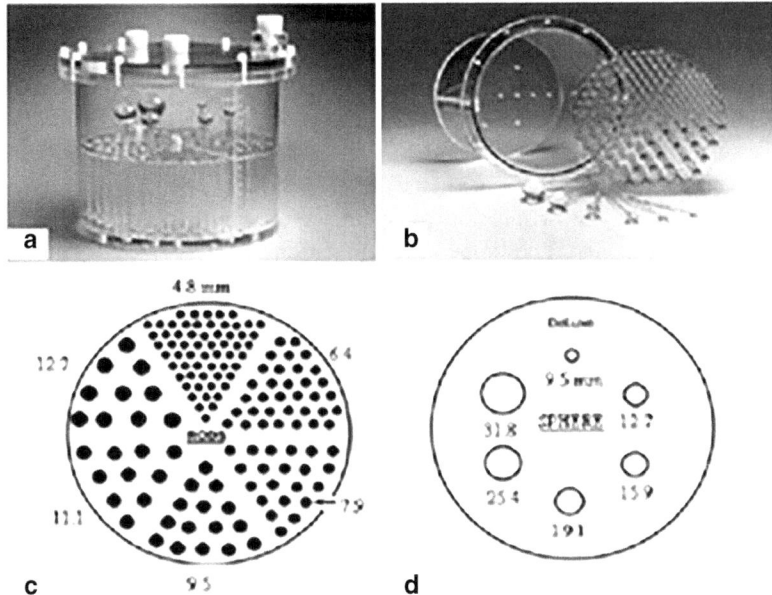

studies. Adjustment of the cutoff frequency may be done to achieve the desired result of images having the highest resolution and contrast with a mid-range of noise level. Do not oversmooth the images.

The reconstructed phantom slices are visually inspected for spatial resolution, contrast, and uniformity (Fig. 9.5).

For the resolution, identify the smallest rod sector that can be visualized in the image slices and record the corresponding diameter of the rods. A sector is considered to be visualized when more than half of the rods in that sector can be identified. Note whether the smallest rods are clearly visualized or visualized with low contrast.

For the contrast detectability, identify the smallest sphere that can be visualized in the image slices and record the corresponding sphere diameter. Note whether the smallest visualized sphere has contrast that is greater or less than that of the noise.

A uniformity index is not calculated for SPECT. Rather, the image slices are inspected for specific artifacts (attenuation, ring, focal) [2].

9.4.6 Routine Tests for 3D-Ring Cadmium-Zinc-Telluride (CZT) System

In nuclear medicine imaging, the introduction of cadmium-zinc-telluride (CZT) detectors is considered one of the most significant innovations of recent years. Semiconductor detectors, such as CZT, convert gamma photons directly into electric signals, offering improved extrinsic energy resolution and count sensitivity as compared to conventional Anger systems which are based on thallium-doped sodium iodide NaI(Tl) detectors. At present, no specific standards for performance measurements for 3D-ring CZT SPECT systems are available. The NEMA NU 1-2018 standard could be used to evaluate the performance of these systems, although not all tests are fully applicable due to the systems' ability to acquire 3D images only, the presence of an integrated collimator, and the pixelated nature of the detectors, so some previously described tests need to be adapted to the different setup of the system.

All measurements can only be performed extrinsically because of the integrated collima-

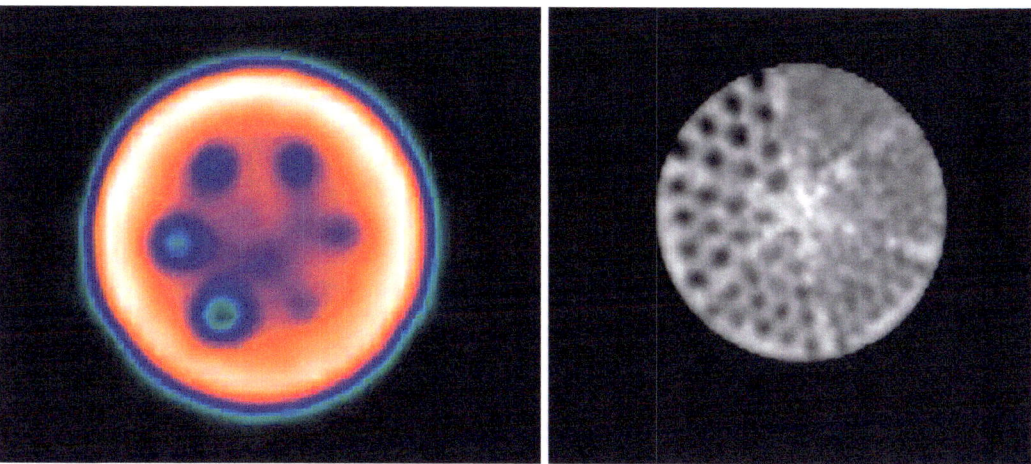

Fig. 9.5 Acquisition images of Jaszczak phantom for spatial resolution and contrast tests

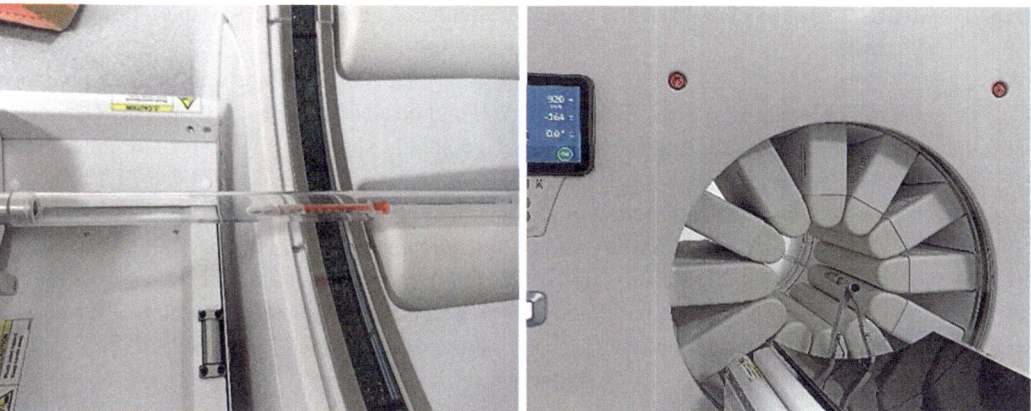

Fig. 9.6 Different sources geometry used for the tests

tors. Some tests are not applicable due to the pixelated nature of the detectors, such as intrinsic spatial resolution, linearity, and multiple window spatial registration. Additionally, the minimal acquisition radius for the 12 detectors is 15 cm, which precludes the measurement of sensitivity and system spatial resolution at a 10 cm distance from the collimator surface. Whole-body spatial resolution is also not applicable, as the system acquires a "step and shoot" mode.

Sources with different geometries than for conventional system must be used. For the mea-surements were used sources with linear geometry suspended in the center of the FOV with an auxiliary tube for energy resolution and system spatial resolution tests, the ^{57}Co sealed linear source for flood-field uniformity test and daily QC, single syringe in the axillary tube for COR and count rate tests (Fig. 9.6).

Acquisitions should be carried out according to the manufacturer's indications and the and analyses for all the parameters already previously described, such as photopeak full width at half maximum (FWHM) to the photopeak center energy, the number of defective pixels and the size of clustered defective pixels for the uniformity test, can be performed according to the NEMA NU 1-2018 instructions.

The NEMA NU 1-2018 standard can then be followed as for tests on conventional systems, adapting them to the characteristics of these new systems. Only few papers have yet been presented on the performance testing of these systems in literature, but the results of performance tests of these systems have shown promising results, particularly in terms of energy resolution, spatial resolution, and volumetric sensitivity, improvements that could potentially lead to higher-quality clinical images [3].

9.5   Additional Test for Hybrid Systems

CT scanners have been added to SPECT and PET systems for the image co-registration of the SPECT/PET and CT images. The CT images are also used to provide attenuation correction of the SPECT/PET. These hybrid systems have separate SPECT/PET and CT acquisition hardware. As such, performance measurements of both modalities are specified and performed separately.

In addition to the routine test for PET and SPECT, additional tests have been performed for the hybrid systems that are SPECT/CT and PET/CT spatial coregistration and the CT dose and image quality assessment [4].

9.5.1   Spatial Coregistration

The alignment between PET or SPECT, CT and patient couch tomographs must be checked. Spatial registration tests measure the accuracy of the spatial registration (or alignment) of the field-of-view between the reconstructed SPECT/PET and CT images. The motivation for SPECT/CT and PET/CT image registration is that spatial registration is critical for accurate image reconstruction using CT-based attenuation correction and the display of fused images for clinical interpretation.

To evaluate the spatial registration, display both SPECT/PET and CT images series from either the manufacturer's test procedure or the SPECT phantom acquisition using available clinical SPECT and CT fusion software. The test must be performed at the time of installation and after any maintenance on the couch or following operations that involve separating the two PET and CT tomographs from the clinical operating position. It is important to note, however, that even if the PET and CT tomographs are not separated for a long period of time, a misalignment between PET and CT images may be revealed as a result of possible movements of the sliding part of the couch, which regularly undergoes stress with each ascent and descent of the patient. It is therefore good practice to periodically check the alignment between the systems and the patient couch.

The location of objects in the test phantoms should be clearly observed within the CT images and should spatially align with the same objects (hot or cold) in the SPECT or PET phantom images. Hot spots of point sources within the manufacturer's test phantom should be centered within the corresponding CT objects.

If there is mismatch in the locations of each source between the CT and SPECT/PET images, use the fusion software to move (translate) the CT images to align them with the SPECT images. Record the absolute value of the offset in each direction in units of pixel shifts or mm for all sources evaluated and calculate the mean deviation between the SPECT/PET and CT images along each direction (x, y, or z).

To perform the coregistration, test is necessary to follow the manufacturer's indications and used a dedicated phantom.

9.5.2   CT Dose and Image Quality Assessment

It is necessary that that the physicist who is responsible for monitoring SPECT/PET performance ensures that certain features of the CT system are evaluated at acceptance testing, annual surveys, and for routine quality control.

In order to ensure optimization of performance and patient protection in CT procedures, the European commission have suggested use of two reference dose quantities; weighted computed tomography dose index (CTDI$_w$) for a single slice, and dose-length product (DLP) for a complete examination. The CT Dose Index (CTDI) is the most common parameter defined to represent the integrated dose to one point in an axial scan and is defined as "the integral along a line parallel to the axis of rotation (z) of the dose profile $D(z)$ for a single slice, divided by the nominal slice thickness T":

$$\text{CTDI} = \frac{1}{T} \bullet \int_{-\infty}^{+\infty} D(z)\, dz \,(\text{mGy}) \qquad (9.3)$$

In practice, a convenient assessment of CTDI can be made using a pencil ionization chamber. Such measurements may be carried out free-in-air on the axis of rotation of the scanner (CTDI$_{air}$), or at the center and peripheries of standard CT dosimetry phantom, (CTDI$_c$), (CTDI$_p$). Such measurements of CTDI in the standard phantom can be used to provide an indication of the average dose over a single slice for each setting of nominal slice thickness. On the assumption that dose in a particular phantom decreases linearly

with radial position from the surface to the center, then the average dose to the slice is approximated by the weighted (CTDI$_w$):

$$\text{CTDI}_w = \left(\frac{1}{3}\text{CTDI}_{100,c} + \frac{2}{3}\text{CTDI}_{100,p} \right) \quad (9.4)$$

where CTDI$_c$ is measured dose at center of the phantom, and CTDI$_p$ is the average dose at different peripheries of the phantom (Fig. 9.7).

The dose-length product for a complete examination is defined by the equation:

$$\text{DLP} = \text{CTDI}_w \bullet \text{Scan Length} \,(\text{mGy cm}) \qquad (9.5)$$

The CT dose index (CTDI$_w$) and DLP for the routinely used CT protocols imaging should be reported. The CT dose measurements are performed using a small thimble chamber, such as a Farmer chamber (see AAPM TG Report 111), or by following the manufacturer's recommendations.

Assessment of the image quality, paying particular attention to CT image artifacts, should be performed routinely. The quality assurance procedures recommended by the manufacturer should be followed.

The main aspects of CT image quality that need to be evaluated are as follows:

Fig. 9.7 CTDI phantom

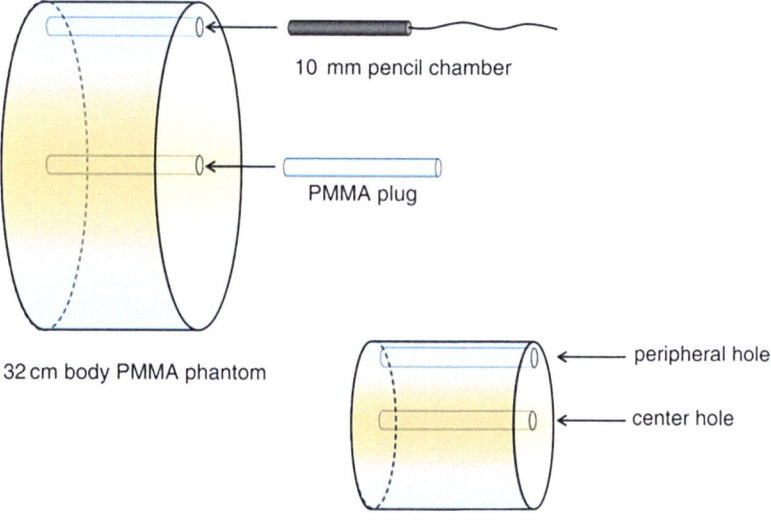

Table 9.2 Routine QC tests for an X-ray CT as part of hybrid system as PET/CT or SPECT/CT

Test	Purpose	Frequency	Description
X-ray CT—daily	Daily procedures	Daily	Follow manufacturer's procedures for daily use, and guidance from the medical physics expert for diagnostic radiology
Linearity	To determine CT number accuracy	Yearly	CT number accuracy: to assign CT numbers according to a linear function with density. At least in water and in air
Uniformity	To determine uniformity on CT images	Yearly	Evaluate the uniformity of CT numbers on an image for water or tissue-equivalent material, at the center and periphery of dummy
X-ray CT—alignment	To determine 3D alignment vector of PET or SPECT and CT field of view	Yearly	Manufacturer provides alignment phantom; to be also performed after major service
X-ray CT—performance	To check CT performance and radiation exposure	As advised by the radiation protection adviser and medical physics expert for diagnostic radiology	The CT scanner is an X-ray device that must be checked according to national radiation safety legislation under the direction of the appropriate radiation protection adviser and medical physics expert for diagnostic radiology

- Laser accuracy and table indexing accuracy
- CT image quality indices (image homogeneity, CT number accuracy, CT resolution, and noise)

These tests are performed with dedicated phantom provided by the manufactures or by commercial phantom specifically designed for these tests [1].

In Table 9.2, the routine QC tests to be performed in a quality assurance program for an X-ray CT as part of hybrid system, such as PET/CT or SPECT/CT, are reported.

References

1. Busemann Sokole E, Płachcínska A, Britten A. Routine quality control recommendations for nuclear medicine instrumentation. Eur J Nucl Med Mol Imaging. 2010;37:662–71.
2. NEMA standards publication NU 1-2018 - performance measurements of gamma cameras.
3. Zorz A, Rossato M, Turco P, Colombo Gomez L, Bettinelli A, De Monte F, Paiusco M, Zucchetta P, Cecchin D. Performance evaluation of the 3D-ring cadmium–zinc–telluride (CZT) StarGuide system according to the NEMA NU 1-2018 standard. EJNMMI Phys. 2024;11:69.
4. EFOMP's guidelines "quality controls in PET/CT and PET/MR", version 02.03.2022;

Quality Control for Hybrid Positron Emission Tomography (PET/CT and PET/MR) Scanners in Nuclear Medicine

10

Vincenzo Rizzo, Federica Savino, Paolo Turco, and Alessandra Zorz

10.1 Introduction

As discussed in the previous chapter regarding quality controls for SPECT/CT scanners, also for PET scanners, establishing a routine quality control (QC) program is mandatory to ensure the correct diagnostic performance and quantitative accuracy.

Several recommendations by national and international agencies exist for periodic PET/CT and PET/MR, such as from the European Association of Nuclear Medicine (EANM), International Atomic Energy Agency (IAEA), American Association of Physicists in Medicine (AAPM), and International Electrotechnical Commission (IEC).

10.2 PET/CT

In Table 10.1, the routine QC tests to be performed in a quality assurance program for a PET/CT are reported [2].

The international references for quality controls for PET tomographs are the 2018 NEMA documents [3].

However, these documents do not provide guidance on the periodic tests necessary to monitor the proper functioning of the system and to acquire the appropriate calibrations. These tests have performance methods, tolerances, and periodicity that depend on the tomograph in question and must be performed (often automatically and using a source inside the tomograph) following the manufacturer's guidelines. Although the NEMA documents allow the evaluation and comparison of different clinical PET scanners, neither document specifies the values of the technical benchmarks and their tolerances.

The purpose of the NEMA document is to provide standard procedures that allow, in an objective manner, the evaluation of the characteristics of PET tomographs so that:

V. Rizzo (✉) · F. Savino
Division of Nuclear Medicine, Azienda Ospedaliera
G. Moscati, Avellino, Italy
e-mail: Vincenzo.rizzo@aornmoscati.it;
Federica.savino@aornmoscati.it

P. Turco
Division of Nuclear medicine, AOU, Padova, Italy
e-mail: Paolo.turco@aopd.veneto.it

A. Zorz
Division of Health Physics, IOV, Padova, Italy
e-mail: Alessandra.zorz@iov.veneto.it

© The Author(s), under exclusive license to Springer Nature Switzerland AG 2025
L. Camoni, L. Mansi (eds.), *Nuclear Medicine Hybrid Imaging for Radiographers & Technologists*,
https://doi.org/10.1007/978-3-031-86228-1_10

Table 10.1 Routine QC tests for a PET/CT

Test	Purpose	Frequency	Description
Physical inspection	To check gantry covers in tunnel and patient handling system	Daily	Inspect for mechanical and other defects that may compromise safety of patient or staff
Daily QC	To test and visualize proper functioning of detector modules; visual inspection of 2D sinograms (automated)	Daily	To be performed with point or rod sources without attenuating object inside scanner field of view
Uniformity	To estimate axial uniformity across image planes 1 − [max] by imaging a uniformly filled object	After maintenance/ new setups/ normalization	To be also performed after software upgrade or changes; the object could be a 20-cm diameter ^{68}Ge cylinder, or a refillable cylinder with ^{18}F
Normalization	To determine system response to activity inside the field of view	Variable (at least six-monthly)	Frequency of test depends on system reliability and service; must be performed after firmware upgrade and hardware service; use phantoms and instructions as recommended by manufacturer
Calibration	To determine calibration factor from image voxel intensity to true activity concentration	Variable (at least six-monthly)	Must follow a new normalization; follow the manufacturer's procedures
Spatial resolution	To measure spatial resolution of point source in sinogram and image space	Yearly	Use a ^{18}F point source (nonstandard) or linear source
Count rate Performance	To measure count rate as a function of (decaying) activity over a wide range of activities	After new setups/ normalization/ recalibrations	To include count loss correction; and specific measurements of: (a) total/random/scatter/net true coincidences, and (b) noise equivalent count rate
Sensitivity	To measure the volume response of the system to a source of given activity concentration	Yearly	Perform according to NEMA NU2 standards with a set of sleeved rod sources [1]; an alternative method is given in NEMA-NU2 1994
Image quality	To check hot and cold spot image quality of standardized image quality phantom	Yearly	According to NEMA NU2 image quality test [1]; required after system installation, not mandatory during clinical operation

- The resulting measurements can be cited by manufacturers to specify the performance levels guaranteed by their tomographs.
- Measurement procedures may be used by users for tomograph acceptance testing.
- Some of the proposed measurements can be used for quality control of the equipment.

Representative parameters of the characteristics of PET tomographs according to the NEMA 2018 are as follows:

- Spatial resolution (transverse, radial and axial resolution)
- Scatter fraction, count losses, and randoms measurement
- Sensitivity measurement
- Accuracy: correction for count losses and randoms
- Image quality, accuracy of attenuation, and scatter corrections

10.2.1 Daily QC

Within the framework of the QC of a PET tomograph, the daily QC (DQC) represents a very important tool in the operational management of the PET system because of the frequency with which this control must be performed. The procedure for DQC should make it possible to:

- Check the correct functioning of the main components of the tomograph.
- Identify significant variations in the response of individual detectors.
- Identify significant variations in the overall system response.
- Optimize system performance prior to the start of clinical activity.

It is also necessary for the DQC to be defined and implemented in such a way as to be practical and simple to perform (possibly automatic) and of simple and unambiguous interpretation with regard to the results it produces (possibly quantitative).

The procedures for CQG implemented today in the various PET tomographs include hardware and software initializations for a general functional check of the system; verification of the status of the system calibration files through comparison with fast calibrations performed during DQC; test acquisitions to check the operation of the main components of the tomograph; test acquisitions to check the response of the detectors.

The different design of PET tomographs for clinical use means that it is not possible to define a standard protocol for DQC because each system requires different conditions for the realization of its DQC with regard to:

- The phantom and the activity used during the test.
- The statistical conditions to be achieved (counts acquired), such as to guarantee the significance of the result obtained.
- The type of measurement (e.g., 2D, 3D, emissive, coincident, single event detection, etc.).

For these reasons, the DQC of the different PET systems has to be proposed by the manufacturer. The DQC must therefore be performed according to the methods described in the respective operating manuals of each PET system, also in compliance with the legal regulations concerning medical devices [4].

10.2.2 Uniformity

The uniformity (U) of a system describes its ability to measure the same activity independently of its position in the field of view (FOV). Nonuniformity in the response may cause artefacts that limit the accuracy of the quantitative determination of the radioactive tracer distribution. The purpose of the test is to provide a measure of the nonuniformity in the response of the detection system. The test is performed using a cylindrical phantom filled with a homogenous solution of ^{18}F and water. The phantom must in all cases cover the entire axial length of the PET system. The radionuclide to be used for the measurement is ^{18}F (alternatively, other positron-emitting radionuclides such as ^{68}Ga or ^{68}Ge can be used). The activity to be used in the test (such that the system percentage count loss is <20%) depends on the specific performance of each PET system.

The data analysis is performed by creating contiguous regions of interest (ROIs) of a square shape with a side length of 1 cm, inscribed in a circle with a diameter of 175 mm, centered on the image of the cylindrical phantom. Tomograph response uniformity is analyzed by calculating the uniformity: intrasection, volume and system (intersection) [4].

10.2.3 Sensitivity

The sensitivity of a tomograph is a parameter that characterizes the frequency of coincidence events detectable by the system in the presence of a low activity radioactive source. The purpose of the test is to determine the detection frequency of

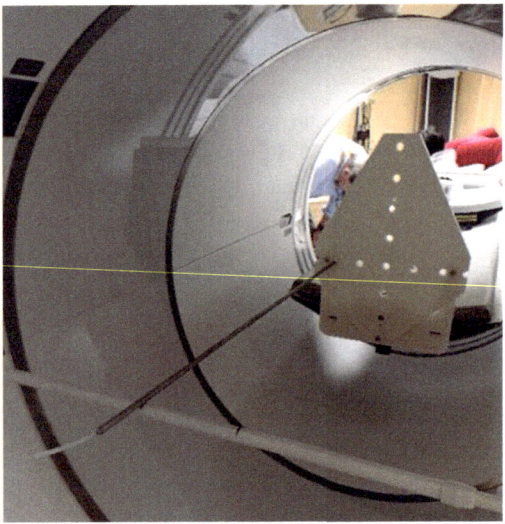

Fig. 10.1 Sensitivity phantom

true coincidences, per unit of activity concentration, corresponding to a standard source of known volume. The test is performed using a cylindrical phantom filled with a homogenous solution of ^{18}F and water. The phantom must in all cases cover the entire axial length of the PET system.

The test is performed using a polyethylene capillary filled with an activity of 2–10 MBq of ^{18}F; this tube is inserted in the center of the five concentric aluminum tubes (Fig. 10.1). The phantom is positioned in air, oriented parallel to the tomograph axis, in the center of the transaxial FOV. Each acquisition lasts 1–4 min. At the end of each measurement, the outermost aluminum tube must be removed. The same set of measurements is repeated by placing the phantom off-axis, 10 cm away from the center of the transaxial FOV. Each PET system includes software that automatically analyses the acquisitions and provides the sensitivity data as cps/kBq [3].

10.2.4 Spatial Resolution

The measurement of the transverse spatial resolution of a PET system represents the ability to reproduce the spatial distribution of a tracer within an object in a reconstructed image. The resolution measurement must be performed by

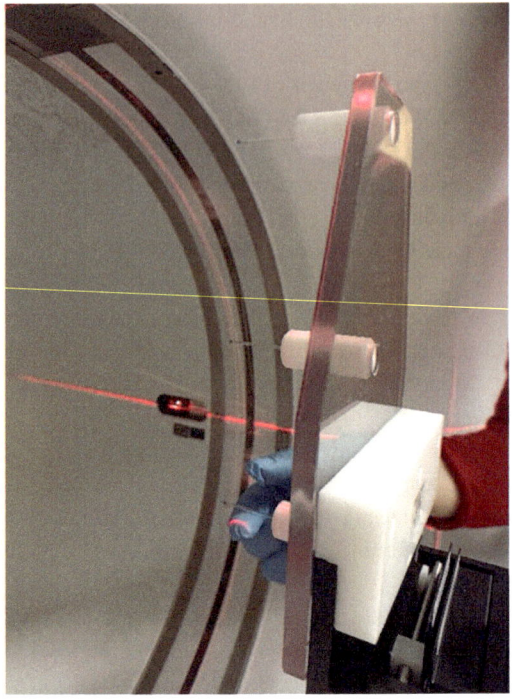

Fig. 10.2 Spatial resolution setup

imaging a point source or a linear source placed in air and reconstructing the images with different reconstruction algorithms. The purpose of this measurement is to qualify the tomograph's ability to detect small sources by characterizing the width of the transverse dispersion functions of point sources or extended linear sources positioned perpendicular to the measurement direction. The width of the dispersion function (generally of Gaussian type) is measured from the full width at half maximum (FWHM). The spatial resolution is also described by the width at one tenth of the height (full width at tenth maximum—FWTM) to account for any deviations from the Gaussian curve particularly at the "tails" of the profile.

The source for the resolution measurement is a steel capillary with an internal diameter of 1 mm (Fig. 10.2). The purpose of the steel capillary is to stop positrons and thus ensure that the test result is not affected by the positron range of the radioisotope used for the test. The radionuclide to be used for the measurement is ^{18}F. If other positron-emitting isotopes are used, it is important to consider that the different emission energy of the positron can influence the result of the spatial resolution test. Within the steel capillary, the distribution of radioactivity must be uniform. Special care must therefore be taken during filling not to leave any air bubbles or areas of discontinuity in the radioisotope. The linear source is acquired at three positions:

1. $X = 0$, $Y = 1$
2. $X = 0$, $Y = 10$
3. $X = 0$, $Y = 20$

Data analysis is performed on each image plane by calculating the FWHM on activity profiles passing through the source in the two orthogonal directions (radial and tangential). The FWHM is determined by linear interpolation between adjacent pixels at half the maximum pixel value of the response function. Finally, the average FWHM (radial and tangential) between all planes is calculated for each source position as an index of the spatial resolution of the system [3].

10.2.5 Image Quality

The image quality test simulates a PET/CT whole-body clinical use case. The test phantom presents different sized hot spheres in a volume of nonuniform attenuation. Additional activity is placed outside the scan FOV, to represent scatter radiation. Image quality is reported in terms of image contrast and signal-noise ratios for the hot spheres.

This test uses an image quality phantom and a line source (to insert in the scatter phantom). Follow the procedures of the manufacturer to calculate the activity levels you need to fill the phantom and the line source. The NEMA NU2 standard recommends multiple measurements to improve the reliability of the results. The durations of the subsequent replicate scans should be adjusted for physical decay in order to acquire the same number of decays.

To evaluate the contrast, the analysis tool of the system plotted circular ROIs of the same diameter on the spheres on the PET images. In the center of the insert simulating the lung, a 5-cm-diameter ROI (in each slice of the phantom) is drawn to consider corrections for attenuation and diffusion [3].

10.2.6 Scatter Fraction, Count Losses, and Randoms Test

The count losses and randoms portion of this test measures the count rate performance of the scanner across a range of radioactivity levels. The scatter fraction portion of this test measures the sensitivity of the scanner to coincidence events caused by scatter.

Scattering of annihilation photons produces false coincidence events. The scatter fraction of a PET scanner is a measure of the sensitivity of the system to scatter events. Scatter sensitivity is measured as the ratio of scatter events to total events, both evaluated, under very low count-rate conditions. In fact, this condition ensures that random coincidences and losses due to system dead time are negligible. In this test, the noise equivalent count rate (NECR) will also be determined. It is defined as the ratio of the square of the trues rate to the total count rate.

This test requires a high amount of activity in a relatively small volume to measure the 3D peak NECR, to assess the count rate performance of the scanner.

To prepare the source, follow the manufacturer's directions. Use the analysis tool to obtain the required data [4].

10.3 Additional Test for Hybrid Systems

For the additional tests for PET systems, such as image coregistration of the PET and CT images and the CT dose and image quality assessment refer to the corresponding paragraph in the previous chapter.

10.4   Quality Control in PET/MR

PET/MR imaging combines the strengths of positron emission tomography (PET) and magnetic resonance imaging (MRI) to provide comprehensive anatomical and functional information in a single examination. This innovative hybrid imaging modality holds great promise in clinical and research settings, offering improved soft tissue contrast, precise anatomical localization, and simultaneous acquisition of metabolic and molecular information. However, the integration of PET and MRI technologies presents unique challenges in terms of quality control (QC) to ensure accurate and reliable imaging results. This chapter explores the importance of QC in PET/MR imaging and discusses key strategies and protocols for maintaining high-quality imaging standards [5–8].

In PET/MR systems, MRI serves multiple roles. It provides high-resolution anatomical images, supports functional imaging (e.g., diffusion-weighted imaging), and in some cases, contributes to attenuation correction for PET data. Magnetic resonance spectroscopy (MRS), a specialized MRI technique, offers additional biochemical information that can complement the metabolic data from PET. The accuracy and reliability of MRI and MRS are crucial to the overall performance of PET/MR systems. Therefore, maintaining stringent QC protocols is necessary to ensure the integrity of the diagnostic information produced [7, 8].

MRI and MRS are advanced diagnostic tools that rely on the principles of nuclear magnetic resonance (NMR) to produce detailed images and spectra of tissues, respectively. As these technologies have become integral to clinical diagnostics and research, ensuring the accuracy and reliability of the images and spectra produced is paramount. Quality control (QC) processes in MRI and MRS are designed to monitor and maintain the performance of these systems. One of the key frameworks guiding QC in Europe is the EUROSPIN protocol, which provides standardized procedures for assessing the quality of MRI systems and MRS sequences [9].

Quality control in PET/MR imaging encompasses a range of procedures aimed at monitoring and optimizing various aspects of system performance, image quality, and data accuracy. These procedures are essential to detect and mitigate potential sources of error that could compromise diagnostic accuracy and affect patient care.

PET had been described in the previous section, the intent of this part is to focus on the quality controls of PET/MR from the point of view of magnetic resonance (MR): EUROSPIN protocols. Another method to ensure high-quality standards is the one used by the American College of Radiology (ACR). ACR has developed a quality control (QC) protocol for MRI systems to maintain high imaging standards and patient safety [10, 11].

10.4.1 The EUROSPIN Protocol

The EUROSPIN (European Standards for Magnetic Resonance Imaging) initiative was established to harmonize MRI quality control across Europe. It provides comprehensive guidelines for routine QC, ensuring that MRI systems consistently produce high-quality images that are reliable for clinical diagnosis. The EUROSPIN protocol emphasizes the importance of regular testing, precise calibration, and rigorous documentation of results [9].

The primary objectives of the EUROSPIN protocol are as follows:

- **Standardization**: To establish consistent QC procedures across different MRI systems and facilities.
- **Optimization**: To ensure that MRI systems operate at their optimal performance, delivering the highest possible image quality.
- **Safety**: To verify that MRI systems are safe for patient use, with no excessive exposure to electromagnetic fields.
- **Reliability**: To ensure that the diagnostic information derived from MRI scans is accurate and reproducible.

Table 10.2 Routine QC tests for a MRI as part of hybrid system as PET/MR

Test	Purpose	Frequency	Description
System performance check	Daily procedures	Daily	Follow manufacturer's procedures for daily use to identify any visible damage or abnormalities in the MRI system or its components
Signal-to-noise ratio (SNR)	Critical factor that influences the clarity of MRI images	Weekly	It quantifies the ratio of the signal (useful information) to the background noise. A stable SNR indicates that the MRI system is performing optimally. The SNR test is conducted by scanning the ACR phantom using a standard protocol
Geometric accuracy	Ensuring the system's geometric accuracy is vital for correctly measuring anatomical structures	Monthly	This test checks for distortions in the image due to inhomogeneities in the magnetic field or gradient inaccuracies
Image uniformity	Image uniformity assesses the evenness of the image signal across the field of view (FOV)	Monthly	Nonuniformity can indicate problems with the RF coil or other system components. Analyze the uniformity of the signal in the phantom's homogenous regions
Magnetic field homogeneity	Magnetic field homogeneity ensures that the field strength is uniform across the imaging volume	Annual	Poor homogeneity can lead to image distortions and inconsistencies in the MR signal. Use the manufacturer's protocol to measure magnetic field uniformity. Obtain readings from multiple points within the MRI bore using the phantom
Slice thickness accuracy	Slice thickness affects both the spatial resolution of images and the ability to distinguish fine anatomical details	Annual	Scan the phantom using a standard slice thickness (depending on the clinical application, please refer to the physicians responsible for the scanner). Measure the thickness of slices using specific test markers on the phantom
High-contrast and low-contrast resolution	Resolution tests are crucial for determining the system's ability to differentiate between structures of varying signal intensity and spatial proximity	Annual	Perform an MRI scan of the phantom, which contains structures designed to test resolution. Visually inspect the image for clarity of the resolution elements or use software to measure the resolution objectively

Quality control in MRI under the EUROSPIN framework involves a series of standardized tests that assess various aspects of the MRI system's performance. These tests are designed to identify potential issues that could compromise image quality or patient safety [2, 5–9].

In Table 10.2, the routine QC tests to be performed in a quality assurance program for a MRI as part of hybrid system, such as PET/MR, are reported.

10.4.1.1 Daily QC Tests

A visual inspection is crucial to identify any visible damage or abnormalities in the MRI system or its components, such as coils, cables, and the scanner itself.

- **Check the magnet room**: Ensure that the environment is clean and free from metallic objects that could interfere with the magnetic field.
- **Inspect the coils**: Look for any physical damage to the coils and cables, ensuring they are free from defects and properly connected.

MRI systems typically have built-in diagnostic tools to verify operational status. Each day, also a quick "system performance check" should be run, and any errors or issues should be noted for immediate troubleshooting [5].

10.4.1.2 Signal-to-Noise Ratio (SNR)

The SNR is a critical parameter in MRI, as it directly affects image clarity. The EUROSPIN protocol outlines specific methods for measuring SNR, typically involving the use of phantoms—standardized objects with known properties that mimic human tissue. Regular SNR measurements help to identify degradation in system performance, such as issues with the RF coil or gradients, which could lead to reduced image quality [7–9].

10.4.1.3 Geometric Distortion

MRI images can suffer from geometric distortions, which may arise due to non-linear gradients or magnetic field inhomogeneities. The EUROSPIN protocol includes procedures for assessing geometric accuracy, often using phantoms with known geometries. Detecting and correcting geometric distortions is essential for applications where precise anatomical measurements are required, such as in neuroimaging or orthopedic assessments [8].

10.4.1.4 Spatial Resolution

Spatial resolution refers to the ability of the MRI system to distinguish between two closely spaced objects. The EUROSPIN protocol recommends regular testing of spatial resolution using phantoms with varying grid sizes. These tests ensure that the MRI system maintains its ability to provide detailed images, which is crucial for accurate diagnosis, particularly in detecting small lesions or structural abnormalities [10].

10.4.1.5 Artifact Detection

Artifacts in MRI images can arise from various sources, including patient motion, hardware malfunctions, or external electromagnetic interference. The EUROSPIN protocol includes guidelines for identifying and mitigating common artifacts. Regular artifact checks help in maintaining image integrity, reducing the likelihood of diagnostic errors [11].

An example of MRI acquisition of the phantom for EUROSPIN Protocol was reported in Fig. 10.3.

10.4.2 Quality Control for MRS

MRS is a specialized application of MRI that provides chemical information about tissues, allowing for the noninvasive study of metabolic changes in conditions such as cancer or neuro-logical disorders. Quality control in MRS is equally important as in conventional MRI, given that the accuracy of the spectral data directly impacts the interpretation of the biochemical environment of tissues [7–9].

10.4.2.1 Frequency and Phase Stability

In MRS, frequency and phase stability are crucial for accurate spectral acquisition. The EUROSPIN protocol advises on methods to assess the stability of these parameters, typically through repeated acquisitions of a known reference signal. Any instability can lead to spectral artifacts or misinterpretation of metabolite concentrations, affecting the reliability of clinical assessments [8].

10.4.2.2 Linewidth and Resolution

The linewidth of a spectral peak in MRS indicates the sharpness of the resonance frequency and is a measure of the system's ability to resolve different chemical species. The EUROSPIN protocol recommends routine checks of linewidth using standard phantoms. A broader linewidth may suggest issues with the magnetic field homogeneity or the RF coil, necessitating further investigation and possible recalibration [7].

10.4.2.3 Quantitative Accuracy

MRS is often used to quantify metabolite concentrations in tissues. The EUROSPIN protocol includes guidelines for validating the quantitative accuracy of MRS, ensuring that the concentrations measured are consistent with known standards. This involves the use of phantoms with predefined concentrations of metabolites, helping to calibrate the MRS system and ensuring that it provides reliable quantitative data [9].

10.4.2.4 Artifact Suppression

Similar to MRI, MRS can be affected by artifacts, such as those from patient movement, scanner drift, or external RF interference. The EUROSPIN protocol recommends regular checks for common artifacts in MRS spectra and provides strategies for their suppression. Ensuring artifact-free spectra is critical for the accurate interpretation of metabolite data [10, 11].

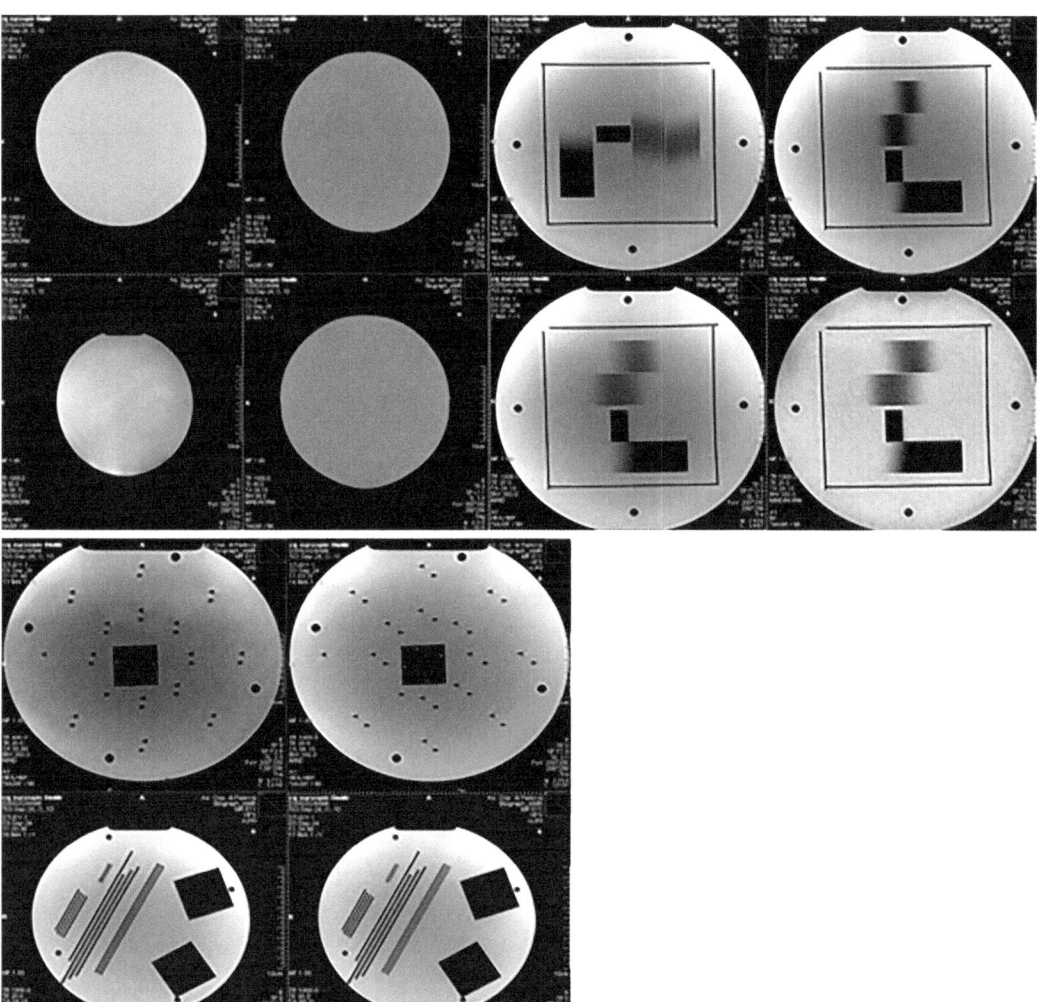

Fig. 10.3 Example of MRI acquisition of the phantom for EUROSPIN protocol

10.4.3 Purpose of ACR Quality Control

As mentioned before, EUROSPIN is not the only QC protocol for MRI. In your country/region or department you can decide to use the ACR QC protocol [11]. The characteristics and steps of this type of protocol are listed below.

The primary objective of the ACR MRI QC program is to ensure:

- High-quality, reproducible images
- Consistent machine performance over time
- Safety for patients and staff

- Compliance with regulatory standards and accreditation requirements

The ACR protocol encompasses routine checks, corrective actions, and preventive maintenance aimed at identifying potential issues before they affect imaging quality or patient safety.

10.4.3.1 Overview of ACR MRI QC Protocol

The ACR MRI QC protocol includes daily, weekly, monthly, and annual tests, depending on the parameter being evaluated. The key parameters include image quality metrics, magnetic field homogeneity, gradient performance, and RF coil integrity. The ACR's guidance provides a framework for how and when to measure these parameters. The essential tests are as follows:

1. Magnetic field homogeneity
2. Geometric accuracy
3. Signal-to-noise ratio (SNR)
4. Image uniformity
5. Slice thickness accuracy
6. High-contrast resolution
7. Low-contrast detectability

The EUROSPIN protocol provides a robust framework for the quality control of both MRI and MRS, ensuring that these systems operate at their highest potential and deliver reliable diagnostic information. By adhering to the EUROSPIN guidelines, healthcare facilities can maintain the integrity of their imaging and spectroscopy data, ultimately leading to improved patient outcomes. As MRI and MRS technologies continue to evolve, ongoing refinement of quality control protocols will be essential to keep pace with technological advancements and emerging clinical applications.

This chapter underscores the importance of maintaining rigorous QC for PET/MR systems, particularly in the MRI and MRS components, where adherence to the EUROSPIN protocols ensures consistent performance and high-quality diagnostic outcomes.

The ACR quality control protocol for MRI ensures the continued performance, reliability, and safety of MRI systems. By performing daily, weekly, monthly, and annual checks, facilities can maintain high image quality, reduce the risk of errors, and extend the life of their MRI equipment. Following these protocols rigorously not only helps with regulatory compliance but also contributes to optimal patient care.

References

1. Jiachen Z, Rao PG. MR artifacts, safety, and quality control. Radiographics. 2006;26:275–97.
2. Busemann Sokole E, Płachcínska A, Britten A. Routine quality control recommendations for nuclear medicine instrumentation. Eur J Nucl Med Mol Imaging. 2010;37:662–71.
3. NEMA Standard Publication NU-2-2018 – Performance of Positron Emission Tomographs (PET).
4. EFOMP's guidelines "quality controls in PET/CT and PET/MR", version 02.03.2022.
5. Klarhöfer M, Dietrich O, Reiser MF. Quality control in clinical magnetic resonance imaging. Eur Radiol. 2004;14(5):857–65. https://doi.org/10.1007/s00330-004-2193-5.
6. Wood ML, Henkelman RM. MR image artifacts from periodic motion. Med Phys. 1985;12(2):143–51. https://doi.org/10.1118/1.595770.
7. Barker PB, Lin DDM. In vivo proton MR spectroscopy of the human brain. Prog Nucl Magn Reson Spectrosc. 2006;49(2):99–128. https://doi.org/10.1016/j.pnmrs.2006.03.002.
8. Steinmetz M, Zaitsev M. Quality assurance in MR spectroscopy: concepts and strategies. MAGMA. 2010;23(6):349–62. https://doi.org/10.1007/s10334-010-0217-2.
9. EUROSPIN Consortium. EUROSPIN standards and protocols for MRI quality control. European Commission Project Report; 2003, p. 1–97. https://cordis.europa.eu/project/id/QLK3-CT-2002-01950.
10. Keenan KE, et al. Recommendations for improved stability and reproducibility in high-resolution MR spectroscopy. J Magn Reson Imaging. 2011;34(2):460–7. https://doi.org/10.1002/jmri.22652.
11. American College of Radiology. MRI quality control manual. ACR. This manual provides the official guidelines for the MRI Quality Control (QC) protocol, outlining the daily, weekly, monthly, and annual tests required to maintain machine performance and ensure patient safety. 2018.

Strategies for Standardization in Hybrid Imaging

Maria Agnese Pirozzi [ID] and Anna Prinster [ID]

11.1 Overview of Hybrid Imaging Towards Standardization

Hybrid imaging technologies represent significant advances in diagnostic imaging by combining the strengths of multiple imaging modalities into a single system, with the potential to enhance medical imaging by providing combined anatomic-metabolic image information [1, 2]. Since the first PET/CT (and SPECT/CT) systems became available, PET examinations have been performed primarily as combined PET/CT due to the highest diagnostic value. Therefore, more recently, hybrid PET/MR scanners have also been introduced and made available, although more expensive and with lower throughput than PET/CT.

Each of these technologies leverages the unique capabilities of its component modalities to provide comprehensive diagnostic information, improving the accuracy and reliability of medical assessments [3, 4]. This section will provide an overview of these hybrid imaging technologies, highlighting their differences and emphasizing the importance of standardization in optimizing performance and interoperability.

11.1.1 PET/CT

PET/CT integrates two powerful imaging modalities into one cohesive system, providing both functional and anatomical information in a single session. This combination leverages the unique strengths of each technology to improve diagnostic accuracy and provide a more complete understanding of a patient's condition. PET provides functional imaging by detecting the distribution of radiotracers within the body, which are indicative of metabolic activity. CT, on the other hand, uses X-rays to generate detailed cross-sectional images of the body's internal structures, providing high-resolution details of bones, organs, and tissues, allowing for precise localization and characterization of anatomical abnormalities. Key applications include oncology where PET/CT is widely used to detect and stage tumors, monitor response to treatment, and identify recurrences. The combination of metabolic and anatomical imaging allows the precise localization of tumors [5, 6]. Furthermore, in cardiology, PET/CT is used to evaluate myocardial perfusion and viability [7], helping to identify areas of reduced blood flow or damaged cardiac tissue, while in neurology it helps in the evaluation of

M. A. Pirozzi (✉)
Department of Advanced Medical and Surgical Sciences, University of Campania "Luigi Vanvitelli", Naples, Italy
e-mail: mariaagnese.pirozzi@unicampania.it

A. Prinster
Institute of Biostructure and Bioimaging, National Research Council, Naples, Italy
e-mail: anna.prinster@ibb.cnr.it

L. Camoni, L. Mansi (eds.), *Nuclear Medicine Hybrid Imaging for Radiographers & Technologists*,
https://doi.org/10.1007/978-3-031-86228-1_11

neurological disorders such as Alzheimer's disease [8], epilepsy [9], and brain tumors [10].

PET/CT involves exposure to both PET radiotracers and CT X-rays, which contributes to a higher overall radiation dose than PET/MR. However, PET/CT generally offers faster imaging times than PET/MR, making it more suitable for certain clinical situations where faster diagnostic results need to be determined. By comparison, PET/CT is more expensive than SPECT/CT due to the need for a cyclotron to produce radiotracers, although it offers greater sensitivity and spatial resolution than SPECT, thus allowing the detection of very low concentrations of radiotracers and providing more detailed images (especially important for the detection of small lesions).

11.1.2 PET/MR

PET/MR combines the metabolic imaging of PET with the superior soft tissue contrast and functional imaging capabilities of MRI. PET/MR is particularly advantageous in brain imaging, providing detailed information about brain metabolism and anatomy, which is crucial for diagnosing neurological conditions [11, 12]. Other advantages are expressed for musculoskeletal disease imaging whereby PET/MR offers added value for the imaging of soft tissue tumors and inflammatory conditions affecting muscles and joints [13, 14]. For oncology it is particularly useful in pediatric oncology [15] and for imaging tumors located in organs, such as the liver [16], prostate [17], and brain [18, 19], thanks to the better soft tissue contrast and lower radiation dose.

PET/MR exposes the patient to a lower dose of radiation than PET/CT, as MRI does not use ionizing radiation. Furthermore, providing better soft tissue contrast than CT is more suitable for the detailed evaluation of soft tissues. However, PET/MR typically requires longer imaging times and is more expensive than PET/CT, which may be a limitation in certain clinical settings.

11.1.3 SPECT/CT

SPECT/CT provides functional imaging by detecting gamma rays emitted by radiotracers, while CT offers anatomical imaging. The combination of the two modalities improves diagnostic accuracy by correlating functional abnormalities with precise anatomical locations. SPECT/CT is often used in cardiology for myocardial perfusion imaging, helping to diagnose and evaluate coronary artery disease [20]; in oncology to aid in the detection and staging of certain cancers, such as neuroendocrine tumors [21]; and in orthopedics [22] for evaluating bone disorders, including fractures, infections, and bone metastases. Compared to the other hybrid technologies, SPECT/CT uses radiotracers which are generally less expensive and have longer half-lives than PET radiotracers, making SPECT/CT more accessible in some settings. However, SPECT typically has lower spatial resolution than PET, which may be a limitation for detecting small lesions [23].

11.2 Importance of Standardization for Hybrid Imaging

In this subchapter, we will analyze in detail the main aspects related to standardization for Hybrid Imaging systems for clinical studies, and experimental and research protocols.

11.2.1 Why Standardization?

The importance of standardization in hybrid imaging (i.e., PET/CT, PET/MR, and SPECT/CT), has been widely recognized both in clinical practice and in research applications [24]. Standardization of the acquisition protocols and equipment calibration procedures is necessary for accurate quantification of PET and SPECT data, which are increasingly used and widespread in diagnostics, especially in the oncology field. It is a well-known problem that differences in patients evaluated by activity quantification parameters can be explained in terms of differences in the use of PET or SPECT imaging methods. This is even more true for hybrid equipment for which it is necessary to establish specific recommendations and guidelines to harmonize the quantitative protocols of ^{18}F-FDG PET and SPECT studies. The introduction of hybrid systems raises the issue of standardization at a level that involves both nuclear medicine physicians and radiologists with their respective societies that have been collaborating for several years to create working groups that facilitate the exchange of expertise and arrive at shared guidelines in the shortest possible time [25]. Furthermore, the increasing diffusion and necessity of creating large databases of data, the so-called biobanks, available for use in radiomics and/or artificial intelligence makes data harmonization essential.

11.2.2 Performance Optimization

Standardized protocols ensure optimal imaging system performance by maintaining consistent calibration and image quality across facilities. This is crucial for accurate diagnostics and treatment planning, as variations in imaging can lead to discrepancies in interpreting metabolic and anatomical data, with a potentially significant impact on diagnostic accuracy.

The performance of hybrid imaging systems is strictly dependent on the instrumentation characteristics of both combined modalities and on the pre- and post-processing applied to the raw data [26].

For SPECT and PET imaging, these characteristics while mainly dependent on detectors, collimators (SPECT imaging), and geometry of the system are also influenced by the acquisition parameters. More importantly, quantitative accuracy and reproducibility of both modalities, in terms of Standardized Uptake Value (SUV) outcomes, especially in a multicenter study, are also heavily influenced by attenuation correction methods necessary to properly reconstruct images (i.e., reconstruction algorithms and

instrument calibrations) [27]. Indeed, image reconstruction algorithms are particularly relevant in hybrid imaging, since the combined simultaneous use of CT or MRI with PET and SPECT has an influence on how data are acquired and/or processed. For example, a combination of MRI and PET in a unique system poses the problems of the mutual distortion effect that each of the two modalities has on the other. Indeed, in PET/MR systems higher spatial resolutions of PET images can be achieved since the strong magnetic field of the MR system deflects the positrons and thus decreases the positron range [28].

The use of CT or MR in combined hybrid systems poses also the question of image attenuation correction since the two systems have different algorithms and consequently different data reconstructions and processing [29, 30].

11.2.3 Interoperability

Hybrid imaging systems can lead to compatibility issues as they incorporate data from multiple modalities, besides generating in some cases fused images, in which data from the different modalities acquired by the scanner are merged to allow appreciation of their complementary information. Standardization enables seamless integration and sharing of imaging data across platforms and institutions, reducing technical barriers and enhancing clinical workflows. The Digital Imaging and Communications in Medicine (DICOM) standard, developed by the National Electrical Manufacturers Association (NEMA), a consortium of manufacturers responsible for issues related to patent and regulatory infringement, for example, is widely used in radiology and is being extended to other areas like pathology to improve cross-system interoperability. DICOM ensures the availability of the data in a common format to be shared across different modalities, vendors, and institutions, enabling multiparametric, multicenter protocols and studies. NEMA is also active in drafting standard protocols to harmonize the sensitivity, spatial resolution, noise, scatter fraction, counting rate linearity, and image quality characteristics of

PET studies [24] across vendors and scanners. Standardization efforts facilitate the seamless integration of different imaging systems and software, enabling consistent data interpretation and comparison across platforms and institutions.

11.2.4 Regulatory Compliance

Following standardized guidelines ensures that imaging facilities meet the necessary regulatory standards for safety and efficacy. This is essential not only for clinical practice but also for adhering to legal and safety requirements. It is therefore necessary to define levels of standardization for hybrid imaging that may depend on different applications and/or applications on multicenter studies. Of note, to date no dedicated standards have been implemented for hybrid imaging applications, that currently rely on the procedures developed for the standalone modalities which are merged in these scanners, substantially ignoring the specificities that their combined use implies and their potentialities.

Dedicated standards in quality assurance and quality controls are thus desirable, which should be realized in straight collaboration with scanner vendors, guaranteeing service-like homogeneous acquisition protocols with a well-defined common output to compare the performances of the different systems [31, 32]. To this end, it also welcomes the use of standard inter- and intra-modality phantoms to properly calibrate hybrid systems.

11.2.5 Research and Development

In the research domain, standardization facilitates reproducibility and comparability across studies. Consistent imaging protocols allow researchers to generate reliable data, which is critical for developing new diagnostic tools and treatment methods.

As machine learning methods become more and more pervasive in this field, data standardization is showing a major impact on the accuracy of these techniques [33], which have a clear potential to boost the inherently multiparametric information provided by hybrid imaging [34].

In the context of hybrid imaging, standardization is thus essential to facilitate reproducibility and comparability in research and clinical applications, as well as in preclinical hybrid imaging, where scanner heterogeneity is even more conspicuous. Without such standardization, variability in image acquisition and analysis can hinder the ability to compare outcomes across studies and institutions, ultimately affecting the development of new diagnostic and therapeutic techniques.

Of note, although it is well known that standardization improves the accuracy and precision of imaging data, thus ensuring that research findings can be translated effectively from preclinical studies to clinical applications, standardization procedures still struggle to be implemented in this field [35]. As the use of hybrid imaging will further increase the heterogeneity of preclinical imaging data, it appears clear that additional efforts must be carried out to promote standardization in this field.

By using harmonized protocols, researchers can generate reliable datasets, reducing biases in the interpretation of results and enhancing the translatability of novel diagnostics, such as radiotracers, across different research settings.

11.3 Standardization Frameworks and Initiatives in Hybrid Imaging

Several organizations and initiatives have established frameworks and guidelines to advance these goals. This section reviews key standardization frameworks and initiatives aimed at achieving uniformity in hybrid imaging systems, such as PET/CT, PET/MR, and SPECT/CT.

However, it should be emphasized that the following are not inflexible rules or requirements of practice and are not intended, nor should they be used, to establish a legal standard of care. The standards/guidelines do not prescind a final judgment on the correctness of a specific procedure or course of action adopted by medical professionals considering, in each case, the unique circumstances of each case [36]. Therefore, there is no implication that an approach different from the standards/guidelines is below the standard of care. On the contrary, it is possible to adhere to the standards of best practice, as well as responsibly adopt a course of action different from that outlined in the standards/guidelines when, in the reasonable judgment of the professional, such a course of action is indicated by the patient's condition, limitations of available resources, or advances in knowledge or technology (after the publication of the standards/guidelines).

The following is a brief overview of the standards that can be used for hybrid imaging evaluations.

11.3.1 Relevant ISO Standards

The International Organization for Standardization (ISO) is a globally recognized entity that develops and publishes international standards across various industries, including medical imaging. ISO standards are instrumental in ensuring quality, safety, and efficiency in imaging practices. Relevant ISO Standards for hybrid imaging should be:

– *ISO9001:2015 (Quality management systems—Requirements).* This standard, although not specific to healthcare, establishes the criteria for a quality management system and is widely used to ensure that organizations consistently provide products and services that meet regulatory and customer requirements.
– *ISO13485:2016 (Medical devices—Quality management systems—Requirements for regulatory purposes).* This standard specifies requirements for a quality management system where an organization needs to demonstrate its ability to provide medical devices and related services that consistently meet customer and applicable regulatory requirements.

– *ISO15189:2022 (Medical laboratories—Requirements for quality and competence).* This standard specifies requirements for quality and competence in medical laboratories. It is particularly relevant for hybrid imaging facilities to ensure reliable and accurate diagnostic results.

11.3.2 Relevant IEC Standards

The International Electrotechnical Commission (IEC) develops international standards for electrical and electronic technologies, including medical imaging equipment. IEC standards focus on the safety, performance, and electromagnetic compatibility of imaging devices. IEC standards that could be considered relevant for hybrid imaging are:

– *IEC 60601 Series (Medical Electrical Equipment).* This series of standards specifies safety and performance requirements for medical electrical equipment. It includes specific parts that address requirements for imaging equipment (such as PET/CT, PET/MR, and SPECT/CT).
– *IEC 61223 Series (Evaluation and routine testing in medical imaging departments).* This series covers the evaluation and routine testing of the image quality of X-ray equipment, including CT scanners used in hybrid imaging systems.

11.3.3 Key SNMMI Guidelines

The Society of Nuclear Medicine and Molecular Imaging (SNMMI) provides guidelines and standards specifically for nuclear medicine practices, including hybrid imaging technologies. SNMMI guidelines are widely adopted in clinical settings to ensure the consistency and safety of imaging procedures, recognizing that the safe and effective use of diagnostic hybrid imaging requires specific training, skills, and techniques [36]. Key SNMMI guidelines include:

- *Imaging Protocols.* SNMMI publishes standardized imaging protocols for various clinical applications, ensuring consistent and reproducible imaging practices.
- *Quality Control.* Guidelines for quality control procedures help maintain the performance of hybrid imaging systems, including routine verification and calibration.
- *Radiation Safety.* SNMMI provides radiation safety guidelines, emphasizing the importance of minimizing radiation exposure to patients and healthcare workers.

11.3.4 Key EANM Guidelines

The European Association of Nuclear Medicine (EANM) is another key organization that develops standards and guidelines for nuclear medicine, including hybrid imaging technologies [37]. The efforts of the EANM complement those of the SNMMI, providing a comprehensive framework for the practice of nuclear medicine in Europe. Key EANM guidelines for hybrid imaging provide:

- *Procedure Guidelines.* EANM publishes procedure guidelines for various nuclear medicine and hybrid imaging applications, promoting standardized imaging protocols across Europe.
- *Quality Control.* Guidelines to ensure that nuclear medicine equipment is functioning properly and constitute an important part of quality management in a nuclear medicine department. The described tests are designed to detect problems before they affect clinical patient studies and are intended to provide a full evaluation of equipment performance and to ensure that equipment is performing properly after service or adjustment.
- *Education and Training.* EANM offers educational programs and training to ensure that healthcare professionals are well-versed in the latest imaging techniques and standards.

11.3.5 Key Features of DICOM

DICOM is the international standard for transmitting, storing, retrieving, printing, process, and displaying medical imaging information [38]. DICOM ensures that medical imaging devices and systems from different manufacturers can communicate and work together seamlessly.

The DICOM standard provides the following key features:

- *Interoperability.* DICOM facilitates the exchange of medical images and associated data between different imaging systems, ensuring compatibility and consistency.
- *Standardized file formats.* DICOM standardizes the format of medical image files, including patient information, image data, and metadata, ensuring complete and accessible imaging records.
- *Network protocols.* DICOM provides network protocols for the transfer of images and related information, enabling efficient and secure data exchange between systems.

11.3.6 Key IHE Initiative

Integrating the Healthcare Enterprise (IHE) is an initiative that promotes the coordinated use of established standards (such as DICOM and Health Level Seven [HL7]), to improve the sharing of information across healthcare systems [39]. IHE develops integration profiles that specify how standards should be used to address specific clinical needs. Potentially, key contributions of IHE to hybrid imaging systems may include:

- *Integration Profiles.* IHE develops detailed integration profiles that guide the implementation of interoperability standards in healthcare systems, ensuring seamless data exchange and integration.

- **Connectathons.** IHE organizes events known as Connectathons [40], where healthcare providers and organizations can test the interoperability of their systems in a controlled environment, promoting the adoption of standardized practices.

11.4 Practical Implications of Standardization in Hybrid Imaging

Equipment calibration, quality control (QC), image reconstruction protocols and data management protocols of hybrid nuclear medicine imaging devices are essential to ensure their proper functioning and to obtain accurate and quantitative results. Indeed, hybrid imaging systems present additional challenges caused by differences between the combined imaging modalities.

11.4.1 Equipment Calibration and Quality Control

Regular calibration of hybrid imaging equipment is essential to maintain optimal performance and ensure accurate imaging results. Calibration involves adjusting the imaging system to known standards, verifying the performance of imaging detectors, and ensuring the alignment of multimodal imaging components. The current EANM guidelines for routine QC of nuclear medicine equipment focus more on the inherent multimodality aspect of state-of-the-art PET/CT and PET/MR scanners. EANM guidelines provide a comprehensive overview of recommended QC procedures to ensure the optimal operating state of a PET system, integrated with a CT or MRI system. For this purpose, they also discuss the rationale for the different tests, provide recommendations on the frequency of each test, and present the relevant MRI and CT tests for an integrated system. In addition, they also recommend a preventive action scheme to prevent QC tests from deviating from the predefined range of acceptable performance values so that optimal performance of the PET system is maintained for routine clinical use [41].

To summarize, key features for calibration and QC to ensure the quality of imaging results are:

- **Frequency.** Equipment should be calibrated periodically, as recommended by the manufacturer and appropriate regulatory agencies. Calibration should also be performed after any significant maintenance or repair.
- **Documentation.** Detailed records of calibration procedures and results should be maintained to track performance trends and identify any deviations from standard performance levels.

11.4.2 Image Reconstruction Protocols

Quantitative hybrid imaging is substantially influenced by the choice of image reconstruction parameters depending on the different scanner technologies and the differences in the implementation of image reconstruction algorithms among vendors, as well as users. To minimize the physical variability of SUV measurements between scanners from different sites or manufacturers, in addition to the acquisition parameters, image reconstruction parameters should be set to minimize the differences. Different sites cannot change the installed systems but with the guidance of image reconstruction parameters, differences between sites can be minimized. For example, several efforts have been implemented to minimize the variability of clinical PET, mainly for 18F-FDG, such as RSNA-QIBA [42], SNMMI-CTN [43], and EANM [44, 45] in the context of PET/CT. These efforts aimed to propose specifications and requirements in patient preparation, injection, and imaging, to ensure comparability and consistency for quantitative FDG-PET across scanners.

Therefore, standardized image reconstruction protocols are critical to producing consistent, high-quality images. In summary, image reconstruction involves processing raw data acquired by the imaging system to create clinically useful images, based on the following key characteristics:

- *Algorithm selection.* Choose reconstruction algorithms that are widely accepted and validated within the medical imaging community. Algorithms should be optimized for the specific hybrid imaging modality and clinical application.
- *Parameter settings.* Establish standard parameter settings for image reconstruction, such as filter types, numbers of iterations, and resolution settings. Standardized parameters help ensure consistency in image quality and diagnostic accuracy.
- *Quality control.* Implement routine QC procedures to monitor the performance of image reconstruction algorithms. Regular testing with phantom studies and comparison with baseline images can help identify any discrepancies or artefacts.

11.4.3 Data Management

Following the standards presented above, it is worth emphasizing here that effective data management is also essential to maintain the integrity, security, and accessibility of hybrid imaging data. Standardized data management practices facilitate efficient data storage, retrieval and sharing (for example, using Picture archiving and communication systems [PACS], as also suggested by IHE). The aspects to consider in the context of hybrid imaging data management may be summarized as follows:

- *Data storage.* Use standardized formats for storing imaging data, such as DICOM. Ensure that data storage systems are secure and comply with regulatory requirements for data protection and privacy.
- *Data retrieval.* Implement standardized procedures for retrieving imaging data, including the use of metadata and indexing systems to facilitate rapid and accurate access to data.

- *Data sharing.* Establish protocols for sharing imaging data between different institutions and systems. Ensure that data-sharing practices comply with relevant regulations and guidelines, such as those related to patient confidentiality and data security.

11.5 Phantom for Standardization in Hybrid Imaging

In hybrid imaging, such as PET/CT, PET/MR, and SPECT/CT, phantoms are essential tools for verification and testing, as well as standardization and QC of imaging systems. Phantoms are test objects with well-defined properties used to simulate both the shape of human tissues/organs and, when possible, their physiological conditions, thus enabling consistent testing, calibration, and validation of imaging systems without involving human subjects. Indeed, by using phantoms, clinicians and researchers can evaluate the performance of imaging systems, optimize image acquisition protocols, and ensure the reproducibility of results across machines and institutions. Therefore, incorporating phantoms into routine quality assurance procedures not only enhances the reliability of hybrid imaging systems but also supports the development of standardized imaging protocols, improving the harmonization and the overall effectiveness of clinical and research applications.

11.5.1 Key Roles of Phantoms for Standardized Hybrid Imaging

The key role of phantoms in nuclear medicine hybrid imaging is mainly in the following aspects:

- *Multimodality validation.* In hybrid systems, phantoms are essential to validate the co-registration of functional and anatomical images. These models are often designed to simulate, for example, both PET and CT or MRI properties, ensuring that images from both modalities are perfectly aligned to be interpreted together accurately.

- **Calibration and quality control.** Phantoms are routinely used in hybrid imaging systems, to ensure that individual PET and CT or MRI components are properly calibrated and that quantitative measurements, such as PET SUVs, are accurate. This is essential to maintain a high standard quality of diagnostic hybrid imaging.
- **Reproducibility and comparability.** Phantoms enable the standardization of imaging procedures by providing a consistent reference point. Phantoms can be used to test the consistency of radiotracer distribution in PET imaging, allowing researchers to compare results between different studies and institutions, thus promoting the reproducibility of research results.

11.5.2 Types

In hybrid imaging, various types of phantoms are used for calibration, validation, and quality control of the measurements. Each phantom is designed to test specific parameters, to guarantee the accuracy and reliability of both the functional (PET/SPECT) and anatomical (CT/MRI) imaging components. The types of phantoms used in hybrid imaging can be categorized as follows, where the purpose, design, and applications are briefly outlined.

11.5.2.1 Uniformity Phantoms

Uniformity phantoms are designed to evaluate the uniformity of signal response across the imaging field in PET, SPECT. These phantoms are essential for quality control and system calibration [46].

- *Purpose*: Used to test the uniformity of radiotracer distribution in PET and SPECT systems. They evaluate the scanner's ability to produce images with consistent radiotracer absorption over a uniform area.

- *Design*: Typically filled with a known concentration of radiotracer solution, uniformity phantoms have a homogeneous composition, allowing the system to be tested for uniformity of response.
- *Applications*: Ensure that no areas of distortion or inconsistent radiotracer absorption occur, which could affect the diagnostic quality of the images.

Common examples of uniformity phantoms used in hybrid imaging are reported below:

- **Jaszczak Phantom.** Also known as the Data Spectrum ECT phantom, it is one of the most widely used phantoms for assessing imaging uniformity in academic centers and hospitals to check the quality of SPECT or some gamma camera systems [47]. It is used for accreditation by clinical and academic facilities for the American College of Radiology (ACR) [48]. It is a cylinder (made of acrylic plastic with several inserts) filled with a radiotracer (such as Technetium-99 m or Fluorine-18) containing uniform and non-uniform sections. The Jaszczak phantom has six hollow spheres and six solid spheres that allow uniformity testing (and contains inserts to assess spatial resolution and contrast). Primarily used for routine quality control and performance evaluation of SPECT systems [49] but can also be adapted for hybrid PET/SPECT systems.
- **NEMA IEC Body Phantom.** It is a standardized tool developed by NEMA and IEC for testing the performance of PET and PET/CT systems. It is widely used in clinical and research settings to evaluate key performance parameters such as image uniformity. The phantom consists of a torso-shaped container filled with a radioactive solution that mimics human tissue attenuation. It also includes 6 spheres of different sizes (typically ranging from 10 to 37 mm in diameter) that can be filled with radiotracers. These spheres are used to simulate lesions of varying sizes and contrast levels [50]. It is primarily used in

PET/CT systems, in both clinical and research settings, to verify the accuracy of hybrid imaging systems, ensuring consistency across different imaging systems and compliance with international standards.

- **Hoffman Brain Phantom.** It is a widely used brain phantom for evaluating the performance of PET and SPECT systems. It simulates the complex structures of the human brain, including the cerebral cortex and ventricles, with regions of varying density and radiotracer concentration to simulate both grey and white matter, thus allowing for the assessment of imaging quality uniformity, spatial resolution, and quantification in brain scans [51]. It can help in validating the accuracy of hybrid brain imaging in PET(CT/MRI) and SPECT/CT systems by assessing image reconstruction algorithms, quantification of radiotracer uptake, and resolution of fine brain structures, especially in multicenter studies [52].
- **Uniform Cylinder Phantom.** It is a basic, yet essential tool used in PET, SPECT, and CT imaging to assess image uniformity and evaluate system calibration. The cylindrical phantom can be filled with a solution that emits radiation uniformly, allowing the imaging system to be tested for consistent signal detection [53, 54].

11.5.2.2 Spatial Resolution Phantoms

Spatial resolution phantoms help calibrate and validate the performance of hybrid imaging systems, ensuring to accurately detect and resolve small features that are critical for diagnostic and research purposes. These phantoms are specialized tools used to evaluate the ability of imaging systems to distinguish between two closely spaced objects (e.g., the ability to accurately detect small lesions or other fine anatomical details).

- *Purpose*: Used to measure the spatial resolution of the imaging system, which determines how well the system can distinguish between two closely spaced objects.
- *Design*: Usually composed of small structures, such as rods or spheres of varying sizes,

positioned at defined distances to assess the resolving power of both the PET/SPECT and CT/MRI components.
- *Applications*: Frequently used to determine how small a lesion the system can detect, which is critical for accurate diagnoses in oncology.

The following are commonly used spatially resolution phantoms:

- **Spheres and Cylinders Phantom.** These geometric phantoms test the system's ability to resolve spherical and cylindrical objects of different sizes, which is important for detecting spherical lesions such as tumors. The model may therefore contain multiple spheres [55] or cylinders [54] of varying diameters arranged in specific patterns. The resolution of the system is then determined by its ability to separate and identify these objects in the resulting image. They are often used in both clinical PET and SPECT to evaluate the scanner's ability to detect small lesions or areas of abnormal uptake. The previously presented NEMA IEC Body Phantom can also be associated with this group of phantoms.
- **Hoffman Brain Phantom.** It can be used also for the assessment of spatial resolution [56].

11.5.2.3 Attenuation Phantoms

Attenuation phantoms are designed to simulate the effects of human tissue on radiation attenuation in nuclear medicine imaging systems and hybrid imaging systems. These phantoms are critical for testing the accuracy of attenuation correction algorithms, which adjust for signal loss as radiation passes through different tissue types. Without proper attenuation correction, images may show false areas of high or low radiotracer absorption, leading to misdiagnosis or misinterpretation of data. By simulating the properties of human tissue, these phantoms help verify and tune attenuation correction algorithms, ensuring that imaging systems produce reliable, high-quality images [57, 58].

- *Purpose*: Used to evaluate the system's ability to correct attenuation (the reduction in signal strength) caused by body tissues. Accurate attenuation correction is critical for accurate quantification in PET and SPECT.
- *Design*: These models simulate different tissue densities (e.g., bone and soft tissue) to test the system's correction algorithms.
- *Applications*: Improving measurement accuracy in PET imaging (e.g., SUV).

The following are commonly used attenuation phantoms:

- **Uniform Cylinder Phantom.** It is also frequently utilized for calibrating the attenuation correction in hybrid imaging systems, ensuring uniform image reconstruction across the entire detector field.
- **NEMA IEC Body Phantom.** It is also used for calibrating the attenuation correction in hybrid imaging systems [59]. The phantom typically includes multiple compartments that can simulate different tissue densities (such as soft tissue, bone, and air). This allows for a comprehensive test of how well the imaging system compensates for attenuation.
- **RSD Alderson Phantoms.** These anthropomorphic phantoms mimic the human body (as well as, for neuroimaging the striatum through the RSD Striatal Phantom) in size, shape, and tissue composition. They are made from tissue-equivalent materials that simulate human organs, bones, and soft tissues, and can be sectioned to allow the insertion of dosimeters and other measurement devices. Primarily used for dosimetry, calibration, and quality assurance in radiation therapy and diagnostic imaging, they can be also used to simulate human attenuation in PET, SPECT, and CT imaging [60].

11.5.3 The StepBrain Phantom

Having a phantom of the brain anatomy to use in hybrid imaging can be considered crucial for equipment validation and testing for neurology studies. Typically, anthropomorphic brain phantoms that attempt to mimic the external anatomy of the brain have reduced sulci depths or only recreate the surface shape of the brain. Even when these phantoms mimic the physical appearance of the human brain, they fail to accurately represent the anatomy and variety of brain tissue. In addition, hybrid imaging of these phantoms is not commonly practical. This may be due to a variety of issues, which are often attributable to the need for structures smaller than the resolution of the imaging method or insufficient contrast (e.g., between the uptake of the structure of interest versus those surrounding it).

The StepBrain phantom aims to improve the interpretation of patient brain studies using nuclear medicine methods (i.e., PET and SPECT). It is a novel multi-compartmental anatomical brain model to simulate in vivo tracer uptake in grey matter (GM), white matter (WM), and striatum. This multi-modal anthropomorphic phantom overcomes the limitations of other available brain phantoms and has been developed by the society Human Shape Technologies (https://www.humanshape.eu/). It was created by fully exploiting the potential of fused deposition modelling 3D printing to replicate the real anatomy of brain compartments. The 3D-printable model was obtained from the MRI of a healthy volunteer, which was segmented and ad hoc processed to associate the deep GM nuclei (pallidum, dentate nucleus, and thalamus) to the GM compartment, whereas the substantia nigra and the red nucleus to the WM compartment. The phantom allows simulating ^{18}F-FDG PET brain studies with a degree of realism never achieved with other available phantoms, as validated in acquisitions obtained using the target activity to obtain the real concentration ratios. The results of the post-processing of the phantom with partial volume effect correction tools developed for human PET studies have indeed confirmed the accuracy of these methods in recovering target activity concentrations [61].

Advantages over other available brain phantoms include the presence of three separate compartments that can be simultaneously filled with different concentrations of arbitrary choice of radiotracer, thus replicating any chosen concentration ratio. This is in comparison to the most widely available anthropomorphic brain PET phantom, the previously presented Hoffman phantom, which consists of a single compartment that has a brain-shaped cavity with flat acrylic glass inserts partially occupying it (to simulate the WM), but which only works well if the PET scanner resolution along the z-axis is low enough to not show the layers that make up the internal slices. The StepBrain model instead provides realistic PET image profiles also along the z-axis. Furthermore, while the Hoffman model has a fixed GM/WM activity ratio, StepBrain can simulate any GM/WM ratio. The ability to independently choose different tracer concentrations in the three compartments allows, in principle, its use to simulate other tracers, including amyloid, tau and dopaminergic innervation tracers (e.g., 6-fluoro-l-dopa), as well as other imaging modalities, by filling the compartments with different suitable solutions (e.g., with different para- and ferromagnetic solutions for simulating MRI studies).

References

1. Cal-Gonzalez J, Rausch I, Shiyam Sundar LK, Lassen ML, Muzik O, Moser E, et al. Hybrid imaging: instrumentation and data processing. Front Phys. 2018;6:47.
2. Hicks R, Lau E, Binns D. Hybrid imaging is the future of molecular imaging. Biomed Imaging Interv J. 2007;3(3):e49.
3. Bockisch A, Freudenberg LS, Schmidt D, Kuwert T. Hybrid imaging by SPECT/CT and PET/CT: proven outcomes in cancer imaging. Semin Nucl Med. 2009;39(4):276–89.
4. Beyer T, Freudenberg LS, Townsend DW, Czernin J. The future of hybrid imaging—part 1: hybrid imaging technologies and SPECT/CT. Insights Imaging. 2011;2(2):161–9.
5. Gallamini A, Zwarthoed C, Borra A. Positron emission tomography (PET) in oncology. Cancers (Basel). 2014;6(4):1821–89.
6. Trotter J, Pantel AR, Teo BKK, Escorcia FE, Li T, Pryma DA, et al. Positron emission tomography (PET)/computed tomography (CT) imaging in radiation therapy treatment planning: a review of PET imaging tracers and methods to incorporate PET/CT. Adv Radiat Oncol. 2023;8(5):101212.
7. Sciagrà R, Lubberink M, Hyafil F, Saraste A, Slart RHJA, Agostini D, et al. EANM procedural guidelines for PET/CT quantitative myocardial perfusion imaging. Eur J Nucl Med Mol Imaging. 2021;48(4):1040–69.
8. Marcus C, Mena E, Subramaniam RM. Brain PET in the diagnosis of Alzheimer's disease. Clin Nucl Med. 2014;39(10):e413–26.
9. Kumar A, Chugani HT. The role of radionuclide imaging in epilepsy, part 1: sporadic temporal and extratemporal lobe epilepsy. J Nucl Med Technol. 2017;45(1):14–21.
10. Galldiks N, Lohmann P, Albert NL, Tonn JC, Langen KJ. Current status of PET imaging in neuro-oncology. Neurooncol Adv. 2019;1(1):vdz010.
11. Catana C, Drzezga A, Heiss WD, Rosen BR. PET/MRI for neurological applications. J Nucl Med. 2012;53(12):1916–25. https://doi.org/10.2967/jnumed.112.105346.
12. Jadvar H, Colletti PM. Competitive advantage of PET/MRI. Eur J Radiol. 2014;83(1):84–94.
13. Kogan F, Broski SM, Yoon D, Gold GE. Applications of PET-MRI in musculoskeletal disease. J Magn Reson Imaging. 2018;48(1):27–47.
14. Seraj SM, Hancin E, Aly M, Werner T, Newberg A, Alavi A, et al. Role of PET/MRI in musculoskeletal diseases. J Nucl Med. 2020;61(Suppl 1):1138.
15. Pedersen C, Aboian M, McConathy JE, Daldrup-Link H, Franceschi AM. PET/MRI in pediatric neuroimaging: primer for clinical practice. Am J Neuroradiol. 2022;43(7):938–43.
16. Guniganti P, Kierans AS. PET/MRI of the hepatobiliary system: review of techniques and applications. Clin Imaging. 2021;71:160–9.
17. Evangelista L, Zattoni F, Cassarino G, Artioli P, Cecchin D, Dal Moro F, et al. PET/MRI in prostate cancer: a systematic review and meta-analysis. Eur J Nucl Med Mol Imaging. 2021;48(3):859–73.
18. Brendle C, Maier C, Bender B, Schittenhelm J, Paulsen F, Renovanz M, et al. Impact of 18F-FET PET/MRI on clinical management of brain tumor patients. J Nucl Med. 2022;63(4):522–7.
19. Smith NJ, Deaton TK, Territo W, Graner B, Gauger A, Snyder SE, et al. Hybrid 18F-fluoroethyltyrosine PET and MRI with perfusion to distinguish disease progression from treatment-related change in malignant brain tumors: the quest to beat the toughest cases. J Nucl Med. 2023;64(7):1087–92.
20. George RT, Mehra VC, Chen MY, Kitagawa K, Arbab-Zadeh A, Miller JM, et al. Myocardial CT perfusion imaging and SPECT for the diagnosis of coronary artery disease: a head-to-head comparison from the CORE320 multicenter diagnostic performance study. Radiology. 2014;272(2):407–16.
21. Maxwell JE, Howe JR. Imaging in neuroendocrine tumors: an update for the clinician. Int J Endocr Oncol. 2015;2(2):159–68.
22. Scharf S. SPECT/CT imaging in general orthopedic practice. Semin Nucl Med. 2009;39(5):293–307.
23. Lu FM, Yuan Z. PET/SPECT molecular imaging in clinical neuroscience: recent advances in the investigation of CNS diseases. Quant Imaging Med Surg. 2015;5(3):433–47.

24. Boellaard R. Standards for PET image acquisition and quantitative data analysis. J Nucl Med. 2009;50(Suppl 1):11S–20S.

25. Coleman RE, Delbeke D, Guiberteau MJ, Conti PS, Royal HD, Weinreb JC, et al. Concurrent PET/CT with an integrated imaging system: intersociety dialogue from the Joint Working Group of the American College of Radiology, the Society of Nuclear Medicine, and the Society of Computed Body Tomography and Magnetic Resonance. J Am Coll Radiol. 2005;2(7):568–84.

26. Nørgaard M, Ganz M, Svarer C, Frokjaer VG, Greve DN, Strother SC, et al. Optimization of preprocessing strategies in positron emission tomography (PET) neuroimaging: a [11C]DASB PET study. NeuroImage. 2019;199:466–79.

27. Morzenti S, Spadavecchia C, Dolci C, Ponti ED, Guerra L, Landoni C, et al. 83. Performance optimization using new PET/CT technology with respect to count statistic variation. Phys Medica. 2018;56:113–4.

28. Kolb A, Sauter AW, Eriksson L, Vandenbrouke A, Liu CC, Levin C, et al. Shine-through in PET/MR imaging: effects of the magnetic field on positron range and subsequent image artifacts. J Nucl Med. 2015;56(6):951–4.

29. Kinahan PE, Townsend DW, Beyer T, Sashin D. Attenuation correction for a combined 3D PET/CT scanner. Med Phys. 1998;25(10):2046–53. https://pubmed.ncbi.nlm.nih.gov/9800714/.

30. Chen Y, An H. Attenuation correction of PET/MR imaging. Magn Reson Imaging Clin N Am. 2017;25(2):245–55.

31. Grant AM, Deller TW, Khalighi MM, Maramraju SH, Delso G, Levin CS. NEMA NU 2-2012 performance studies for the SiPM-based ToF-PET component of the GE SIGNA PET/MR system. Med Phys. 2016;43(5):2334–43.

32. Delso G, Fürst S, Jakoby B, Ladebeck R, Ganter C, Nekolla SG, et al. Performance measurements of the Siemens mMR integrated whole-body PET/MR scanner. J Nucl Med. 2011;52(12):1914–22.

33. Cobo M, Menéndez Fernández-Miranda P, Bastarrika G, Lloret Iglesias L. Enhancing radiomics and deep learning systems through the standardization of medical imaging workflows. Sci Data. 2023;10(1):732.

34. Castiglioni I, Gallivanone F, Soda P, Avanzo M, Stancanello J, Aiello M, et al. AI-based applications in hybrid imaging: how to build smart and truly multiparametric decision models for radiomics. Eur J Nucl Med Mol Imaging. 2019;46(13):2673–99.

35. Tavares AAS, Mezzanotte L, McDougald W, Bernsen MR, Vanhove C, Aswendt M, et al. Community survey results show that standardisation of preclinical imaging techniques remains a challenge. Mol Imaging Biol. 2023;25(3):560–8. https://pubmed.ncbi.nlm.nih.gov/36482032/.

36. Morbelli S, Esposito G, Arbizu J, Barthel H, Boellaard R, Bohnen NI, et al. EANM practice guideline/SNMMI procedure standard for dopaminergic imaging in Parkinsonian syndromes 1.0. Eur J Nucl Med Mol Imaging. 2020;47(8):1885–912.

37. Guedj E, Varrone A, Boellaard R, Albert NL, Barthel H, van Berckel B, et al. EANM procedure guidelines for brain PET imaging using [18F]FDG, version 3. Eur J Nucl Med Mol Imaging. 2022;49(2):632–51.

38. DICOM. [cited 2024 Oct 7]. DICOM. https://www.dicomstandard.org.

39. IHE International. [cited 2024 Oct 7]. Integrating the Healthcare Enterprise (IHE). https://www.ihe.net/.

40. IHE International. [cited 2024 Oct 7]. Connectathon. https://www.ihe.net/testing/connectathon/.

41. Koole M, Armstrong I, Krizsan AK, Stromvall A, Visvikis D, Sattler B, et al. EANM guidelines for PET-CT and PET-MR routine quality control. Z Med Phys. 2022;33(1):103–13.

42. Kinahan PE, Perlman ES, Sunderland JJ, Subramaniam R, Wollenweber SD, Turkington TG, et al. The QIBA profile for FDG PET/CT as an imaging biomarker measuring response to cancer therapy. Radiology. 2020;294(3):647–57.

43. Sunderland J, Kinahan P, Karp J, Byrd D, Scheuermann J, Panetta J, et al. Development and testing of a formalism to identify harmonized and optimized reconstructions for PET/CT in clinical trials. J Nucl Med. 2015;56(Suppl 3):563.

44. Aide N, Lasnon C, Veit-Haibach P, Sera T, Sattler B, Boellaard R. EANM/EARL harmonization strategies in PET quantification: from daily practice to multicentre oncological studies. Eur J Nucl Med Mol Imaging. 2017;44(Suppl 1):17–31. https://pubmed.ncbi.nlm.nih.gov/28623376/.

45. Boellaard R, Delgado-Bolton R, Oyen WJG, Giammarile F, Tatsch K, Eschner W, et al. FDG PET/CT: EANM procedure guidelines for tumour imaging: version 2.0. Eur J Nucl Med Mol Imaging. 2015;42(2):328–54.

46. Fahey F, Christian P, Zukotynski K, Sexton-Stallone B, Kiss C, Clarke B, et al. Use of a qualification phantom for PET brain imaging in a multicenter consortium: a collaboration between the pediatric brain tumor consortium and the SNMMI Clinical Trials Network. J Nucl Med. 2019;60(5):677–82.

47. Tazegul TE, Polemi AM, Snyder A, Snyder C, Collins PG. Automated phantom analysis for gamma cameras and SPECT: a methodology for use in a clinical setting. J Appl Clin Med Phys. 2020;21(11):205–14.

48. Accreditation support. [cited 2024 Oct 8]. Phantom testing: nuclear medicine (revised 9-4-2024). https://accreditationsupport.acr.org/support/solutions/articles/11000062798-phantom-testing-nuclear-medicine-revised-9-4-2024-.

49. Agency IAE. Quality assurance for SPECT systems. International Atomic Energy Agency; 2009 [cited 2024 Oct 8]. pp. 1–249. https://www.iaea.org/publications/8119/quality-assurance-for-spect-systems.

50. Oliveira CM, da Silva TA, Vieira IF, Lima FRA, Vieira JW, de Sa LV. Characterization of a PET-NEMA/IEC body phantom for quality control tests of PET/

CT equipment. In: Brazil; 2011. http://inis.iaea.org/search/search.aspx?orig_q=RN:43056338.

51. Hoffman EJ, Cutler PD, Digby WM, Mazziotta JC. 3-D phantom to simulate cerebral blood flow and metabolic images for PET. IEEE Trans Nucl Sci. 1990;37(2):616–20.

52. Shekari M, Verwer EE, Yaqub M, Daamen M, Buckley C, Frisoni GB, et al. Harmonization of brain PET images in multi-center PET studies using Hoffman phantom scan. EJNMMI Phys. 2023;10(1):68.

53. Rahmim A, Lodge MA, Crabb AH, Zhou Y, Wong DF, Gottesman RF. Simultaneous monitoring of PET image resolution, noise, uniformity and quantitative accuracy using uniform cylinder phantom measurements in the multi-center setting. In: 2014 IEEE nuclear science symposium and medical imaging conference (NSS/MIC). 2014 [cited 2024 Oct 8]. pp. 1–3. https://ieeexplore.ieee.org/abstract/document/7430840.

54. Lodge MA, Leal JP, Rahmim A, Sunderland JJ, Frey EC. Measuring PET spatial resolution using a cylinder phantom positioned at an oblique angle. J Nucl Med. 2018;59(11):1768–75.

55. Kolthammer JA, Su KH, Grover A, Narayanan M, Jordan DW, Muzic RF. Performance evaluation of the ingenuity TF PET/CT scanner with a focus on high count-rate conditions. Phys Med Biol. 2014;59(14):3843.

56. Vonderen KV, Leonard S, Linscheid L, Gruchot M, Dillehay G. Image quality assessment of Hoffman brain phantom scans performed on a next generation and previous generation PET/CT scanners. J Nucl Med. 2019;60(Suppl 1):2052.

57. Rausch I, Valladares A, Sundar LKS, Beyer T, Hacker M, Meyerspeer M, et al. Standard MRI-based attenuation correction for PET/MRI phantoms: a novel concept using MRI-visible polymer. EJNMMI Phys. 2021;8(1):18.

58. Mizuta T, Yamakawa Y, Minagawa S, Kobayashi T, Ohtani A, Takenouchi S, et al. Attenuation correction for phantom tests: an alternative to maximum-likelihood attenuation correction factor-based correction for clinical studies in time-of-flight PET. Ann Nucl Med. 2022;36(11):998–1006.

59. Ziegler S, Jakoby BW, Braun H, Paulus DH, Quick HH. NEMA image quality phantom measurements and attenuation correction in integrated PET/MR hybrid imaging. EJNMMI Phys. 2015;2(1):18.

60. Kim JS, Kim HS, Ryu JK, Jung WY, Dong KR, Chung WK. Optimization of low dose CT based attenuation correction for brain PET/CT protocols. J Nucl Med. 2014;55(Suppl 1):2609.

61. Pirozzi MA, Gaudieri V, Prinster A, Magliulo M, Cuocolo A, Brunetti A, et al. StepBrain: a 3-dimensionally printed multicompartmental anthropomorphic brain phantom to simulate PET activity distributions. J Nucl Med. 2024;65(9):1489–92. https://jnm.snmjournals.org/content/early/2024/07/18/jnumed.123.267277.

State of the Art in Pre-clinical Imaging

12

Guido Rovera, Gianluca Destro, Edoardo Dighero,
Martina Cioffi, Maria Luce Mangia,
Alessandra Agosti, Gloria Garelli,
Matteo Bauckneht, Gianmario Sambuceti,
Enzo Terreno, and Silvia Morbelli

12.1   Introduction

Preclinical research utilizing animal models is a crucial part of biomedical science, serving to investigate and validate new biomarkers, imaging agents, and therapeutic interventions prior to clinical trial initiation. Today, an extensive variety of animal models is available, effectively replicating various human diseases, including cancer, cardiovascular, neurological, and inflammatory conditions [1, 2]. Nuclear medicine molecular imaging offers three-dimensional, functional visualization of biological activity within living organisms through the use of radioactive tracers, revealing how these processes are spatially distributed in both animal models and human bodies. In preclinical research, molecular imaging has become increasingly valuable, as it allows to translate findings from animal models to the human setting. The availability of precise metabolic information significantly enhances drug development and facilitates the assessment of therapeutic efficacy by monitoring the drug impact on the underlying mechanisms of diseases at molecular level.

Preclinical molecular imaging offers several benefits, notably the ability to explore both anatomical and molecular aspects of biological processes. This is made possible through hybrid imaging technologies that merge functional imaging, such as positron emission tomography (PET) or single-photon emission computed tomography (SPECT), with structural imaging techniques like magnetic resonance imaging (MRI) or computed tomography (CT). Another key advantage is the capability of preclinical imaging to deliver quantitative data while preserving the natural biological processes being studied: Indeed, it allows for the examination of complex interactions between physiological/biochemical mechanisms within living animals, where immune, hormonal, and systemic

G. Rovera · M. Cioffi · M. L. Mangia · A. Agosti
G. Garelli · S. Morbelli (✉)
Nuclear Medicine Division, Department of Medical
Sciences, University of Turin, Turin, Italy
e-mail: guido.rovera@unito.it;
martina.cioffi@unito.it; marialuce.mangia@unito.it;
alessandra.agosti@unito.it; gloria.garelli@unito.it;
silviadaniela.morbelli@unito.it

G. Destro · E. Terreno
Molecular and Preclinical Imaging Centers,
Department of Molecular Biotechnology and Health
Sciences, University of Turin, Turin, Italy
e-mail: gianluca.destro@unito.it;
enzo.terreno@unito.it

E. Dighero
Department of Health Sciences (DISSAL), University
of Genoa, Genoa, Italy
e-mail: edoardo.dighero@edu.unige.it

M. Bauckneht · G. Sambuceti
Department of Health Sciences (DISSAL), University
of Genoa, Genoa, Italy

IRCCS Ospedale Policlinico San Martino,
Genoa, Italy
e-mail: matteo.bauckneht@unige.it;
gianmario.sambuceti@unige.it

© The Author(s), under exclusive license to Springer Nature Switzerland AG 2025   147
L. Camoni, L. Mansi (eds.), *Nuclear Medicine Hybrid Imaging for Radiographers & Technologists*,
https://doi.org/10.1007/978-3-031-86228-1_12

responses remain fully functional. Moreover, preclinical imaging supports non-invasive, longitudinal monitoring of animal models, enabling the observation of changes over time. This enhances the statistical robustness of research by minimizing biological variability, as each animal can act as its own baseline control. Importantly, preclinical imaging also promotes ethical research practices since it allows for repeated, non-invasive assessment of disease progression and treatment responses, significantly reducing the need to sacrifice animals at different stages of the study. In contrast to molecular imaging, conventional investigative methods in preclinical research, such as histology and tissue sampling, present significant drawbacks [3]. First, in vitro techniques cannot provide a comprehensive, whole-boy assessment across different time points. Second, these methods involve extracting cells or tissues thus disrupting the original microenvironment and potentially leading to results that may not accurately reflect real pathophysiological conditions. Due to their invasive nature, these techniques also typically necessitate sacrificing animals at each data collection point, making longitudinal analysis unfeasible and significantly increasing the number of animals required for experimental and control groups. To address these challenges, preclinical imaging has emerged as an essential tool for conducting non-invasive, in vivo longitudinal studies in animal models, offering a more efficient and ethically responsible approach to research.

The demand for more personalized cancer therapies continues to drive significant advancements in preclinical imaging for oncological research. The vast diversity of molecular alterations underlying neoplastic transformation and the unpredictable response to treatment of cancer cells make the quest for personalized and effective cancer therapy particularly challenging. Non-invasive in vivo imaging techniques, such as positron emission tomography (PET), are instrumental in deepening our understanding of tumor behavior and progression, facilitating the development of more targeted therapies. Additionally, molecular imaging offers insights into the biodistribution of novel tumor-targeting ligands, unin-tended off-target interactions, as well as tumor and extracellular matrix characteristics. Beyond oncology, preclinical imaging also provides valuable insights for neurological research by allowing the assessment of brain perfusion and oxygenation, metabolic activity, synaptic density, protein accumulation, and receptor binding. This technology also enhances our ability to study inflammatory and infectious diseases by enabling the early, non-invasive detection and quantification of inflammation. In cardiology, molecular imaging can be used to investigate myocardial perfusion and metabolism, advancing our understanding of heart conditions. Furthermore, preclinical molecular imaging significantly aids in drug development by non-invasively evaluating target expression, whole-body biodistribution, and organ-specific toxicity.

As reported by the European Association of Nuclear Medicine (EANM) guidelines on preclinical imaging [4], according to a recent market report on preclinical imaging, the global market (including PET, SPECT, MRI, CT, ultrasound, and optical imaging) is projected to grow at a rate of 6.5% from 2022 to 2028. Considering the potential of small animal imaging, advancements in SPECT/PET technologies are crucial for facilitating the seamless translation of preclinical research into clinical applications.

12.2 Scanners for Pre-clinical Molecular Imaging

Today, a wide range of preclinical imaging scanners is available from various manufacturers. Although these systems share some features with their clinical counterparts, significant adjustments are necessary to appropriately scale down clinical imaging technologies for preclinical applications. The performance of PET scanners, in particular, is defined by parameters such as spatial resolution, detection sensitivity, and timing accuracy. Preclinical PET scanners must achieve a much higher spatial resolution than clinical systems, given the considerably smaller dimensions of anatomical structures in small animals. Additionally, preclinical systems necessitate superior temporal resolution in order to register physiological processes with greater precision. Advancements in PET system performance focus on several key areas [5]: the choice and configuration of detector materials, improvements in sensor technologies, optimization of data acquisition techniques, and multimodal hybrid imaging integration, as outlined in the following sections. These enhancements are critical for meeting the stringent requirements of high-resolution and high-sensitivity imaging in pre-clinical research.

Crystal Material PET detector materials must meet several critical requirements, including high detection efficiency (achieved through a high attenuation coefficient), excellent energy resolution to effectively distinguish between scattered radiation and the photopeak, and fast timing to minimize random events and enable time-of-flight measurements. While a variety of scintillation materials are available, such as sodium iodide (NaI:Tl) and bismuth germanate (BGO), lutetium oxyorthosilicate (LSO) and lutetium-yttrium oxyorthosilicate (LYSO) have become the materials of choice for both clinical and pre-clinical PET scanners [6]. In addition to traditional inorganic scintillators, alternative materials such as cadmium zinc telluride (CZT) are also utilized. CZT detectors offer several advantages: compactness, high energy resolution and spatial resolution, and reduction of parallax errors thanks to their capability for three-dimensional event localization. However, these benefits come with trade-offs, as CZT detectors have poor timing resolution and a relatively low atomic number, limiting their effectiveness in certain applications.

Depth of Interaction (DOI) A key factor influencing spatial resolution in PET imaging is accurately determining the depth at which photons interact within the crystal elements. If a single depth assumption is used, parallax errors can introduce image blurring, especially in the compact geometries of preclinical imaging systems. Thus, integrating DOI capabilities is highly advantageous. Monolithic detector designs naturally incorporate DOI information, and semiconductor detectors can also provide such information. Instead, for traditional scintillators made of discrete crystals, the main methods to determine DOI are phoswitch detectors, differential light sharing, and dual-sided readout approaches.

Photosensors PET systems utilizing scintillators require photosensors to convert photons into electrical signals. Small-animal PET systems have traditionally used position-sensitive photomultiplier tubes (PSPMTs) for this purpose. However, PMTs present several drawbacks, such as dead zones around their peripheries, large size, and incompatibility with the strong magnetic fields used in MRI. Solid-state photomultipliers (SiPMs) have now become the preferred technology for high-resolution PET systems. SiPMs are cost-effective to manufacture, significantly more compact, capable of operating in magnetic environments, and exhibit high gain and rapid response times. This technology has rapidly improved, and most modern clinical [7, 8] and preclinical PET systems are equipped with SiPM technology.

Signal Multiplexing With the increasing adoption of SiPMs over PSPMTs, signal multiplexing has emerged as a critical area of innovation. One challenge posed by SiPMs is the large number of output channels generated by their arrays, which can hinder scalability. To address this, multiplexing techniques are used to strategically combine SiPM outputs, thereby reducing the number of channels and simplifying data processing while maintaining system performance.

Multimodality Scanner Configurations One of the drivers for innovation in preclinical PET technology is the increased interest in multimodality imaging systems. These systems, such as PET/CT, facilitate the integration of functional imaging from PET with anatomical imaging from CT scans, enabling comprehensive insights into biological processes. Additionally, PET can be paired with magnetic resonance imaging (MRI), which provides soft tissue morphological imaging. PET/MR systems are increasingly popular in preclinical research because—beyond the high-resolution soft tissue visualization—they do not require ionizing radiation and allow for multiparametric imaging.

12.2.1 PET/MR Imaging

While the advent of SiPM technology has been pivotal in the development of PET/MR scanners, such devices lack the capability for direct photon attenuation measurement provided by CT. However, in small-animal imaging, this issue is less critical, and the advantages of MRI—such as superior soft tissue contrast—more than compensate for the lack of direct PET attenuation correction.

12.2.2 PET/SPECT Imaging

The advancement of preclinical SPECT/CT technology has followed a similar trajectory to that of PET/CT, ultimately leading to the creation of integrated tri-modality PET/SPECT/CT systems [9, 10]. Some of these innovative scanners employ the same detector for both PET and SPECT modalities, enabling simultaneous imaging with dual tracers. This capability unlocks new research possibilities, including the differential imaging of perfusion and metabolism in neurodegenerative diseases or dual receptor-binding studies.

12.2.3 PET/Optical Imaging

The integration of PET with optical imaging techniques arises from the need to investigate multiple molecular targets simultaneously. While optical imaging, which employs fluorescent probes, is widely used in preclinical research, it remains largely non-translatable to clinical applications. Combining optical methods with nuclear radiotracer imaging helps bridge the gap between preclinical and clinical studies. Research efforts are directed towards the development of simulta-

neous PET/optical imaging systems, enhancing the ability to study complex biological processes in real time.

12.2.4 Multiple Animal Imaging and Artificial Intelligence

Several PET scanners now have the capability to image multiple mice simultaneously addressing the high relative cost associated with imaging a single animal per scan session. This advancement helps mitigate the financial challenges that often limit the broader adoption of preclinical PET. Additionally, innovations that streamline data and image analysis, such as the integration of artificial intelligence, are poised to further reduce costs and improve the efficiency of preclinical PET studies.

Beyond technical advancements, there is a strong need for rigorous quality standards. While quality control (QC) measures in preclinical imaging may seem less critical since they do not yield direct diagnostic information, their importance becomes clear when considering the translational potential of preclinical research for clinical applications. The European Association of Nuclear Medicine (EANM) has recently released guidelines [4] that outline best practices for implementing robust QC programs for SPECT and PET systems in preclinical imaging laboratories. These guidelines are designed to enhance the translational reliability of preclinical imaging data by ensuring consistent, reproducible, and accurate imaging practices, as well as the precision of SPECT and PET quantification.

12.3 Preclinical Applications of Molecular Imaging

Preclinical in vivo molecular imaging techniques are invaluable for advancing our understanding of disease mechanisms and the underlying biology of both animals and humans. Indeed, molecular imaging can play a crucial role across various stages of drug development and validation, as detailed below.

12.3.1 Analysis of Tumor Biology

Preclinical molecular imaging plays a crucial role in understanding tumor biology by assessing receptor expression, tumor-specific biomarkers, and metabolic activity. Specifically, ^{18}F-fludeoxyglucose ([^{18}F]FDG), a radiolabeled glucose analogue, helps to measure glucose uptake in tumors, providing insights into their growth and aggressiveness. More specialized PET agents have been developed to target specific molecules or gene products, offering deeper insights into tumor biology and therapy responses. A prime example is the PET radiopharmaceutical [^{68}Ga]Ga-PSMA, which has significantly advanced prostate cancer imaging by enabling the detection of Prostate-Specific Membrane Antigen (PSMA) overexpression on prostate cancer cells. Additionally, tumor vascularization and blood flow serve as important indicators of tumor behavior, and can be visualized using radiotracers that easily diffuse through the vascular system and tumor cell membranes, such as ^{15}O-water, ^{13}N-ammonia, and ^{82}Rb-chloride.

12.3.2 ImmunoPET

ImmunoPET imaging is a non-invasive molecular imaging technique that combines the high specificity of antibodies for targeting specific antigens with the sensitivity and quantitative capabilities of PET systems. A preclinical study conducted by Wang et al. [11] explored the use of immunoPET to assess receptor expression in cancer models, specifically focusing on triple-negative breast cancer (TNBC). The treatment of TNBC is particularly challenging due to its heterogeneity and the absence of actionable therapeutic targets, highlighting a significant clinical need for novel molecular targets. AXL, a member of the receptor tyrosine kinase subfamily, has been implicated in TNBC and other cancers and is a potential therapeutic target. In this study, the expression of AXL and its downregulation through treatment with 17-allylamino-17-demethoxygeldanamycin (17-AAG), a potent inhibitor of heat shock protein 90 (HSP90), were evaluated using preclinical PET/CT imaging. The researchers utilized a copper-64-labeled anti-human AXL antibody (^{64}Cu-anti-hAXL) as a radioactive probe, enabling the imaging and quantification of AXL expression and assessing the therapeutic efficacy of AXL-targeted molecular therapies. The short half-life (~13 h) of ^{64}Cu, along with its β+ and β− emissions, makes it an ideal PET radionuclide for labeling antibodies and nanoparticles. The in vivo experiments demonstrated that ^{64}Cu-anti-hAXL selectively binds to AXL-expressing tumor cells and it can non-invasively assess AXL expression in TNBC. This approach could be used to predict drug resistance and therapeutic response to AXL-targeted treatments, potentially advancing the development of theranostic agents.

12.3.3 Evaluation of Drug Delivery Systems

Multi-modal PET imaging is increasingly being utilized for innovative pharmaceutical applications, such as tracking the in vivo behavior of drug formulations to enhance targeted drug delivery. For instance, a recent study explored the movement and disintegration of four distinct devices, each with different release profiles (immediate release, water-soluble, insoluble polymer, pH-dependent), in the gastrointestinal tracts of rats using [^{18}F]FDG radiolabeling [12]. Molecular imaging provided valuable in vivo data on the behavior of these formulations, aiding in the optimization of their design to develop targeted release dosage forms for personalized treatment. Moreover, this approach can support with fine-tuning administration schedules, assess therapeutic efficacy, and predict potential toxicity.

12.3.4 Targeting and Biodistribution

Target validation, along with pharmacokinetics and pharmacodynamics, are critical aspects of drug and therapeutic development. PET imaging serves as a highly effective tool for in vivo therapeutic tracking studies due to its ability to provide dynamic tomographic distribution data over time, with both high temporal and spatial resolution. Thanks to dynamic imaging, blood sampling, and kinetic modeling techniques, molecular imaging can offer crucial insights into distribution kinetics and receptor densities. Exemplary dynamic PET images of neuroinflammation captured during the injection of the Translocator Protein (TSPO) radiotracer [^{18}F]DPA-714 are presented in Fig. 12.1. The choice of the most suitable isotope depends on the specific compound requirements, as well as its biodistribution profiles over time. For example, ^{11}C has a relatively short half-life, making it well-suited for studies of small molecules with brief biodistribution periods. However, it may not be ideal for larger compounds, which typically exhibit longer biodistributions. In such cases, antibodies, which generally have prolonged biodistribution, are often paired with isotopes with longer half-lives,

such as ^{89}Zr and ^{124}I. Preclinical dynamic PET applications have been employed to identify brain-penetrant PET tracers for poly(ADP-ribose) polymerase (PARP) [13]. Currently, several clinical trials are exploring PARP inhibitors as potential treatments for glioblastoma. Noninvasive quantification of baseline PARP expression through PET imaging could offer valuable prognostic insights and help tailor more effective treatments. However, there is a lack of brain-penetrant PARP imaging agents capable of providing accurate in vivo measurements of PARP in the brain. Chen et al. developed a brain-penetrant PARP PET tracer ([^{11}C]PyBic) and assessed its biodistribution, brain kinetics, and binding specificity in both a rat glioblastoma model and healthy nonhuman primates using dynamic PET imaging. The PET results revealed higher tracer uptake in glioblastoma tissue compared to the surrounding brain tissue. Furthermore, the uptake of [^{11}C]PyBic was significantly reduced when

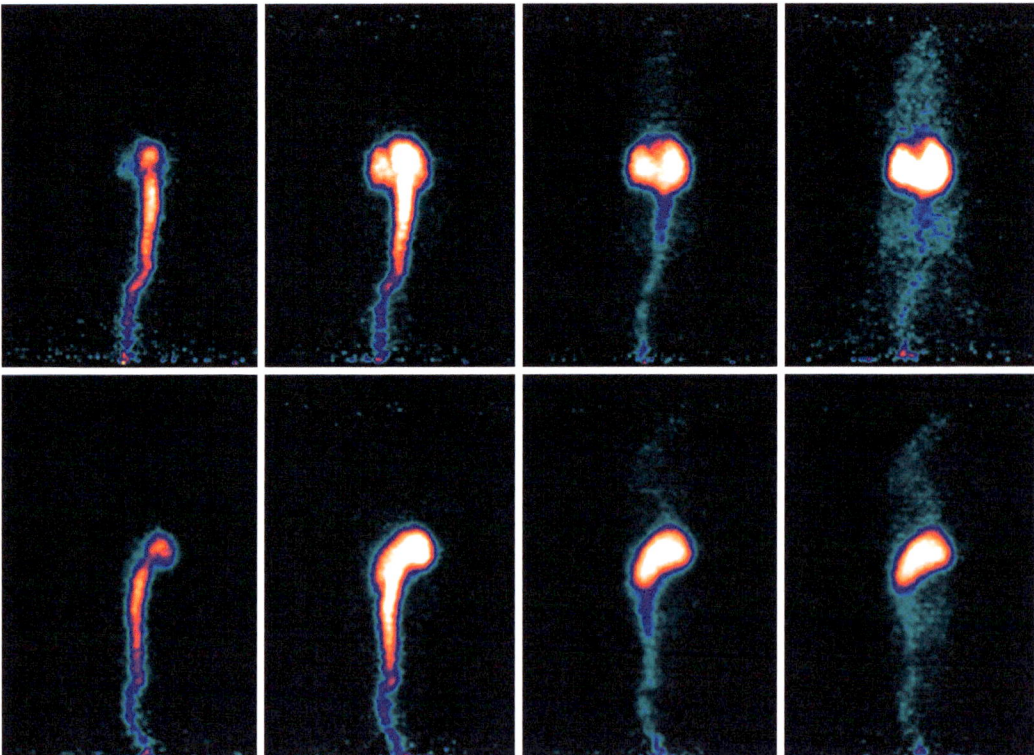

Fig. 12.1 Wild-type mouse, dynamic PET images (left: coronal view, right: sagittal view) captured during the injection of the Translocator Protein (TSPO) radiotracer [18F]DPA-714

other PARP1/2 inhibitors were administered, demonstrating the in vivo binding specificity of the tracer. The tracer exhibited a high brain-to-plasma ratio, indicating its excellent brain permeability and specific binding properties. These findings highlighted the potential use of [^{11}C] PyBic for non-invasive quantification of PARP binding in the brain, making it a promising tool for applications in oncology and neuroimaging.

12.3.5 Monitoring Drug Activity and Interaction

Ensuring that a drug reaches its specific target tissue is a critical aspect of drug development. To evaluate this, absorption, distribution, metabolism, and excretion (ADME), studies are performed to track how drugs and their metabolites travel through the body, crossing cellular membranes to exert their effects. This membrane passage is often an active process facilitated by transmembrane transporter proteins. Many drugs are administered alongside others, and when both are substrates for the same transporter proteins, drug-drug interactions (DDIs) may occur. In such cases, one drug can influence the pharmacokinetics of the other, often altering its tissue distribution. These transporter-mediated DDIs are important for both drug safety and efficacy. Identifying clinically relevant DDIs between an investigational drug and other medications should be a priority during drug development. A recent study [14] examined the role of transporters in the disposition of erlotinib, a drug used to treat advanced metastatic non-small cell lung cancer (NSCLC) and pancreatic cancer, using PET imaging in combination with MRI. Erlotinib is a reversible tyrosine kinase inhibitor (TKI) targeting the epidermal growth factor receptor (EGFR) and is known to be a substrate for several transporter proteins, including breast cancer resistance protein (BCRP), P-glycoprotein (P-gp), organic anion transporter 3 (OAT3), and organic cation transporter 2 (OCT2). The study used serial PET/MRI imaging to assess the influence of transporters on the tissue distribution and excretion of ^{11}C-erlotinib in four different mouse groups (wild-type, co-injected with unlabeled erlotinib, pretreated with a dual P-gp/BCRP inhibitor, and P-gp/BCRP knockout). The results confirmed that BCRP, P-gp, and SLC transporters affect the in vivo distribution of ^{11}C-erlotinib both in normal and tumor tissue. Moreover, the study showed that erlotinib could cause transporter-mediated DDIs when co-administered with other drugs utilizing the same transporters. Additionally, the brain distribution of erlotinib could be enhanced by inhibiting P-gp and BCRP at the blood-brain barrier (BBB), as previous studies have shown that efflux transport by P-gp and BCRP reduces erlotinib's brain distribution. Thus, the inhibition of these transporters could improve the drug's effectiveness in treating NSCLC brain metastases.

12.3.6 Evaluation of Therapeutic Efficacy

Preclinical PET imaging is frequently used in studies evaluating therapeutic responses since PET tracers enable quantitative assessments of tumor response. While [^{18}F]FDG (which tracks glucose metabolism) is the most widely used radiotracer, [^{18}F]FLT (which indicates cell proliferation), [^{18}F]FAZA/[^{18}F]FMISO (which detect hypoxia), and other tracers have been utilized to examine processes like perfusion/hypoxia, protein synthesis, cell proliferation, and receptor density. As an example of the use of [^{18}F]FDG, previous research has explored the anti-cancer effects of metformin using [^{18}F]FDG PET imaging [15]. Metformin, a widely prescribed medication for type 2 diabetes, alters normal glucose metabolism. In addition to its primary use in diabetes management, a secondary effect of metformin—discovered serendipitously—is its ability to suppress tumor growth. Although the precise mechanism is still debated, one of the key pathways of the anti-cancer effect is through AMP-activated protein kinase (AMPK), which regulates metabolism and cell growth. The study investigated the combined impact of short-term starvation (STS), known for its ability to significantly slow cancer growth while inducing toxic levels of reactive oxygen species (ROS), and metformin on tumor progression. Using in vivo FDG-PET imaging in murine models of colon and breast carcinomas, the researchers observed that tumor growth was most effectively halted when metformin was combined with STS.

12.3.7 Theranostics

Theranostics is an emerging field of medicine that combines diagnostic and therapeutic approaches, marking a significant step towards more personalized treatment strategies. Advances in molecular biology have greatly enhanced our understanding of the receptors expressed by tumor cells. In theranostics, these molecular targets can be leveraged to both image the tumor and deliver targeted cytotoxic agents directly to cancerous tissues. The development of new theranostic radiotracers is a key focus of preclinical imaging research, advancing the potential of theranostics for a wide range of cancers.

One area of focus in theranostics involves targeting the Fibroblast Activation Protein α (FAP), which is abundantly expressed on cancer-associated fibroblasts in epithelial-derived cancers. Tumors in the breast, colon, and pancreas often exhibit prominent desmoplastic reactions, leading to an increased presence of stromal cells, making FAP an attractive target for molecular imaging and targeted therapies. Single-domain antibodies (sdAbs) are the smallest antibody fragments, offering advantageous pharmacokinetic properties for both imaging and therapy. A study by Dekempeneer et al. [16] described the development of an sdAb targeting FAP in a mouse model, suitable for both imaging and therapeutic applications through radiolabeling with ^{131}I and ^{68}Ga for SPECT/PET imaging as well as ^{131}I and ^{225}Ac for targeted radionuclide therapy. The radiolabeled sdAbs showed rapid and specific accumulation in FAP-positive glioblastoma tumors at preclinical PET/SPECT imaging, while the therapeutic compounds demonstrated dose-dependent therapeutic effects in FAP-positive tumor-bearing mice thus highlight the potential of radiolabeled sdAb as an effective radiotheranostic agent for FAP-positive cancers.

12.3.8 Non-oncological Applications

Preclinical molecular imaging techniques have been used in the field of neuroscience to acquire valuable metabolic insights into the brain, such as detecting changes in brain activity that might be indicative of conditions such as Alzheimer's Disease (AD) and Parkinson's Disease (PD). PET/MR imaging holds particular significance in neurology, as it delivers concurrent soft-tissue and metabolic imaging, allowing for detailed investigations of brain anatomy, pathologies, and metabolic dysfunctions in animal models. PET imaging allows to investigate the pathological hallmarks of neurodegenerative diseases, such as the alteration of brain glucose metabolism, the accumulation of amyloid-β (Aβ) and tau proteins in AD models and the presence of neuroinflammation. Glucose metabolism represents a useful biomarker for numerous neurological conditions, given that brain glucose metabolism is often altered in various diseases, and this can be effectively monitored using [^{18}F]FDG PET. As for neuroinflammation, the tracer [^{18}F]DPA-714 binds to the Translocator Protein (TSPO) which becomes upregulated in activated microglia and macrophages during inflammatory processes, thus allowing the visualization of neuroinflammatory processes. Representative PET images acquired in an animal model using [^{18}F]FDG and [^{18}F]DPA-714 are shown in Fig. 12.2. Preclinical molecular imaging also plays a pivotal role in neuro-oncological studies, aiding in the optimization of PET-guided therapies within the framework of multimodal cancer treatments. For instance, Verhoeven et al. [17] explored the feasibility of using PET-guided subvolume boosting in glioblastoma animal models, as an accurate definition of the tumor volume is of utmost importance for guiding RT.

Beyond neurology, researchers have employed multi-modal PET imaging to gain comprehensive insights into cardiovascular physiology and

Fig. 12.2 *Top row:* wild type (WT) mouse, static PET images (left: coronal view, right: sagittal view) captured 35 min after the injection of the glucose analogue radiotracer [^{18}F]FDG, with a 5-min acquisition time. *Bottom row:* WT mouse, static PET images (left: coronal view, right: sagittal view) captured 40 min after the injection of the Translocator Protein (TSPO) radiotracer [18F]DPA-714, with a 5-min acquisition time

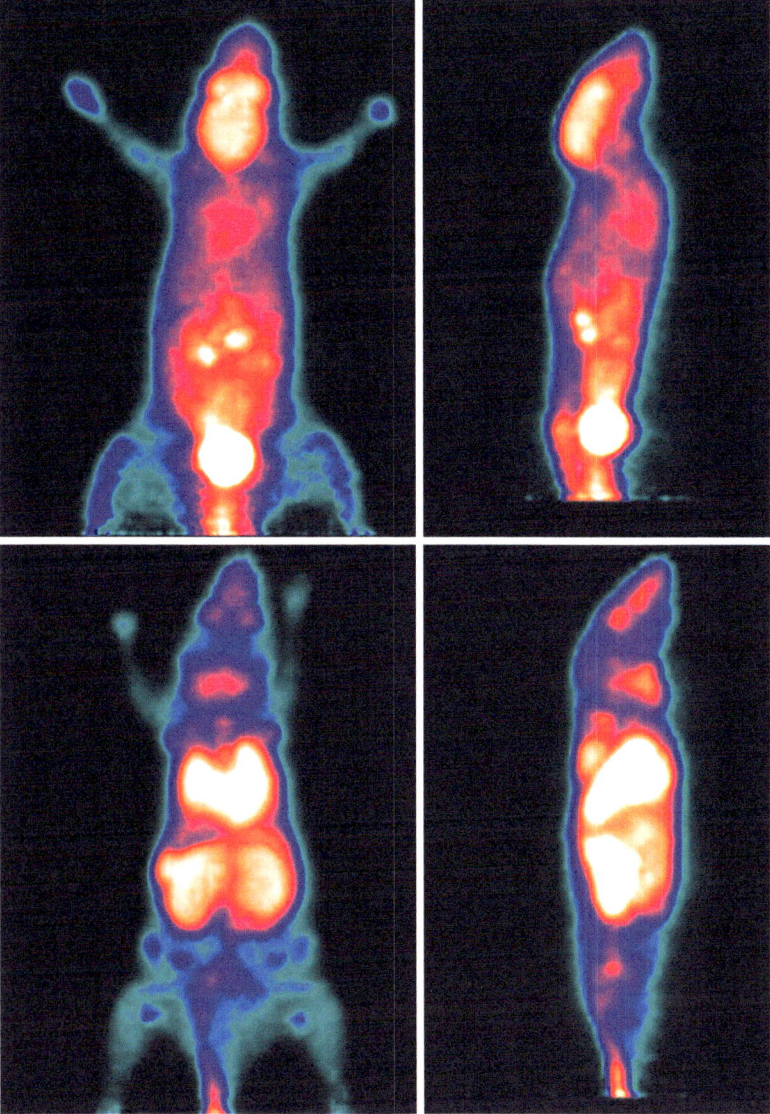

pathology. In preclinical cardiac imaging, the investigated parameters often include myocardial metabolic viability and perfusion, but additional aspects like inflammation, neural innervation, apoptosis, and neovascularization can also be assessed using PET [18]. The advanced spatial and temporal resolution of preclinical molecular imaging scanners is essential for visualizing cardiac disease features, such as plaques and ischemic lesions, in small animal models. Moreover, the CT functionality of state-of-the-art PET/CT scanners complements PET by providing detailed information on vessel calcification, cardiac structure, and fine anatomical features in murine models. PET/MR is also gaining traction in cardiovascular research, where MRI data can provide insights into tissue metabolic states, structural integrity, perfusion, and global or localized function. This dual-modality approach is particularly advantageous for imaging plaques and characterizing inflammatory processes at the molecular level. Additionally, molecular imaging stands out as one of the few technologies capable of assessing cardiac autonomic denervation, a parameter shown to correlate with the risk of cardiovascular events, thus offering valuable prognostic information.

12.4 Conclusion

Overall, as biotechnology advances and new discoveries deepen our understanding of disease pathophysiology, the need to translate these scientific breakthroughs into practical clinical applications is anticipated to grow even more in the future. Preclinical hybrid imaging of animal models can help to bridge the gap between in vitro studies and clinical applications. Thanks to highly precise metabolic data, this imaging technology aids in developing more personalized therapeutic strategies by enhancing our understanding of disease mechanisms and biological responses to treatments.

References

1. Lauber DT, Fülöp A, Kovács T, Szigeti K, Máthé D, Szijártó A. State of the art in vivo imaging techniques for laboratory animals. Lab Anim. 2017;51:465–78.
2. Kiessling F, Pichler BJ, Hauff P, editors. Small animal imaging. Cham: Springer International Publishing; 2017. http://link.springer.com/10.1007/978-3-319-42202-2.
3. James ML, Gambhir SS. A molecular imaging primer: modalities, imaging agents, and applications. Physiol Rev. 2012;92:897–965.
4. Vanhove C, Koole M, Fragoso Costa P, Schottelius M, Mannheim J, Kuntner C, et al. Preclinical SPECT and PET: joint EANM and ESMI procedure guideline for implementing an efficient quality control programme. Eur J Nucl Med Mol Imaging. 2024;51:3822–39.
5. Lehnert AL, Miyaoka RS. Innovations in small-animal PET instrumentation. PET Clin. 2024;19:59–67.
6. Moses WW, Janecek M, Spurrier MA, Szupryczynski P, Choong W-S, Melcher CL, et al. Optimization of a LSO-based detector module for time-of-flight PET. IEEE Trans Nucl Sci. 2010;57:1570–6.
7. Rovera G, Urso L, Stracuzzi F, Laudicella R, Frantellizzi V, Cottignoli C, et al. Advantages of SiPM-based digital PET/CT technology in nuclear medicine clinical practice: a systematic review—part 1 oncological setting. Clin Transl Imaging. 2024;12:769. https://doi.org/10.1007/s40336-024-00653-0.
8. Rovera G, Urso L, Stracuzzi F, Laudicella R, Frantellizzi V, Cottignoli C, et al. Advantages of SiPM-based digital PET/CT technology in nuclear medicine clinical practice: a systematic review—part 2. Clin Transl Imaging. 2024;12:743. https://doi.org/10.1007/s40336-024-00650-3.
9. Goorden MC, van der Have F, Kreuger R, Ramakers RM, Vastenhouw B, Burbach JPH, et al. VECTor: a preclinical imaging system for simultaneous submillimeter SPECT and PET. J Nucl Med. 2013;54:306–12.
10. Yao R, Deng X, Beaudoin J-F, Ma T, Cadorette J, Cao Z, et al. Initial evaluation of LabPET/SPECT dual modality animal imaging system. IEEE Trans Nucl Sci. 2013;60:76–81.
11. Wang W, Zhao J, Wen X, Lin CC-J, Li J, Huang Q, et al. MicroPET/CT imaging of AXL downregulation by HSP90 inhibition in triple-negative breast cancer. Contrast Media Mol Imaging. 2017;2017:1686525.
12. Goyanes A, Fernández-Ferreiro A, Majeed A, Gomez-Lado N, Awad A, Luaces-Rodríguez A, et al. PET/CT imaging of 3D printed devices in the gastrointestinal tract of rodents. Int J Pharm. 2018;536:158–64.
13. Chen B, Ojha DP, Toyonaga T, Tong J, Pracitto R, Thomas MA, et al. Preclinical evaluation of a brain penetrant PARP PET imaging probe in rat glioblastoma and nonhuman primates. Eur J Nucl Med Mol Imaging. 2023;50:2081–99.
14. Wanek T, Traxl A, Kuntner-Hannes C, Langer O. Investigation of transporter-mediated drug-drug interactions using PET/MRI. In: Kuntner-Hannes C, Haemisch Y, editors. Image fusion in preclinical applications. Cham: Springer International Publishing; 2019. p. 117–33. https://doi.org/10.1007/978-3-030-02973-9_6.
15. Marini C, Bianchi G, Buschiazzo A, Ravera S, Martella R, Bottoni G, et al. Divergent targets of glycolysis and oxidative phosphorylation result in additive effects of metformin and starvation in colon and breast cancer. Sci Rep. 2016;6:19569.
16. Dekempeneer Y, Massa S, Santens F, Navarro L, Berdal M, Lucero MM, et al. Preclinical evaluation of a radiotheranostic single-domain antibody against fibroblast activation protein α. J Nucl Med. 2023;64:1941–8.
17. Verhoeven J, Bolcaen J, De Meulenaere V, Kersemans K, Descamps B, Donche S, et al. Technical feasibility of [18F]FET and [18F]FAZA PET guided radiotherapy in a F98 glioblastoma rat model. Radiat Oncol. 2019;14:89.
18. Nekolla SG, Rischpler C, Paschali A, Anagnostopoulos C. Cardiovascular preclinical imaging. Q J Nucl Med Mol Imaging. 2017;61:48–59.

Dose Optimization in Hybrid Imaging

13

Tomoaki Yamamoto ⓘ, Mitsuha Fukami,
Norikazu Matsutomo ⓘ, and Kohei Hanaoka ⓘ

13.1 Introduction

Tomoaki Yamamoto

Single-photon emission computed tomography (SPECT)/computed tomography (CT) and positron emission tomography (PET)/CT are crucial for improving the quality of diagnostic imaging in nuclear medicine. These hybrid imaging modalities can simultaneously provide both functional and anatomical information by combining nuclear medicine images (SPECT or PET) with anatomical images (CT).

Moreover, CT both enhances diagnostic accuracy and contributes to improving the quantitative accuracy of SPECT and PET. Attenuation correction based on tissue attenuation coefficients obtained from CT images increases the reliability of nuclear medicine images and enhances the precision of quantitative evalua-

tions. Without this correction, the distribution of radiotracers would be difficult to assess accurately, potentially compromising the reliability of the diagnosis.

CT also plays a key role in the optimization of treatment planning through image guidance. This is particularly important in radiopharmaceutical therapy, where CT is essential for determining the precise location of tumors and their relationship with surrounding tissues.

However, the use of CT in SPECT/CT and PET/CT comes with the challenge of increased radiation exposure to patients. Therefore, from the perspective of radiation protection, it is necessary to optimize not only the dose from radiopharmaceuticals but also the CT dose, depending on the clinical application. Recent advances, such as the introduction of low-dose CT techniques and adaptive filtering technologies, have enabled the reduction of radiation exposure while maintaining diagnostic quality.

In sum, CT in SPECT/CT and PET/CT are indispensable tools for improving diagnostic accuracy, enhancing the precision of quantitative evaluations, and optimizing treatment planning. Appropriate dose management and technological advancements will continue to be critical issues in balancing diagnostic efficacy with patient safety.

T. Yamamoto (✉) · M. Fukami · N. Matsutomo
Faculty of Health Sciences, Department of Medical Radiological Technology, Kyorin University,
Mitaka-Shi, Tokyo, Japan
e-mail: tyamamoto@ks.kyorin-u.ac.jp;
mitsuha-f@ks.kyorin-u.ac.jp;
nmatsutomo@ks.kyorin-u.ac.jp

K. Hanaoka
Division of Positron Emission Tomography, Institute of Advanced Clinical Medicine, Kindai University,
Osaka, Japan
e-mail: khanaoka@med.kindai.ac.jp

© The Author(s), under exclusive license to Springer Nature Switzerland AG 2025
L. Camoni, L. Mansi (eds.), *Nuclear Medicine Hybrid Imaging for Radiographers & Technologists*,
https://doi.org/10.1007/978-3-031-86228-1_13

13.2 Medical Internal Radiation Dose (MIRD) Method

The Medical Internal Radiation Dose (MIRD) method, first described in 1968 in MIRD Pamphlet No. 1 [1], has long been used for estimating internal radiation exposure in nuclear medicine, evolving to the present day. The method is described in detail by Zanzonico [2], including new findings. To explain the principle briefly, the source region (r_s) and target region (r_t) are selected from among several organs, and the dose to the target region (D_{r_t}) is determined. The dose can be calculated using Eq. (13.1).

$$D_{r_t} = \sum_s \int_0^\infty A_s \, dt \, S\left(r_s \rightarrow r_t\right) \qquad (13.1)$$

Here, $\int_0^\infty A_s \, dt$ is the accumulated radioactivity, which is the integral of radioactivity from the time of administration to the time of complete elimination in all source regions; and S is the dose delivered to the target region in the source region (Gy). Monte Carlo simulations are used for these calculations, where estimates are calculated using male and female model phantoms for several age groups, from newborns to adults. However, what all these methods have in common is that they all use models that mimic healthy subjects to derive estimates, and not data from individual subjects with different metabolic functions.

In accordance with the "as low as reasonably achievable (ALARA)" principle, radiation exposure should be kept as low as possible, while at the same time avoiding any negative impact on examination results from reducing exposure. Therefore, the relationship between radiation dose and physical image quality metrics should be considered. While adult doses are provided for each radiopharmaceutical, in children the doses are currently adjusted according to body weight. Guidelines for determining these doses have been released by nuclear medicine societies in several countries. Since each of these guidelines has their own characteristics, it is advisable to refer to guidelines that are appropriate for your region.

Recently, in addition to estimating internal exposure resulting from examinations and exposure from computed tomography (CT) with hybrid imaging systems, there is a strong need to accurately predict the dose delivered to target organs in nuclear medicine therapy. This can be achieved, as shown in Fig. 13.1, by organ segmentation and determining time activity curves for each organ with hybrid imaging, from which three-dimensional physical dosimetry and bioeffective dosimetry based on pharmacokinetics can be derived so that the dose delivered to the target and surrounding organs in nuclear medicine therapy can be determined with high accuracy. Toward this goal, it is expected that methods utilizing deep learning and other technologies will be widely introduced.

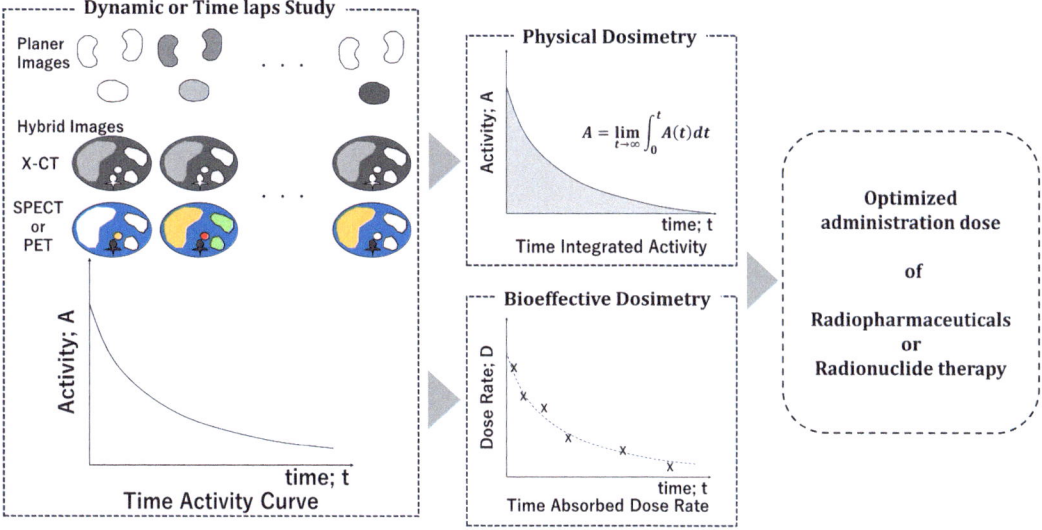

Fig. 13.1 Imaging-based optimal dose calculation algorithm for nuclear medicine examination/therapy

13.3 Dosage Guidelines

Tomoaki Yamamoto

Traditionally, the dose of radiopharmaceuticals administered to children has been adjusted according to their age, using Eq. (13.2). However, there is a large difference in body weight among children of the same age, suggesting that weight-based adjustment is more appropriate.

$$\text{Pediatric dose} (\text{MBq}) = \text{adult dose} \times \frac{(\text{age} + 1)}{(\text{age} + 7)} \quad (13.2)$$

The European Association of Nuclear Medicine (EANM), Society of Nuclear Medicine and Molecular Imaging (SNMMI), Japan Society of Nuclear Medicine (JSNM), and other societies have published guidelines on their websites regarding the dosage of radiopharmaceuticals. The dosage for examinations in children, who are particularly sensitive to radiation exposure, should be determined according to the guidelines appropriate for each country. In 2014, the EANM and SNMMI jointly published a guideline document [3], based on which the JSNM issued a guideline document [4] in 2014. This section provides an overview of the guidelines.

The names of radiopharmaceuticals differ among countries and regions. Table 13.1 shows a combined dosage card based on the EANM/SNMMI and JSNM guidelines. Table 13.2 shows the class- and body weight-specific coefficients proposed by the JSNM.

Based on this table, the optimal dose for children is calculated using the following equation.

Administered activity (MBq) = Baseline activity in Table 13.1 × Body weight - specific coefficient in Table 13.2

If the result is less than the minimum activity, the minimum activity should be used. If the result is higher than the adult dose, the adult dose should be used.

Below is an example calculation:

If a fludeoxyglucose-18 (FDG) scan is performed on a child weighing 10 kg, the baseline activity according to the JSNM guidelines is 14.0 MBq regardless of the site, whereas the EANM/SNMMI guidelines specify 14.0 and

Table 13.1 Dosage card based on the JSNM and EANM/SNMMI guidelines

Nuclides	Radiopharmaceuticals EANM/SNMMI	JSNM	Class	Baseline activity (MBq) EANM/JSNM	Minimum activity (MBq) EANM/JSNM
I-123	(Thyroid)	NaI	C	0.6	3
	Amphetamine (brain)	Iofetamine	B	13.0	18
	Hippuran (abnormal)		B	5.3/---	10/---
	Hippuran (normal)		A	12.8/---	10/---
	MIBG	MIBG (tumors)	B	28.0/28.0	37/40
		MIBG (myocardium)	B	---/7.9	---/16
		Iomazenil	B	---/11.9	---/24
		BMIPP	B	---/7.9	---/16
F-18	(torso)		B	25.9/---	26/---
	(brain)	FDG	B	14.0	14
	Sodium fluoride		B	10.5/---	14/---
Ga-67	Citrate	Citrate	B	5.6	10
Tc-99m	Albumin (cardiac)	Albumin (cardiac pool)	B	56.0	80
	Colloid (gastric reflex)		B	2.8/---	10/---
	Colloid (liver/spleen)	Sn colloid (liver/spleen)	B	5.6	15
	Colloid (marrow)	Sn colloid (bone marrow)	B	21.0	20
		Phytate (liver/spleen)	B	---/5.6	---/15
	MDP	MDP/HMDP (bone)	B	35.0	40
	DMSA	DMSA	B	6.8/25.6	18.5/15
	DTPA (abnormal)		B	14.0/---	20/---
	DTPA (normal)	DTPA	A	34.0	20
	MAG3	MAG3	A	11.9/34.0	15/20
	ECD (brain perfusion)	ECD	B	32.0	110
	HMPAO (brain)	HMPAO	B	51.8	100
	HMPAO (WBC)		B	35.0/---	40/---
	IDA (biliary)	PMT	B	10.5	20
	Spleen (denatured RBC)		B	70.0/---	100/---
	MAA/microsheres	MAA	B	5.6/13.2	10/10
	Pertechnetate (cystography)		B	1.4/---	20/---
	Pertechnetate (gastric mucosa)	Pertechnetate (gastric mucosa)	B	10.5	20
	Pertechnetate (cardiac first pass)		B	35.0/---	80/---
	Pertechnetate (thyroid)	Pertechnetate (thyroid)	B	5.6	10
	RBC (blood pool)	RBC	B	56.0	80
	Sestamibi/tetrofosmin (cancer)	MIBI/tetorofosmin (tumor)	B	63.0	80
	Sestamibi/tetrofosmin (cardiac rest 2-day min)	MIBI/tetorofosmin (myocardium rest/stress 2-day max)	B	42.0/---	80/---
	Sestamibi/tetrofosmin (cardiac rest 2-day max)		B	63.0/---	80/---
	Sestamibi/tetrofosmin (cardiac stress 2-day min)		B	42.0/---	80/---
	Sestamibi/tetrofosmin (cardiac stress 2-day max)		B	63.0/---	80/---
	Sestamibi/tetrofosmin (cardiac rest 1-day)	MIBI/tetorofosmin (cardiac first scan 1-day)	B	28.0	80
	Sestamibi/tetrofosmin (cardiac stress 1-day)	MIBI/tetorofosmin (cardiac second scan 1-day)	B	84.0/84.0	80/160
		GSA	B	---/5.3	---/11
	Technegas (lung ventilation)		B	70.0/---	100/---
Tl-201		Chloride (tumor)	B	---/5.3	---/11
In-111		Chloride	B	---/5.3	---/11

Table 13.2 Body weight- and class-specific weight coefficients proposed by the JSNMT

Body weight (kg)	Class		
	A	B	C
3	1	1	1
4	1.12	1.14	1.33
6	1.47	1.71	2
8	1.71	2.14	3
10	1.94	2.71	3.67
12	2.18	3.14	4.67
14	2.35	3.57	5.67
16	2.53	4	6.33
18	2.71	4.43	7.33
20	2.88	4.86	8.33
22	3.06	5.29	9.33
24	3.18	5.71	10
26	3.35	6.14	11
28	3.47	6.43	12
30	3.65	6.86	13
32	3.77	7.29	14
34	3.88	7.72	15
36	4	8	16
38	4.18	8.43	17
40	4.29	8.86	18
42	4.41	9.14	19
44	4.53	9.57	20
46	4.65	10	21
48	4.77	10.29	22
50	4.88	10.71	23
52–54	5	11.29	24.67
56–58	5.24	12	26.67
60–62	5.47	12.71	28.67
64–66	5.65	13.43	31
68	5.77	14	32.33

25.9 MBq for the brain and torso, respectively. Therefore, the calculation results are as follows:

JSNM : $14 \times 2.71 = 140\,\text{MBq}$
EANM (Brain) : $14 \times 2.71 = 140\,\text{MBq}$
EANM (Torso) : $25.9 \times 2.71 = 259\,\text{MBq}$

For example, if the optimal dose for an adult is standardized at 370 MBq, then the calculated value should be used in the above example. Figure 13.2 shows a graph comparing doses based on the different guidelines in the body weight range of

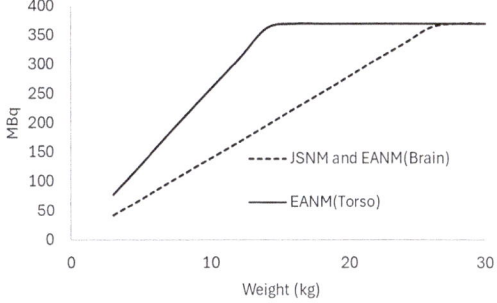

Fig. 13.2 Optimal dose by body weight

3–30 kg. If most FDG scans are performed on tumors throughout the body, there are differences in doses between the guidelines in the lower weight range. The dosage should be determined in consideration of the situation in each country.

13.4 Metrics for Radiation Exposure from CT in Hybrid Imaging

Mitsuha Fukami

In nuclear medicine, hybrid imaging systems are increasingly used to identify lesion sites as well as for attenuation correction. Hybrid imaging involves radiation exposure, which cannot be measured directly. It is therefore necessary to evaluate the exposure using exposure metrics. This section describes the exposure metrics for X-ray CT used in hybrid imaging and their evaluation methods. The CT exposure metrics currently standardized by organizations such as the International Atomic Energy Agency (IAEA) and the International Electrotechnical Commission (IEC) include the computed tomography dose index (CTDI), dose-length product (DLP), size-specific dose estimate (SSDE), and organ dose estimation (ODE). Below are detailed descriptions of these metrics.

13.4.1 CTDI and DLP

CTDI represents air collision kerma measured using an ionization chamber and a phantom (Fig. 13.3), and is expressed in units of Gy. CTDI metrics include $CTDI_{100}$, weighted $CTDI_{100}$ ($CTDI_w$), and volume $CTDI_w$ ($CTDI_{vol}$).

$CTDI_{100}$ is calculated from the measurements at the center and four marginal sites of the phantom, and $CTDI_w$ is a weighted average of $CTDI_{100}$ at the center and five marginal sites of the phantom (Fig. 13.4). $CTDI_{vol}$ is $CTDI_w$ divided by the pitch factor. These metrics are given by Eqs. (13.3)–(13.5) below:

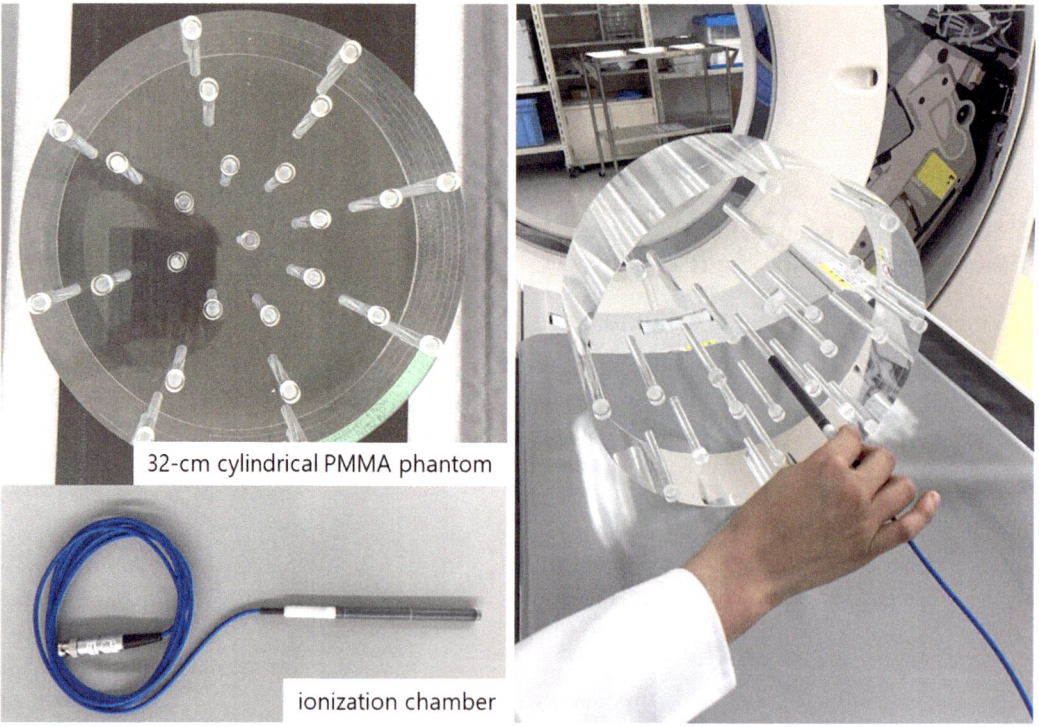

32-cm cylindrical PMMA phantom

ionization chamber

Fig. 13.3 Photographs of an ionization chamber and a phantom for CTDI measurement

$$\text{CTDI}_{100} = \frac{1}{\text{BW}} \int_{-50}^{+50} D_1(Z)\,dz \qquad (13.3)$$

BW represents the X-ray beam width and $D_1(Z)$ represents the dose profile at the center of the gantry.

$$\text{CTDI}_{\text{w}} = \frac{1}{3}\text{CTDI}_{100\,\text{center}} + \frac{2}{3}\text{CTDI}_{100\,\text{peripheral}} \quad (13.4)$$

$$\text{CTDI}_{\text{vol}} = \frac{1}{\text{PF}}\text{CTDI}_{\text{w}} \qquad (13.5)$$

Pitch factor (PF) is the table displacement divided by the X-ray beam width.

DLP is CTDI_{vol} taking into account the scan length and is calculated by multiplying CTDI_{vol} by the scan length (L) as follows:

$$\text{DLP} = \text{CTDI}_{\text{vol}} \times L \qquad (13.6)$$

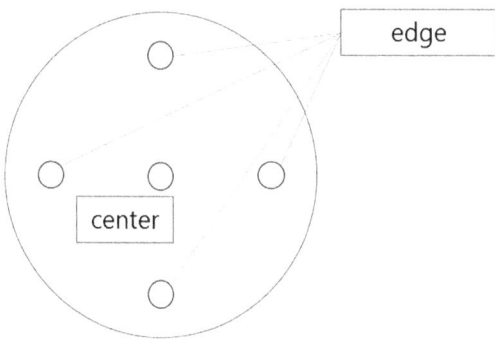

Fig. 13.4 Phantom position during CTDI measurement

CTDI_{vol} and DLP are required to be displayed on the console to allow for radiation dose management in CT.

13.4.2 Size-Specific Dose Estimates

CTDI_{vol} has been used for dosimetry. However, it was recently found to be underestimated in patients with a small body size. As a solution to the problem of size dependence of this metric, SSDE was developed as a new metric by the AAPM in 2011. SSDE is obtained by multiplying CTDI by a conversion factor known as effective diameter (ED), allowing the determination of radiation exposure taking the patient's size into account [5].

SSDE can be calculated by the following formula based on Eq. (13.7):

$$\text{SSDE} = \text{Conversion factor}_{\text{ED}} \times \text{CTDI}_{\text{vol}} \quad (13.7)$$

Here "Conversion factor$_{\text{ED}}$" is a conversion factor based on the effective diameter calculated from the longest and shortest diameters of the CT axial cross-section (Fig. 13.5).

For detailed values, refer to the AAPF report [5].

Although the use of SSDE eliminated the problem of size dependence, this metric did not consider the density of the human body, raising concerns about underestimation of exposure in

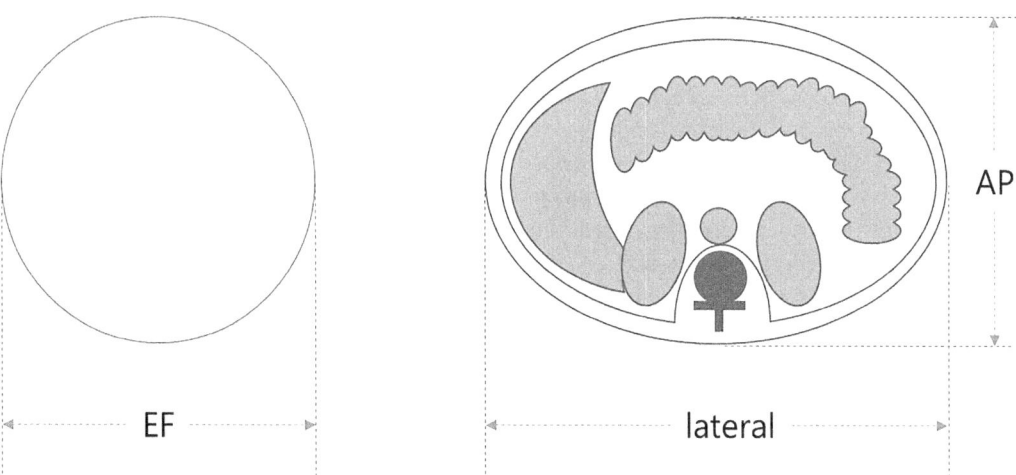

Fig. 13.5 Concept of the effective diameter

the thoracic region compared with the abdominal region. Then, the AAPM in 2014 proposed a method for calculating SSDE based on water-equivalent diameters [6].

$$SSDE = \text{conversion factor}_{Dw} \times CTDI_{vol} \quad (13.8)$$

The conversion factor $_{Dw}$ is determined according to the water-equivalent diameter, which is calculated from the water-equivalent area calculated from the pixel values of a CT image.

Rajaraman et al. calculated and compared $CTDI_{vol}$ and SSED, which takes into account the effective diameter, in 111 patients weighing an average of 62 kg who underwent myocardial perfusion single-photon emission computed tomography (SPECT)/CT. The results showed that $CTDI_{vol}$ was lower than SSDE, indicating that the radiation dose may be underestimated in patients with a small size [7]. Shah et al. calculated SSDE using a conversion factor that takes into account water-equivalent diameters and found that the thoracic SSDE was greater than the abdominal SSDE, concluding that the use of SSDE would allow more accurate estimation of radiation exposure [8]. Thus, SSDE has become the primary radiation exposure metric as it allows for more accurate estimation.

13.4.3 Radiation Exposure in Different Organs

The aforementioned metrics, such as $CTDI_{vol}$ and SSED, are physical quantities and cannot be used directly as measures of radiation exposure in different organs. Accordingly, exposure in each organ needs to be estimated by simulation or other methods. These estimation methods include measuring absorbed doses using a human phantom and simulation using a digital phantom. The method using human phantoms can estimate doses in only patients with a standard size, while the simulation-based method using digital phantoms can provide customized estimates for individual patients.

Various dosimetry software products have been released by academic societies and companies. CT-Expo (SASCRAD) is software developed in Germany and uses phantoms that only assume male patients. ImPACT (National Radiological Protection Board: NRPB) is a software developed in the UK and uses MIRD-type phantoms to construct an organ exposure dose database. VirtualDose is a software released by Virtual Phantoms Inc. Recently, an increasing number of reports have been published comparing these software products. Gao et al. compared ImPACT, CT-Expo, and VirtualDose and reported that the difference in effective dose between Impact and VirtualDose was 32% [9]. Saeed also compared dose estimates in different organs using these three software products and reported that the between-software differences were larger in the colon, brain, esophagus, and thyroid gland [10]. These reports suggest that when using software for dose estimation, it is important to understand the characteristics of each software. In nuclear medicine, hybrid imaging systems equipped with CT are becoming increasingly popular. Therefore, it is important to accurately determine CT-related radiation exposure and thereby optimize protocols and reduce exposure.

13.5 Dose Reduction Technologies

Norikazu Matsutomo

X-ray CT technology has brought tremendous benefits to nuclear medicine and molecular imaging, contributing to improved diagnostic accuracy by enabling precise attenuation correction as well as providing accurate anatomical information and uptake locations. However, the use of X-ray CT technology inevitably increases medical radiation exposure to patients, making the appropriate use of the technology essential. Based on the ALARA principle, we need to effectively utilize technologies to reduce

Table 13.3 CT exposure reduction technologies available for nuclear medicine systems

	GE	CANON	SIEMENS	United Imaging
AEC	3D mA modulation	Volume EC	CARE dose 4D	Auto ALARA kVp Auto ALARA mA
Hybrid iterative reconstruction	ASiR ASiR-V	AIDR 3D AIDR 3D Enhanced	SAFIRE/ ADMIRE	KARL 3D iterative denoising reconstruction algorithm
Model-based iterative reconstruction				
Deep learning reconstruction	TrueFidelity	AiCE		DELTA (Deep Learning Trained Algorithm) uAI AIIR (Artificial Intelligence Iterative Reconstruction)

exposure as much as possible while optimizing protection and maintaining image quality and attenuation correction accuracy. Table 13.3 lists major X-ray CT exposure reduction technologies for currently available SPECT/CT and positron emission tomography (PET)/CT systems. This section provides an overview of these CT exposure reduction technologies and their features.

13.5.1 Automatic Exposure Control (AEC)

AEC is an important feature of X-ray CT systems. It automatically adjusts the tube current to obtain proper images with the minimum necessary X-ray dose according to the patient's size and the target region. The principles of AEC vary from manufacturer to manufacturer, including modulating the tube current for each slice based on the positioning images (AP and lateral views), modulating the tube current according to the shape and size of the patient during one rotation of the X-ray tube, and having the user set the reference image (standard deviation: SD) and modulating the tube current according to its image quality (Fig. 13.6). AEC works based on settings that take into account the imaging area and the patient's size. When used appropriately, AEC can minimize the radiation dose to the patient while maintaining the clinically necessary image quality. However, inappropriate settings can cause not only increased radiation dose, but also increased image noise, unwanted artifacts, and reduced image contrast. Therefore, the user should be fully aware of the characteristics of each AEC system. Especially in ^{18}F-FDG PET scans, it is important to understand the response characteristics of the AEC system because of the large variation in body thickness in the imaging range from the parietal to inguinal regions. When scanning children, setting the image quality level and reference body weight differently from those for adults can help prevent excessive doses (Fig. 13.7).

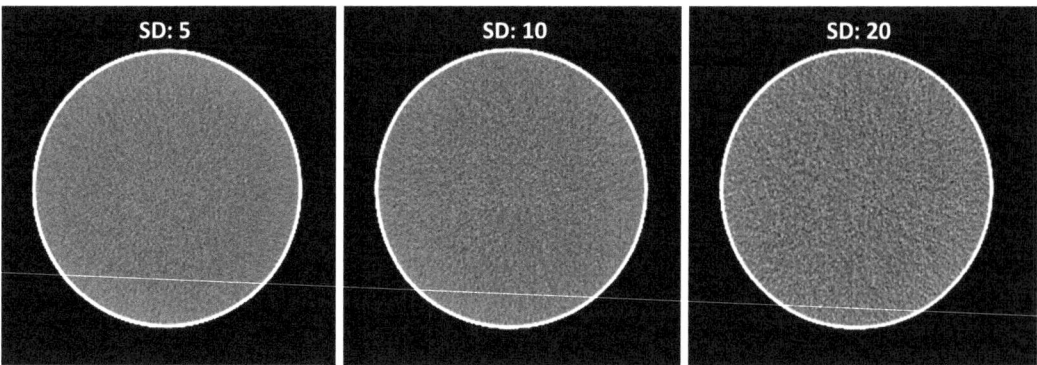

SD: automatic exposure control tube current SD

Fig. 13.6 Differences in CT images according to SD settings. Changing the SD of the volume EC (CANON) changes the quality of the CT image

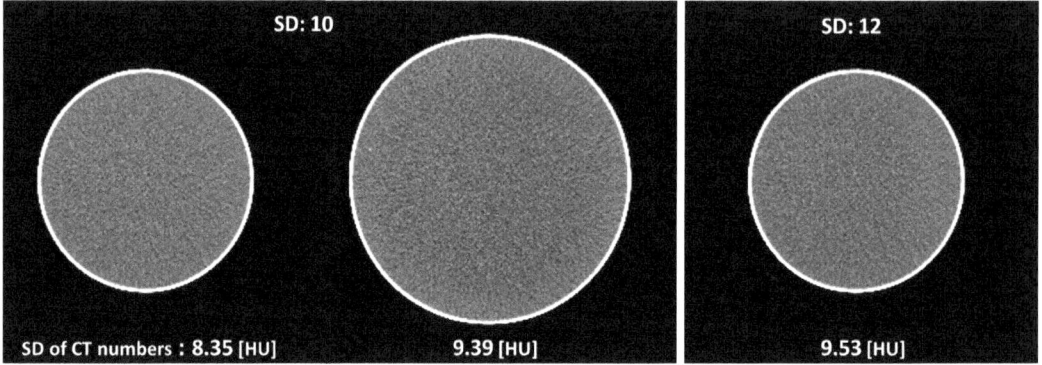

Fig. 13.7 Patient size and SD settings. When the same SD is applied, smaller patient sizes result in a lower actual SD. Thus, the same SD setting as for adults may result in an excess dose for children, necessitating different SD settings for children and adults

13.5.2 Statistical Iterative Image Reconstruction

Norikazu Matsutomo

Filtered back projection (FBP) is a long-standing, analytical CT image reconstruction method. However, the image noise characteristics limited how much the dose could be reduced during imaging. To overcome this limitation, the statistical iterative image reconstruction (hybrid iterative reconstruction) was introduced to reduce image noise. This reconstruction method is based on FBP with the introduction of successive approximation processing and has been reported to provide a certain level of dose reduction while maintaining low contrast resolution [11]. However, this method has been associated with reduced resolution and different image texture from FBP images depending on parameters, suggesting the need for careful consideration of the dose reduction.

Model-based iterative reconstruction (MBIR), an image reconstruction method based solely on successive approximation processing, is also used in CT. MBIR, like statistical iterative image reconstruction used in nuclear medicine, minimizes discrepancies between measured (observed) data and image-derived projected (calculated) data by iterative calculations. These discrepancies

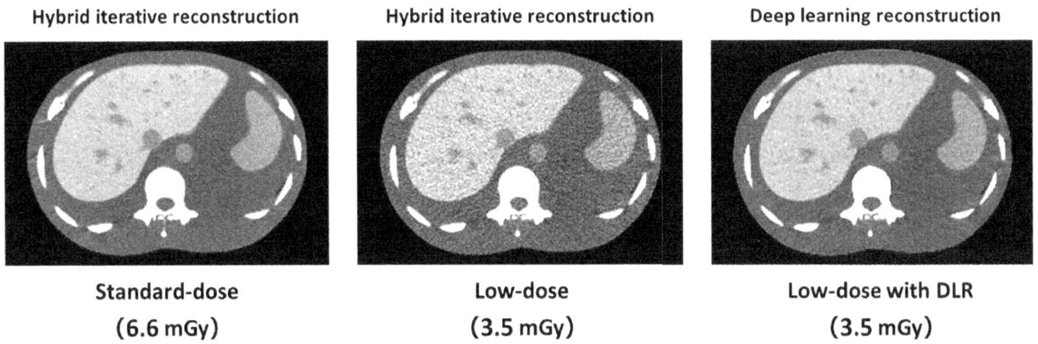

Hybrid iterative reconstruction	Hybrid iterative reconstruction	Deep learning reconstruction
Standard-dose (6.6 mGy)	Low-dose (3.5 mGy)	Low-dose with DLR (3.5 mGy)

Fig. 13.8 Effect of deep learning reconstruction. DLR provides noise reduction while maintaining higher sharpness compared with hybrid iterative reconstruction

are due to statistical noise, device-related geometric blurring, and artifacts. Thus, reflecting these error factors in the corrected data allows for the reduction of statistical noise and artifacts. MBIR is more effective in reducing statistical noise than statistical iterative image reconstruction, thus enabling imaging with a reduced radiation dose. In nuclear medicine, MBIR has also been shown to reduce radiation dose in CT scan without affecting SPECT/PET image quality and quantitativity [12]. It is expected that the use of statistical iterative image reconstruction and MBIR will become the norm in the future.

13.5.3 Deep Learning Reconstruction

Deep learning reconstruction (DLR) is a method for reducing statistical noise using deep learning technology, and is more like a filter-based noise reduction method than an image reconstruction method. In general, DLR uses a deep convolution neural network (DCNN) to reduce noise. The DCNN is constructed through a learning process in which images with low statistical noise are used as training data, and the corresponding low-dose (low-quality) images are made as close to the training data as possible. Although network structures vary among manufacturers, learning with images from high-end imaging systems as training data ensures that high-quality images can be obtained even on general-purpose systems (Fig. 13.8). Although DLR is limited in its range of use because it is only available on high-end

systems, it is considered to be useful in SPECT/CT and PET/CT scans as it is more effective than MBIR in reducing noise and provides less discrepancies in image texture [13].

13.5.4 Other Technologies (Low-kV Technology, Tin-Filter, Organ Dose Modulation, Etc.)

Other dose reduction technologies include low-kV imaging, optimization of the X-ray spectrum by combining additional filters such as Bowtie filters with tin filters, and organ dose modulation, in which the tube current at the front side of the body is lowered to reduce the dose to radiation-sensitive superficial organs, such as the lens and mammary gland. It remains to be determined whether these technologies can be applied to SPECT/CT and PET/CT scans without problems, necessitating the establishment of new evidence to reduce radiation exposure in patients.

13.6 CT-Based Attenuation Correction (CTAC)

Kohei Hanaoka

In nuclear medicine examinations, as γ-rays emitted from the source inside the body are detected outside of the body to produce images, they are subject to attenuation and scattering due to interactions as they pass through the human body and reach the detector. There are several methods to correct for this attenuation. In SPECT, correction methods that assume a homogeneous absorber (e.g., Chang's method and Sorenson's method) have conventionally been used. In some PET systems, transmission scanning with ^{68}Ge-^{68}Ga external sources has been used to correct for heterogeneous absorbers. In the PET/CT and SPECT/CT systems commonly used currently, CTAC, in which the CT image is converted into an attenuation coefficient distribution (μ-map), is in widespread use [14]. In PET and PET/MR systems dedicated to specific areas, such as the head and breast, special algorithms or CT images taken separately are used for attenuation correction, rather than CT-AC [15].

Figure 13.9 shows a comparison of images and profile curves with and without attenuation correction in ^{18}F-FDG PET/CT scan. Without attenuation correction, high counts are observed around the human body, with some counts also observed outside the body. In contrast, the results with attenuation correction show that these effects can be diminished. Corrections are important to obtain an accurate radioactivity distribution in nuclear medicine examinations, and in particular, attenuation correction is essential in obtaining accurate quantitative values such as SUV.

13.7 Optimization of CTAC

Kohei Hanaoka

Figure 13.10 shows different types of CT images taken and reconstructed from ^{18}F-FDG PET/CT scans and their characteristics. With a typical PET/CT imaging protocol, two CT images are reconstructed from the raw data obtained by a single CT scan, one for attenuation correction CT (ACCT) and the other for site localization. If the field of view (FOV) of the PET data is larger than that of the ACCT data, care must be taken in setting the FOV because no correction is made in the area outside the FOV of CT, possibly causing truncation artifacts (the FOV of CT for site localization should match that of the PET) [16]. It is also effective to have both arms raised in patients

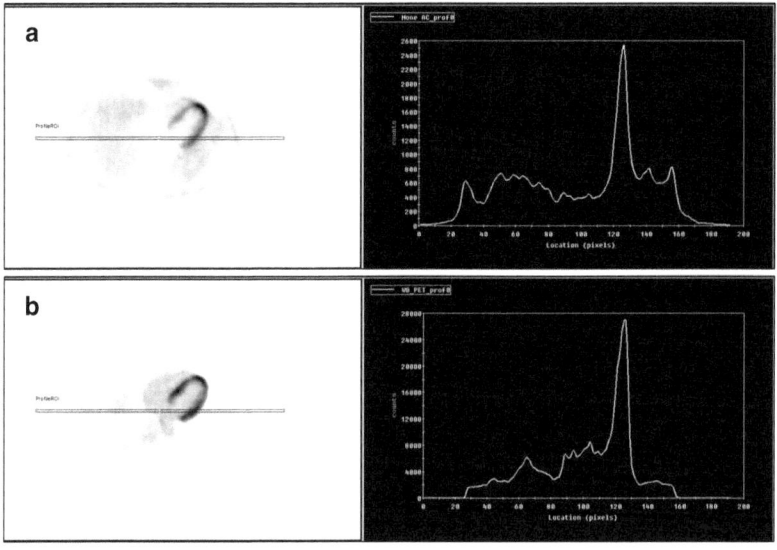

Fig. 13.9 Comparison of ^{18}F-FDG PET images (left) and profile curves (right) without CTAC (top) and with CTAC (bottom). (**a**) None-AC, (**b**) AC with CT

who have no problem doing so based on diagnosis, in order to take advantage of the benefits of reduced exposure by AEC. The current value and scan pitch are set based on the clinically required image quality for CT images for site identification.

SPECT and PET images are often scanned under free-breathing conditions, except when special acquisition techniques are used. Therefore, if a CT scan taken under deep breathing is used as an ACCT scan, discrepancies in organ positions will occur, which will interfere with accurate attenuation. When adding a diagnostic CT scan taken under breath-hold as shown in Fig. 13.10d, additional imaging should be done separately from (b) and (c) to the minimum extent necessary.

CT data obtained with SPECT/CT and PET/CT systems are used not only for anatomical diagnosis or accurate site localization by combining CT, SPECT, and PET images, but also for attenuation correction of nuclear medicine images. To reduce radiation exposure, imaging conditions such as CT dose and imaging range should be considered based on their impact on CT image quality and quantitative values.

13.8 Automatic Organ Segmentation and Dose Estimation by Deep Learning

Tomoaki Yamamoto

It is impossible to actually measure the accumulated dose to all organs separately; the key is to estimate the dose with high accuracy. MIRD is one of the methods used for this purpose and is currently being developed for improved accuracy. Although the accumulated dose associated with nuclear medicine examinations is strongly affected by the biological factors of each patient, it is possible to estimate the accumulated dose for individual organs by hybrid imaging in nuclear medicine. Recently, deep learning has been made available free of charge or at affordable prices. U-Net [17, 18] is often used for organ segmentation. U-Net typically uses (1) fully convolutional network (FCN), (2) deconvolution, and (3) skip connection. Figure 13.11 shows a schematic algorithm of U-Net, which may be familiar to many readers, and is named after its overall shape resembling a "U." The first half of the algorithm performs convolution, and the second half performs deconvolution.

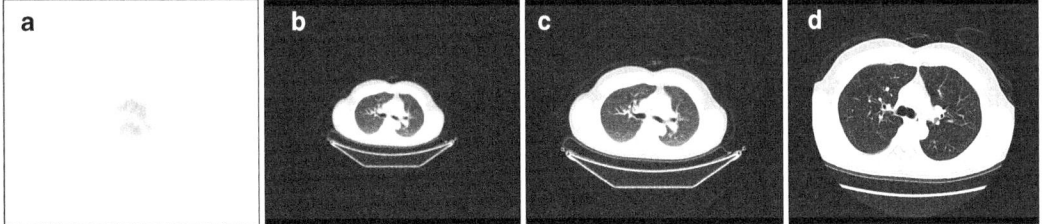

Role of CT	Attenuation correction CT	Localization CT	Diagnosis CT
Axial FOV (cm)	70	50	35
Tube current (mA)	150		200
CTDI vol (mGy)	5.24		9.44
DLP (mGy · cm)	527.9		340.5

Fig. 13.10 Examples of CT images taken and reconstructed by ^{18}F-FDG PET/CT scanning, with exposure-related features image quality improving in the order (**a**) → (**b**) → (**c**). The radiation dose is greater in (**d**) than in (**a**) and (**c**). (**a**) PET image. (**b**) Attenuation correction CT. (**c**) Localization CT. (**d**) Diagnosis CT

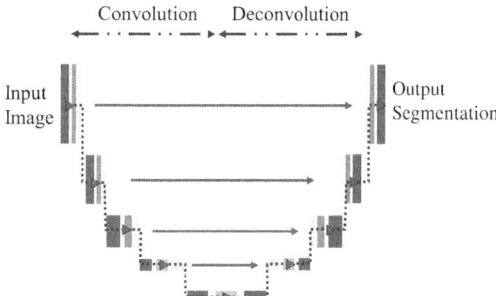

Fig. 13.11 U-Net algorithm

Hybrid imaging uses CT images with high spatial resolution for accurate organ segmentation, which can be fused with SPECT or PET images to determine the organ-specific accumulation rate of radiopharmaceuticals, along with precise positional information on their three-dimensional distribution. These data can then be used to determine physical and biological doses, potentially allowing accurate organ-specific doses to be estimated for individual patients. Although still in the developmental stages, these methods could be used for both managing radiation dose from examinations and performing nuclear medicine therapy, based on more accurate evidence.

References

1. Lassmann M, Treves ST, EANM/SNMMI Paediatric Dosage Harmonization Working Group. Paediatric radiopharmaceutical administration: harmonization of the 2007 EANM paediatric dosage card (version 1.5.2008) and the 2010 North American consensus guidelines. Eur J Nucl Med Mol Imaging. 2014;41(5):1036–41.
2. The Japanese Society of Nuclear Medicine, Optimization Committee for Pediatric Nuclear Medicine Studies. Japanese consensus guidelines for pediatric nuclear medicine. Ann Nucl Med. 2014;28:498–503.
3. Loevinger R, Berman M. A schema for absorbed dose calculations for biologically distributed radionuclides, MIRD pamphlet no. 1. J Nucl Med. 1968;Suppl 1:9–14.
4. Zanzonico P. The MIRD schema for radiopharmaceutical dosimetry: a review. J Nucl Med Technol. 2024;52(2):74–85. https://doi.org/10.2967/jnmt.123.265668.
5. American Association of Physicists in Medicine (AAPM). Size-specific dose estimates (SSDE) in pediatric and adult body CT examinations. AAPF report; 2011.
6. McCollough C, Bakalyar DM, Bostani M. Use of water equivalent diameter for calculating patient size and size-specific dose estimates (SSDE) in CT: the report of AAPM Task Group 220. AAPM Rep. 2014;2014:6–23.
7. Rajaraman V, Ponnusamy M, Halanaik D. Size specific dose estimate (SSDE) for estimating patient dose from CT used in myocardial perfusion SPECT/CT. Asia Ocean J Nucl Med Biol. 2020;8:58–63.
8. Shah MA, Ahmad M, Khalid S, et al. Multivariate analysis of effective dose and size-specific dose estimates for thorax and abdominal computed tomography. J Med Phys. 2023;48:210–8.
9. Gao Y, Quinn B, Mahmood U, et al. A comparison of pediatric and adult CT organ dose estimation methods. BMC Med Imaging. 2017;17(1):28.
10. Saeed MK. A comparison of the CT-dosimetry software packages based on stylized and boundary representation phantoms. Radiography (Lond). 2022;26:e214–22.
11. Jia Q, Zhuang J, Jiang J, Li J, Huang M, Liang C. Image quality of CT angiography using model-based iterative reconstruction in infants with congenital heart disease: comparison with filtered back projection and hybrid iterative reconstruction. Eur J Radiol. 2017;86:190–7.
12. Matsutomo N, Nagaki A, Sasaki M. Validation of the CT iterative reconstruction technique for low-dose CT attenuation correction for improving the quality of PET images in an obesity-simulating body phantom and clinical study. Nucl Med Commun. 2015;36(8):839–47.
13. Higaki T, Nakamura Y, Zhou J, Yu Z, Nemoto T, Tatsugami F, et al. Deep learning reconstruction at CT: phantom study of the image characteristics. Acad Radiol. 2020;27:82–7. https://doi.org/10.1016/j.acra.2019.09.008.
14. Kinahan PE, Hasegawa BH, Beyer T. X-ray-based attenuation correction for positron emission tomography/computed tomography scanners. Semin Nucl Med. 2003;33(3):166–79.
15. Ishii K, Hanaoka K, Watanabe S, et al. High-resolution silicon photomultiplier time-of-flight dedicated head PET system for clinical brain studies. J Nucl Med. 2023;64(1):153–8.
16. Burger C, Goerres G, Schoenes S, et al. PET attenuation coefficients from CT images: experimental evaluation of the transformation of CT into PET 511 keV attenuation coefficients. Eur J Nucl Med. 2002;29(922):927.
17. Ronneberger O, Fischer P, Brox T. U-net: convolutional networks for biomedical image segmentation. arXiv:1505.04597v1; 2015. https://arxiv.org/pdf/1505.04597.
18. Zhou Z, Siddiquee MMR, Tajbakhsh N, et al. UNet++: a nested U-Net architecture for medical image segmentation. Deep Learn Med Image Anal Multimodal Learn Clin Decis Support (2018). 2018;11045:3–11.

Hybrid Imaging in Radionuclide Therapy

14

Pedro Fragoso Costa ⓘ,
Henry-Aravinth Devendranath,
and Alexandros Moraitis

14.1 Introduction

Nuclear medicine (NM) therapy is at a pivotal moment, with an unprecedented number of patients undergoing treatment and an ever-increasing armoury of radiopharmaceuticals in development. Imaging and dosimetry have been crucial since the inception of these treatments, playing a key role in optimizing procedures and enhancing their safety and efficacy. To guide the future of this field, it is essential to reflect on the scientific and technological progress made since its early days.

14.2 The Evolution of Hybrid Imaging in NM Therapy

The origins of NM can be traced back to the early twentieth century with the discovery of radioactivity by Henri Becquerel and the pioneering work of Marie and Pierre Curie. The application of radioactive substances for medical purposes began to take shape in the 1930s and 1940s [1, 2].

P. Fragoso Costa (✉) · H.-A. Devendranath
A. Moraitis
Department of Nuclear Medicine, University Hospital
Essen, Essen, Germany
e-mail: pedro.fragosocosta@uk-essen.de;
pedro.fragoso-costa@uni-duisburg-essen.de;
henry.devendranath@uk-essen.de;
alexandros.moraitis@uk-essen.de

The first significant technical breakthrough was the development of the rectilinear scanner and the scintillation camera by Benedict Cassen and Hal Anger, respectively, in the 1950s [3, 4]. These devices were the first to allow for the visualization of radioactive tracers within the body.

See what you treat

While early NM imaging provided valuable functional data in a two-dimensional manner, it lacked the anatomical context needed for precise localization of tracer accumulation. This limitation led to the first crucial development for hybrid imaging: the development of three-dimensional imaging techniques. The first notable imaging technique dedicated to NM was single photon emission computed tomography (SPECT), introduced in the 1970s [5]. SPECT provided three-dimensional images by rotating the gamma camera around the patient. Yet, this imaging modality was still missing the anatomical information.

The second crucial step that marked the era of hybrid imaging began with the integration of computed tomography (CT). This was first achieved in the context of positron emission tomography (PET). The development of PET/CT in the early 2000s marked a significant milestone [6]. This innovation was driven by the recognition that combining PET's high-sensitivity functional imaging with CT's high-resolution anatomical imaging could provide more accurate and comprehensive diagnostic information. The first commercial PET/CT scanner was introduced in 2001, and its success spurred the development of SPECT/CT systems.

From grey to glow

Since then, hybrid imaging has profoundly affected NM. In radionuclide therapy, precise targeting of lesions is crucial to maximize therapeutic efficacy while minimizing damage to healthy tissues. Hybrid imaging enables the precise delineation of target areas and the identification of critical structures, enhancing the planning and delivery of therapies via careful patient selection and optimization of inclusion criteria (more in Sect 14.4) [7].

Pretherapeutically, it provides comprehensive diagnostic information by correlating functional with anatomical findings. This is particularly evident in oncology, where PET/CT and SPECT/CT can distinguish between benign and malignant lesions and detect metastatic disease with high sensitivity and specificity [8].

Treat what you see

In the future, this may reduce the need for invasive procedures such as biopsies and exploratory surgeries, which not only lowers the risk to patients but also reduces healthcare costs and facilitates patient management.

The field of hybrid imaging continues to evolve, with ongoing advancements aimed at improving image quality and quantification accuracy, reducing patient radiation exposure, and expanding the range of clinical applications. Developments in algorithms for reliable and robust image reconstruction, as well as the incorporation of artificial intelligence, hold promise for enhancing the capabilities of hybrid imaging [9, 10]. Its history in NM is a testament to the continuous quest for better diagnostic and therapeutic tools. From the early days of functional imaging to the sophisticated hybrid systems of today, each advancement has contributed to moving towards personalized medicine.

14.3 Theranostic Concept

Theranostics, a fusion of therapy and diagnostics, represents a revolutionary approach in modern medicine. By combining targeted therapeutic interventions with precise diagnostic techniques, theranostics aims to personalize treatment and improve patient outcomes (Fig. 14.1). This integrated strategy allows for real-time monitoring of the treatment's effectiveness and adjustments tailored to the individual's response [11].

A cornerstone of theranostics is hybrid imaging, which merges different imaging modalities to provide comprehensive insights into the underlying biological processes at play [12]. Techniques such as PET/CT, SPECT/CT [13], and PET/MR [14] combine the functional imaging capabilities of PET or SPECT with the detailed anatomical information provided by CT or MRI. This integrated approach enhances the accuracy of disease diagnosis, staging, and treatment monitoring [15].

Hybrid imaging not only enables precise localization of disease but also aids in assessing the distribution and efficacy of therapeutic agents in the body. By visualizing the interaction between the therapeutic agents and their targets, clinicians can make informed decisions about treatment plans and adjustments [16]. This dual capability of diagnosing and treating in a single, seamless process is what positions theranostics at the frontier of personalized medicine, offering new hope for improved patient care and outcomes.

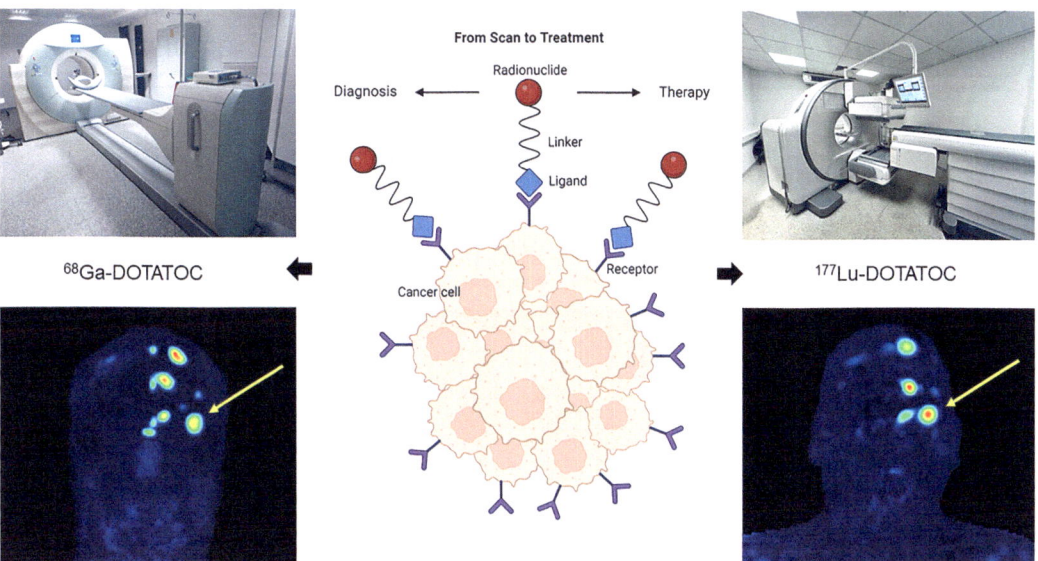

Fig. 14.1 The theranostic concept exemplified by somatostatin receptor directed diagnostic imaging (^{68}Ga-DOTATOC, left panel, Courtesy of Siemens Medical Solutions USA, Inc.) and therapy (^{177}Lu-DOTATOC, right panel) in meningioma

14.4   Therapeutic Nuclear Medicine Imaging

Besides attenuation correction, which is pivotal for accurate three-dimensional imaging of activity distributions, hybrid imaging allows for a precise assessment of disease extent. This enables physicians to monitor disease status and to guide treatment throughout the course of several treatment cycles depending on treatment response from previous cycles. In addition, the combination of metabolic and anatomical imaging allows for response assessment in both anatomical and functional manner, which is important to differentiate between metabolically active and necrotic tumour tissues. In the following, several use-cases of hybrid imaging in the context of NM therapies will be described, focusing on the use of the established radionuclides Iodine-131 (^{131}I), Lutetium-177 (^{177}Lu), and Yttrium-90 (^{90}Y) (Fig. 14.2). For those radionuclides, decay characteristics and production are summarized in Table 14.1.

The use of ^{131}I in the treatment of thyroid cancer and benign thyroid diseases is well established. In addition, when labelled with metaiodobenzylguanidine (mIBG), [^{131}I]I-mIBG is used in the treatment of tumours deriving from neuronal crests such as pheochromocytomas and neuroblastomas [17]. [131]I decays by beta emission (606 keV maximum beta energy of primary decay mode, with a branching fraction [= probability to occur per decay] of 89.6%) and is associated with the prompt emission of gamma rays (364 keV, 81.5% yield). These make ^{131}I suitable for intratherapeutic imaging. For performing SPECT/CT with ^{131}I, high-energy collimators are required to handle the penetrating, high-energy gammas. Typically, high-energy general purpose (HEGP) or high-energy parallel hole (HEPH) collimators are used to optimize image quality. Acquisition times may vary based on the administered activity and patient-specific factors but generally range from 15 to 30 min per bed-position.

Peptide receptor radionuclide therapy (PRRT) using somatostatin receptor-targeting tracers, such as ^{177}Lu labelled [^{177}Lu]Lu-DOTATATE or [^{177}Lu]Lu-DOTATOC, has become a cornerstone in treating advanced, progressive, midgut neuroendocrine tumours [18]. In parallel, prostate-specific membrane antigen (PSMA) targeting

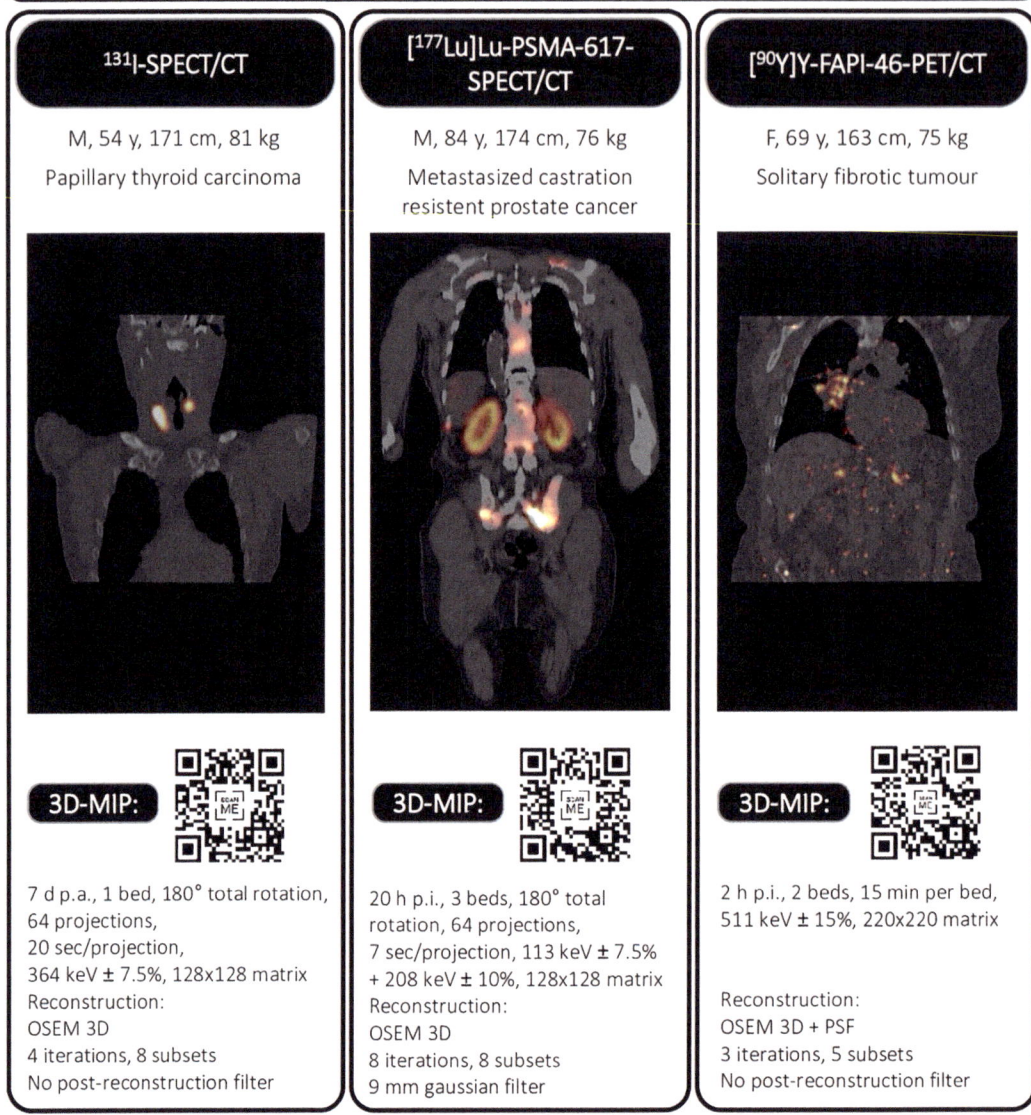

Fig. 14.2 Clinical examples of intra-therapeutic I-131 SPECT/CT, Lu-177-PSMA SPECT/CT and Y-90-PET/CT imaging

tracers, such as [^{177}Lu]Lu-PSMA-617 and [^{177}Lu]Lu-PSMA-I&T have revolutionized the treatment of metastatic castration-resistant prostate cancer [19]. ^{177}Lu decays by beta emission with a high branching fraction of 79.4% directly into stable Hafnium-177 (^{177}Hf, 497 keV maximum beta energy). However, 21.6% of decays result in intermediate excited states of ^{177}Hf. During relaxation into the ground state (stable ^{177}Hf), gamma rays are emitted. The two most dominant emissions have an energy of 208 and 113 keV and yield of 10.4% and 6.2%, respectively. Despite lower photon yield than ^{131}I, these gamma emissions are used clinically for SPECT/CT imaging. Theoretically, low-energy collimators would be sufficient for imaging of the 113-keV photopeak.

Table 14.1 Decay characteristics and production of the most relevant radionuclides for radioligand therapy

Radionuclide	Chemical characteristics	Diagnostic pairs	Endpoint beta-minus energy (prob. %)	Gamma emissions (prob. %)	Half-life	Approved radiopharmaceutical therapies
Iodide-131	Non-metallic solid	Iodine-123 (SPECT) Iodine-124 (PET)	606.3 keV (89.6)	364.5 keV (81.5)	8.0 d	[131I]NaI [131I]I-mIBG
Lutetium-177	Silvery white metal	Radiometals (PET Ga-68; SPECT In-111)	497 keV (79.4)	208 keV (10.4) 113 keV (6.2)	6.6 d	[177Lu]Lu-DOTATATE [177Lu]Lu-PSMA-617
Yttrium-90	Silvery-metallic transition metal	Radiometals (PET Ga-68; SPECT In-111)	2.28 MeV (~100)	Bremsstrahlung 511 keV (0.0006%)	2.67 d	[90Y]-Zevalin [90Y]-microspheres

However, Compton-scattered contribution from the higher 208-keV gammas leads to image blurring and impedes image quantification. Therefore, medium energy low penetration (MELP) or medium energy general purpose (MEGP) collimators are typically used, primarily focussing on the 208-keV photopeak. Acquisition times vary based on the system sensitivity and the administered activity but generally range from 10 to 20 min per bed-position.

^{90}Y decays by beta emission and with a branching fraction of almost 100% into stable Zirconium-90 (2.28 MeV maximum beta energy). These high-energy beta particles dissipate their kinetic energy while travelling through tissue producing a significant amount of bremsstrahlung. This radiation spectrum is used clinically for bremsstrahlung-SPECT/CT [20]. Bremsstrahlung-SPECT/CT is commonly used in the context of selective internal radiotherapy (SIRT) of primary liver malignancies (mostly hepatocellular carcinoma) and liver metastases (mostly from colorectal carcinoma). SIRT relies on the delivery of microscopic (20–60 μm), ^{90}Y labelled resin or glass microspheres directly into the vascular supply of the tumour via an intraarterial catheter.

In addition, ^{90}Y decays through a small transition to an excited state of ^{90}Zr at 1.75 MeV along with a positron emission with a maximum energy of 0.8 MeV. The positron then interacts with an electron and annihilates, emitting two 511-keV-photons. In fact, 32 out of 1 million ^{90}Y disintegrations result in electron-positron annihilation,

therefore, enabling low-count PET/CT imaging [21]. Importantly, ^{90}Y-PET/CT acquisition times may lie between 10 and 20 min per bed, which is untypical for PET/CT imaging, but necessary to compensate for the low positron yield [22]. Because of the quantitative nature of PET/CT, ^{90}Y-PET/CT is used for dosimetry purposes (more about dosimetry in Sect. 14.7) in exploratory studies in the context of fibroblast activation protein (FAP) targeted therapies. FAP is overexpressed in the tumour microenvironment of various cancer types. Early data from the use of [^{90}Y]Y-FAPI-04 and [^{90}Y]Y-FAPI-46 have shown effective treatment results with manageable adverse events in difficult-to-treat end stage cancer patients [23, 24]. In the future, it is expected that FAP targeted therapies will play a dominant role in NM.

14.5 Single-Photon Emission Computed Tomography/X-Ray Computed Tomography

With the growing field of radionuclide therapy, there is an increasing interest in its accurate quantification, serving to assess the efficacy and toxicity of the therapy by determining the dose to the lesion and healthy tissues. For example, in dose-finding studies, researchers are interested in finding the highest possible activity that is tolerable by a group of patients included in the study [25]. This means that the approved prescribed dose is the one that the most fragile member of the study can endure, not a patient-specific dose. To perform patient-specific therapies, a concept introduced in precision medicine [26], patient-specific dosimetry must be accurate and reliable. Dosimetry can be performed using various scintillation-based imaging modalities, including planar views, SPECT, or SPECT/CT [27]. The hybrid SPECT/CT offers the most accurate quantification and should therefore be preferred to the others [28].

Planar-based imaging is generally less accurate for internal dosimetry compared to SPECT/CT-quantification due to physical, physiological and anatomical factors [28]. First, planar acquisition does not allow for precise gamma-ray attenuation correction. A correction can be approximated with conjugated planar views [29] combined with planar transmission scans, which is only valid for infinitely thin organs. Anatomically, critical organs may be partially or fully covered by tissues with higher uptake. Corrections need to be precise and determined by phantom measurements covering all possible scenarios with partial and full tissue overlap, different biological half-life for different tissue and with moving activity (bowel for radioligand therapy) [30]. Lastly, some organs at risk are multi-compartmental, exhibiting different uptake, half-life and radiosensitivity in separate compartments [31]. These compartments need to be assessed independently, which is not possible in planar view.

In contrast to above-mentioned modalities, the hybrid SPECT/CT stand out due to its higher level of accuracy, as it allows for co-registration within a single study rather than in two systems independently in different patient studies [27]. This improves activity quantification and enables precise correlation between observed activity and the corresponding tissue. For precise attenuation correction, it is necessary to know the attenuation map of the patient, which is mostly done using a CT [32]. External transmission sources are gradually being used less for generating attenuation maps as CT-based attenuation maps offer lower noise, better spatial resolution, improved contrast and faster and easier acquisition, leading to more accurate quantification. The additional radiation exposure due to the CT (specially low-dose CT) is negligible when compared to the much higher absorbed dose received during therapy.

SPECT imaging techniques for quantification in radionuclide therapy are characterized by the measurement of gamma energy peaks from single or multiple emissions [33]. Those images are reconstructed, with the goal of achieving precise and reliable quantification in radionuclide therapy. For this, a sensitivity factor must be determined to translate detected counts into activity [34]. This requires a sensitivity calibration which must be assessed on a periodic basis. Additionally, accurate measurement of the injected activity is necessary, which involves pre- and post-syringe activity measurement including decay correction.

Beyond the injected activity, ensuring the accuracy of measured activity concentration in SPECT images requires selecting appropriate acquisition parameters. These include physical corrections such as attenuation-, scatter-, dead time- and partial volume-correction, as well as accounting for the collimator-detector-response. Existing reconstruction algorithms are optimized for the measurement conditions observed in therapeutic imaging. The choice of collimator is radionuclide-dependent and already mentioned above in Sect. 14.4. Continuous gantry-rotation for SPECT-data acquisition is preferred over step-and-shoot due to the large number of projections. To prevent counting losses, the width of the acquisition energy window should be at least twice the energy resolution (FWHM) of the detector. For radionuclides with multiple gamma emissions, it is recommended to consider all emissions to minimize noise with consistent accuracy, as it was shown in studies with Indium-111 [35]. In bremsstrahlung-imaging, energy window settings must be optimized individually for each radionuclide through simulations and phantom experiments. An energy window <100 keV impairs quantification due to down-scatter and significant contributions from lead X-rays originating from the collimator, making it unsuitable for use.

In radionuclide therapy, injected activities often exceed 4 GBq, potentially leading to significant counting losses due to dead time effects. Dead time correction is essential and should be incorporated before image reconstruction. This is particularly important for radionuclides with multiple photon emissions such as I-131, as even photons which are not included in the energy window contribute to the dead time. A study on the dosimetric impact of dead time correction after administering 4 GBq of I-131 showed that applying dead time correction increased whole body time-integrated activity to 8–11% [36].

The quality of the reconstructed image is degraded by Compton scatter of photons within the patient, camera or surrounding materials [37, 38]. Scatter correction can be based on energy or spatial distribution. In a clinical setting, dual energy or triple energy window (TEW) methods are commonly used for scatter estimation, with TEW scatter correction being the preferred approach for radionuclide therapy imaging with radionuclides presenting multiple photon emissions [33]. This method estimates the number of scattered photons contaminating the photopeak, based on the counts of two scatter windows of defined energy window width.

The reconstruction of the SPECT images can be performed using either filtered backprojection or on an iterative algorithm. The latter offers to minimize image degrading physical effects and improves noise suppresion, leading to a more accurate quantification [33, 39]. Iterative algorithms rely on mathematically simulated activity distributions that are iteratively approximated to the actual determined activity using forward projection, this process is repeated until calculated and measured activity distribution converges [33, 40, 41]. Since projected data is affected by statistical noise, statistical criteria are preferred. The most widely used algorithm in commercial SPECT systems is the ordered subset expectation maximization (OS-EM) algorithm, which updates the estimate multiple times per iteration using a different subset of the projections in each update [42].

The Collimator-Detector-Response (CDR) describes the image generated from a point source, with its shape being the predominant factor determining the spatial resolution of the SPECT system [33, 43]. Uncorrected, it results in image blurring and shape distortions in the reconstructed image. CDR-compensation is characterized by a point spread function, which consists of the detector's intrinsic response and the collimator response. This is further subdivided into geometric response, septal penetration and scatter component [44]. The intrinsic and geometric response are typically modeled using a Gaussian distribution, while the geometric response additionally incorporates a source-to-collimator-depended FWHM. Convolving both functions leads to an approximation which accounts primarily for low energy photons [33, 45]. For therapeutic radionuclides, septal penetration and scatter components have a significant contribution to the CDR and are determined either by Monte Carlo simulations or experimentally [45]. The determination of the energy-dependent total CDR must be established for each radionuclide by measuring the in-air point source response at various distances of the collimator.

The partial volume effect (PVE) is more evident in small structures or at the edges of large objects due to spill-in or spill-out [46], affecting activity quantification in these regions. Although a CDR correction within the iterative reconstruction reduces the PVE, partial volume correction (PVC) still needs to be applied for accurate quantification. Corrections can be approached by empirical, or anatomy-based methods [47, 48]. The latter is the most robust approach, using co-registered high-resolution CT (or MRT) images and can be applied to the whole object, assuming a homogenous uptake within that volume, or at a voxel-by-voxel level.

14.6 Positron Emission Computed Tomography/X-Ray Computed Tomography

At the forefront of molecular imaging is Positron Emission Computed Tomography combined with X-ray Computed Tomography (PET/CT). With unparalleled spatial resolution, timing resolution, and sensitivity, PET/CT is currently a key driver of molecular imaging.

PET involves the injection of beta-plus emitting radioligands. This imaging modality relies on scanners with ring-shaped detectors that are designed specifically to accommodate the detection of two simultaneously arriving 511 keV gamma rays (coincidence detection), which result from the annihilation of a positron (positively charged electron) and an electron present in the patient's cells and tissues.

In its clinical applications, PET is predominantly used for diagnostic imaging. The short physical half-life of the most commonly used radionuclides, such as Fluorine-18 (F-18), Carbon-11 (C-11), Nitrogen-13 (N-13) and Oxygen-15 (O-15), which ranges from about 2 to 110 min, dictates that the kinetic coefficient of the functional ligands should also fall within this range. This rapid decay also allows for frequent scanning sessions within a short period, making it easier to monitor disease progression or treatment effectiveness. The short half-life of radionuclides also enables real-time imaging of dynamic processes within the body, providing valuable insights into organ and tissue function. However, if the ligand displays slower dynamics (such as in the case of antibodies), longer-lived radionuclides should be used (e.g. Zr-89, Cu-64 or I-124). These can also be used for therapy planning and prospective dosimetry, as seen in I-124 PET/CT or PET/MR in prospective lesion dosimetry and personalized treatment planning [49, 50].

Few radionuclides display beta-plus emission and simultaneous sufficient beta-minus or alpha emission for an effective therapy effect. The most prominent case of this combination is Y-90 (see Sect. 14.4).

14.7 Radiopharmaceutical Dosimetry (The MIRD Concept)

In NM therapies, where ionizing radiation is used to induce a cytotoxic effect in tumour cells, physical radiation dosimetry is an objective measure to estimate the amount of radiation deposited in tissues of interest. Here, the absorbed dose—defined as the amount of radiation energy deposited per unit mass of tissue—is measured in gray (Gy).

The Medical Internal Radiation Dosimetry (MIRD) concept is a systematic framework designed to calculate the radiation dose delivered to tissues and organs by radiopharmaceuticals [51]. A key characteristic of the MIRD concept is the role of *source* and *target* organs or tissues. The source is where the radiopharmaceutical accumulates, while the target is the region that receives radiation from the source. The target organ can either be the same as the source organ (self-irradiation) or a different one (cross-irradiation).

To calculate radiation doses according to MIRD, first, the total number of disintegrations in a source organ—the cumulated activity $(\tilde{A})$—needs to be determined. This is calculated by integrating the time-activity curve $(A(t))$ over time.

$$\tilde{A} = \int_0^\infty A(t)\mathrm{d}t$$

The time-activity curve is a function describing the activity inside an organ or tumour over time. The activity in an organ or tumour varies over time due to:

(a) Physical decay
(b) Biological redistribution (accumulation and excretion processes) of the radiopharmaceutical (Fig. 14.3).

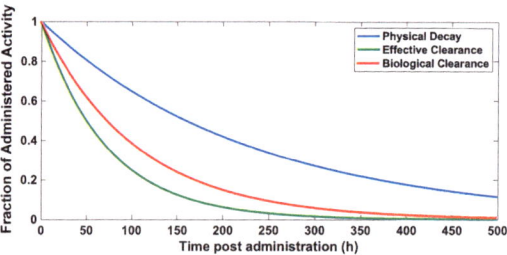

Fig. 14.3 Following administration of a radiopharmaceutical, the activity is eliminated following an effective decay (green line). This is a combination of physical decay (blue line), which occurs at a constant rate regardless of the radionuclide's form or location, and biological clearance (orange line), which is independent of radioactive decay

Typically, the time-activity curve is fitted from serial imaging data. For instance, in PSMA targeting ^{177}Lu-therapy of metastatic prostate cancer, serial SPECT/CT imaging provides valuable data on the distribution and kinetics of the radiopharmaceutical of tumour tissues, as well as of exposed organs such as the kidneys and the salivary glands [52]. This data is used to derive the time-activity curves, which are then integrated to obtain the cumulated activity.

As soon as the cumulated activity is determined, the absorbed dose (D) is calculated using following equation:

$$D = \sum_i \left(\frac{\varepsilon_i}{m} \right) \tilde{A}$$

Here, i is a specific type of radiation (α-, β- or γ, of known energy and branching fraction) that is emitted during radioactive decay, ε_i is its respective energy per disintegration deposited into the target organ and m is the mass of the target organ. For radionuclides with known decay properties and given source-target pairs the sum can be substituted by the so-called S-values—the specific absorbed dose fraction. These values are derived from computational phantom models that simulate human anatomy, are available in standardized tables and provide the dose per unit cumulated activity for a given source-target pair [53]. Using S-values, the absorbed dose can be simplified to:

$$D = S \cdot \tilde{A}$$

For medical technologists, understanding the MIRD concept is essential for several reasons. Accurate dosimetry ensures that the patient receives a dose that is effective for treatment but within safe limits to avoid radiation toxicity. Proper dose calculation helps maximize the therapeutic effect of the radiopharmaceutical, ensuring that the treatment is both safe and effective. Additionally, adhering to dosimetry guidelines and protocols is necessary to meet regulatory standards and ensure quality control.

Acknowledgements The authors would like to thank technologists and nurses of nuclear medicine for their ongoing logistic support.

References

1. Distinguished nuclear pioneer—1970 John Hundale Lawrence, M.D. J Nucl Med. 1970;11(6):292–3.
2. Hertz S, Roberts A. Radioactive iodine as an indicator in thyroid physiology. V. The use of radioactive iodine in the differential diagnosis of two types of Graves' disease. J Clin Invest. 1942;21(1):31–2.
3. Blahd WH. Ben Cassen and the development of the rectilinear scanner. Semin Nucl Med. 1996;26(3):165–70.
4. Anger HO. Scintillation camera with multichannel collimators. J Nucl Med. 1964;5:515–31.
5. Hutton BF. The origins of SPECT and SPECT/CT. Eur J Nucl Med Mol Imaging. 2014;41(Suppl 1):S3–16.
6. Beyer T, Townsend DW, Brun T, Kinahan PE, Charron M, Roddy R, et al. A combined PET/CT scanner for clinical oncology. J Nucl Med. 2000;41(8):1369–79.
7. Ljungberg M, Pretorius PH. SPECT/CT: an update on technological developments and clinical applications. Br J Radiol. 2018;91(1081):20160402.
8. Delbeke D, Schoder H, Martin WH, Wahl RL. Hybrid imaging (SPECT/CT and PET/CT): improving therapeutic decisions. Semin Nucl Med. 2009;39(5):308–40.
9. Ritt P. Recent developments in SPECT/CT. Semin Nucl Med. 2022;52(3):276–85.
10. Seifert R, Weber M, Kocakavuk E, Rischpler C, Kersting D. Artificial intelligence and machine learning in nuclear medicine: future perspectives. Semin Nucl Med. 2021;51(2):170–7.
11. Bodei L, Herrmann K, Schoder H, Scott AM, Lewis JS. Radiotheranostics in oncology: current challenges and emerging opportunities. Nat Rev Clin Oncol. 2022;19(8):534–50.
12. Hicks R, Lau E, Binns D. Hybrid imaging is the future of molecular imaging. Biomed Imaging Interv J. 2007;3(3):e49.
13. Bockisch A, Freudenberg LS, Schmidt D, Kuwert T. Hybrid imaging by SPECT/CT and PET/CT: proven outcomes in cancer imaging. Semin Nucl Med. 2009;39(4):276–89.
14. Quick HH, von Gall C, Zeilinger M, Wiesmuller M, Braun H, Ziegler S, et al. Integrated whole-body PET/MR hybrid imaging: clinical experience. Investig Radiol. 2013;48(5):280–9.
15. Wibmer AG, Hricak H, Ulaner GA, Weber W. Trends in oncologic hybrid imaging. Eur J Hybrid Imaging. 2018;2(1):1.
16. Weber WA, Czernin J, Anderson CJ, Badawi RD, Barthel H, Bengel F, et al. The future of nuclear medicine, molecular imaging, and theranostics. J Nucl Med. 2020;61(Suppl 2):263S–72S.
17. Sharp SE, Trout AT, Weiss BD, Gelfand MJ. MIBG in neuroblastoma diagnostic imaging and therapy. Radiographics. 2016;36(1):258–78.
18. Harris PE, Zhernosekov K. The evolution of PRRT for the treatment of neuroendocrine tumors; what comes next? Front Endocrinol (Lausanne). 2022;13:941832.

19. Wang F, Li Z, Feng X, Yang D, Lin M. Advances in PSMA-targeted therapy for prostate cancer. Prostate Cancer Prostatic Dis. 2022;25(1):11–26.
20. Siman W, Mikell JK, Kappadath SC. Practical reconstruction protocol for quantitative (90)Y bremsstrahlung SPECT/CT. Med Phys. 2016;43(9):5093.
21. Selwyn RG, Nickles RJ, Thomadsen BR, DeWerd LA, Micka JA. A new internal pair production branching ratio of 90Y: the development of a nondestructive assay for 90Y and 90Sr. Appl Radiat Isot. 2007;65(3):318–27.
22. Kersting D, Jentzen W, Jeromin D, Mavroeidi IA, Conti M, Buther F, et al. Lesion quantification accuracy of digital (90)Y PET imaging in the context of dosimetry in systemic fibroblast activation protein inhibitor radionuclide therapy. J Nucl Med. 2023;64(2):329–36.
23. Ferdinandus J, Costa PF, Kessler L, Weber M, Hirmas N, Kostbade K, et al. Initial clinical experience with (90)Y-FAPI-46 radioligand therapy for advanced-stage solid tumors: a case series of 9 patients. J Nucl Med. 2022;63(5):727–34.
24. Prive BM, Boussihmad MA, Timmermans B, van Gemert WA, Peters SMB, Derks YHW, et al. Fibroblast activation protein-targeted radionuclide therapy: background, opportunities, and challenges of first (pre)clinical studies. Eur J Nucl Med Mol Imaging. 2023;50(7):1906–18.
25. Schmidt R. Dose-finding studies in clinical drug development. Eur J Clin Pharmacol. 1988;34(1):15–9.
26. Duan H, Iagaru A, Aparici CM. Radiotheranostics—precision medicine in nuclear medicine and molecular imaging. Nanotheranostics. 2022;6(1):103–17.
27. Jacene HA, Goetze S, Patel H, Wahl RL, Ziessman HA. Advantages of hybrid SPECT/CT vs SPECT alone. Open Med Imag J. 2008;13(2):67–79.
28. Walrand S, Hesse M. SPECT/CT for dosimetry. In: Clinical applications of SPECT-CT. Berlin: Springer; 2022. p. 37–55.
29. King M, Farncombe T. An overview of attenuation and scatter correction of planar and SPECT data for dosimetry studies. Cancer Biother Radiopharm. 2003;18(2):181–90.
30. Fendler WP, Rahbar K, Herrmann K, Kratochwil C, Eiber M. (177)Lu-PSMA radioligand therapy for prostate cancer. J Nucl Med. 2017;58(8):1196–200.
31. De Jong M, Valkema R, Van Gameren A, Van Boven H, Bex A, Van De Weyer EP, et al. Inhomogeneous localization of radioactivity in the human kidney after injection of [(111)In-DTPA]octreotide. J Nucl Med. 2004;45(7):1168–71.
32. Patton JA, Turkington TG. SPECT/CT physical principles and attenuation correction. J Nucl Med Technol. 2008;36(1):1–10.
33. Dewaraja YK, Frey EC, Sgouros G, Brill AB, Roberson P, Zanzonico PB, et al. MIRD pamphlet no. 23: quantitative SPECT for patient-specific 3-dimensional dosimetry in internal radionuclide therapy. J Nucl Med. 2012;53(8):1310–25.
34. Dickson J, Ross J, Voo S. Quantitative SPECT: the time is now. EJNMMI Phys. 2019;6(1):4.
35. Ljungberg M, Frey E, Sjogreen K, Liu X, Dewaraja Y, Strand SE. 3D absorbed dose calculations based on SPECT: evaluation for 111-In/90-Y therapy using Monte Carlo simulations. Cancer Biother Radiopharm. 2003;18(1):99–107.
36. Ferrer L, Delpon G, Lisbona A, Bardies M. Dosimetric impact of correcting count losses due to deadtime in clinical radioimmunotherapy trials involving iodine-131 scintigraphy. Cancer Biother Radiopharm. 2003;18(1):117–24.
37. Hutton BF, Buvat I, Beekman FJ. Review and current status of SPECT scatter correction. Phys Med Biol. 2011;56(14):R85–112.
38. Chuanyong B, Babla H, Conwell R. Emission-based scatter correction in SPECT imaging. Tsinghua Sci Technol. 2010;15(1):1–10.
39. Vandenberghe S, D'Asseler Y, Van de Walle R, Kauppinen T, Koole M, Bouwens L, et al. Iterative reconstruction algorithms in nuclear medicine. Comput Med Imaging Graph. 2001;25(2):105–11.
40. Lyra M, Ploussi A. Filtering in SPECT image reconstruction. Int J Biomed Imaging. 2011;2011:693795.
41. Bruyant PP. Analytic and iterative reconstruction algorithms in SPECT. J Nucl Med. 2002;43(10):1343–58.
42. Köchle G, Unterhumer G, König F, Leitha T. Einfluss des OSEM-3D-Algorithmus auf die Bildqualität bei der SPECT: Eine Phantomstudie an der Siemens Symbia T6-Gammakamera. Radiopraxis. 2010;3(3):137–48.
43. Frey EC, Tsui BMW. Collimator-detector response compensation in SPECT. In: Zaidi H, editor. Quantitative analysis in nuclear medicine imaging. Boston, MA: Springer US; 2006. p. 141–66.
44. Mahani H, Raisali G, Kamali-Asl A, Ay MR. Collimator-detector response compensation in molecular SPECT reconstruction using STIR framework. Iran J Nucl Med. 2017;25(Suppl 1):26–34.
45. Chun SY, Fessler JA, Dewaraja YK. Correction for collimator-detector response in SPECT using point spread function template. IEEE Trans Med Imaging. 2013;32(2):295–305.
46. Marquis H, Willowson KP, Bailey DL. Partial volume effect in SPECT & PET imaging and impact on radionuclide dosimetry estimates. Asia Ocean J Nucl Med Biol. 2023;11(1):44–54.
47. Erlandsson K, Buvat I, Pretorius PH, Thomas BA, Hutton BF. A review of partial volume correction techniques for emission tomography and their applications in neurology, cardiology and oncology. Phys Med Biol. 2012;57(21):R119–59.
48. Shcherbinin S, Celler A. Assessment of the severity of partial volume effects and the performance of two template-based correction methods in a

SPECT/CT phantom experiment. Phys Med Biol. 2011;56(16):5355–71.

49. Jentzen W, Freudenberg L, Eising EG, Sonnenschein W, Knust J, Bockisch A. Optimized 124I PET dosimetry protocol for radioiodine therapy of differentiated thyroid cancer. J Nucl Med. 2008;49(6):1017–23.

50. Plyku D, Hobbs RF, Wu D, Garcia C, Sgouros G, Van Nostrand D. I-124 PET/CT image-based dosimetry in patients with differentiated thyroid cancer treated with I-131: correlation of patient-specific lesional dosimetry to treatment response. Ann Nucl Med. 2022;36(3):213–23.

51. Loeevinger R, Berman M. A schema for absorbed-dose calculations for biologically-distributed radionuclides. J Nucl Med. 1968;Suppl 1:9–14.

52. Sjogreen Gleisner K, Chouin N, Gabina PM, Cicone F, Gnesin S, Stokke C, et al. EANM dosimetry committee recommendations for dosimetry of 177Lu-labelled somatostatin-receptor- and PSMA-targeting ligands. Eur J Nucl Med Mol Imaging. 2022;49(6):1778–809.

53. Snyder WS. MIRD pamphlet no 11: "S" absorbed dose per unit cumulated activity for selected radionuclides and organs; 1975.

Patient's Tailored Hybrid Imaging and Problem Solving

15

Giorgio Testanera, Carolina Rodrigues, Sara Ferreira, Luigi Mansi, and Luca Camoni

15.1 Introduction

The evolution of hybrid imaging modalities in Nuclear Medicine (NM) has significantly transformed the landscape in which imaging professionals operate, as well as the expectations of patients. In this dynamic environment, the role of Nuclear Medicine Technologists (NMTs)[1] has developed from mere support to the medical act to full independent professionals, capable (and

required) to make assessments and act based on this to ensure quality and safety in the imaging procedures. This has been tackled in the EANM Benchmark document [1] for competencies as a key factor for advancing the practice of professionals. Imaging professionals must integrate theoretical knowledge with practical applications and be able to consciously modify fundamental parameters based on clinical indications, patient conditions, and examination types to ensure the best compromise to include image quality, safety, and patient comfort. Mastery of these modifications allows NMTs to enhance diagnostic outcomes and tailor procedures to individual patient needs. Another critical aspect of modern Nuclear Medicine is the ability to manage urgent diagnostic situations efficiently, optimising

---

[1] Nuclear Medicine Technologists (NMTs) are members of a healthcare specialists' team who can undertake the whole range of conventional and modern NM procedures that can have different title or qualifications (Radiographer, Technician e.g.) For the purpose of this book, we used this term referring to convention established by EANM in Benchmark documents [1].

G. Testanera (✉)
Faculty of Life Sciences and Medicine, King's College London and Guy's and St Thomas' PET Centre, School of Biomedical Engineering and Imaging Sciences, London, UK
e-mail: Giorgio.testanera@kcl.ac.uk

C. Rodrigues
Nuclear Medicine and PET/CT Department, Imperial College Healthcare NHS Trust, Hammersmith Hospital and Charing Cross Hospital, London, UK
e-mail: Carolina.Rodrigues@nhs.net

S. Ferreira
Department of PET/CT, Royal Brompton and Harefield Specialist Care, London, UK
e-mail: sara.ferreira4@nhs.net

L. Mansi
Interuniversity Research Center for Sustainability (CIRPS), Rome, Italy

Medicina Futura, Acerra (NA), Italy
e-mail: Luigi.mansi@unicampania.it

L. Camoni
Department of Nuclear Medicine, University of Brescia and ASST Spedali Civili di Brescia, Brescia, Italy
e-mail: luca.camoni@unibs.it

© The Author(s), under exclusive license to Springer Nature Switzerland AG 2025
L. Camoni, L. Mansi (eds.), *Nuclear Medicine Hybrid Imaging for Radiographers & Technologists*,
https://doi.org/10.1007/978-3-031-86228-1_15

equipment use and patient's workflow to meet clinical priorities. This competence ensures that decision-making processes in urgent cases and unexpected situations are handled promptly and effectively, maintaining high standards of patient care even under pressure. Another challenge is maintaining patient comfort and cooperation, vital aspects for the success of NM hybrid imaging scans. NMTs must possess the knowledge and skills to address challenges posed by patients who may move during scans or those with psychiatric conditions using strategies to enhance their cooperation, such as effective communication, use of immobilisation techniques, and creating a calming environment. Ensuring patient comfort not only improves the quality of the images obtained but also enhances the overall patient experience. This chapter will investigate more deeply into providing a comprehensive guide on how to balance risks and optimise resources to tailor the NM diagnostic provisions in different aspects. The breadth of the topics covered in the chapter has also led us to avoid going into detail on some less significant aspects or those already explored in other chapters, especially regarding issues related to paediatrics (Chapter 16) and PET/MR (Chapter 6) and communication (Chapter 17). This also includes the role and challenges faced by nurses or other healthcare professionals, which are particularly relevant for example in the pediatric setting. Likewise, we have chosen to exclude some minor issues, such as contamination (e.g. in ventilation studies and vesicoureteral reflux examinations) or those that have become rare, such as muscle contractions caused by psychological stress or chewing gum, which were critical during the era of stand-alone PET.

15.2 Person-Centred Care (PCC)

Person-centred care (PCC) emphasises the need for healthcare professionals to prioritise individual patient needs, fostering a collaborative and empathetic environment that empowers patients to actively participate in decision making on their own care [2]. This approach cascaded to NM

with the idea to enhance patient experience and outcomes by focusing on the specific needs and circumstances of each patient. It involves optimising the technical aspects of imaging based on each patient's unique clinical situation while ensuring patients feel informed, comfortable, and involved throughout their care journey. Many factors play a role in the requirement to tailor scanning protocols, like body size, medical conditions, and specific diagnostic requirements. The caring aspects of PCC involve clear, empathetic communication while explaining procedures, addressing patient concerns, and obtaining informed consent. Patients should be well-informed about what to expect during their imaging study, the reasons for specific protocols, and any preparatory steps they need to follow. Effective communication helps alleviate anxiety and builds trust between patients and healthcare providers. Recently a scoping review was conducted in accordance with the Joanna Briggs Institute methodology using Keywords and Medical Subject Headings (MeSH) related to PCC in Diagnostic examination [3]. The research showed a wide range of consensus of NM professionals' ability to improve patient care pathways and increase patient satisfaction, leading to enhanced clinical outcomes. At the same time, it highlighted the lack of consistency in strategy to implement PCC in Nuclear Medicine.

15.2.1 NMTs Role in PCC

NMTs work in collaboration with all other professional groups and play a crucial role in patient care with patients undergoing diagnostic imaging procedures. The initial patient assessment to determine appropriateness, approve radioactive administration, and collect informed consent is typically the responsibility of the physician. This can happen with different modalities according to practice and regulations. In some countries deputised to other healthcare, professional NMTs are essential in managing the technical aspects of imaging, in particular explaining exam's procedure, address patient concerns about technical details, and ensure that imaging protocols are correctly implemented. In the context of hybrid imaging modalities like PET/CT and PET/MR, the expertise of NMTs becomes even more significant. NMTs do not face limitations in this field and can act as experts in defining radiological protocols. Their proficiency with hybrid equipment allows them to optimise imaging procedures and contribute to better diagnostic outcomes. Moreover, NMTs play a dynamic role in managing relationships with patients and caregivers, particularly in pediatric cases, enhancing communication and supports patient care.

Effective communication is essential for reducing patient anxiety and ensuring cooperation, involving clear explanations of the procedure and its purpose. Based on the patient's medical history, condition, and specific diagnostic needs, technologists actively participate in customising imaging protocols. This includes adjusting radiotracer dosage, selecting appropriate imaging modalities, and determining the best positioning techniques to ensure optimal image quality. Decisions regarding protocol modifications are made based on patient-specific factors, such as age, weight, medical history, and the presence of comorbidities. This process involves balancing the need for high-quality diagnostic images with the imperative to minimise radiation exposure. An important aspect of this balance is the role of the NMT in deciding on rapid acquisition techniques, especially when dealing with critically ill patients such as psychiatric patients, severely debilitated individuals, or in emergency situations. Additional considerations such as claustrophobia mitigations must also be addressed to ensure patient comfort and compliance. They work closely with NM physicians and a wider multidisciplinary team to interpret clinical indications and determine the most appropriate imaging strategies, contributing to decisions about radiopharmaceuticals, scan parameters, and imaging techniques. These decisions need to be made in real time, in particular when facing unexpected challenges, such as patient discomfort or illness. NMTs also play a crucial role in deciding whether to prematurely terminate an examination due to patient movement or deteriorating critical conditions. This involves being responsible for monitoring acute medical events that may occur during the study, such as epileptic seizures or cardiopulmonary problems, ensuring prompt response and patient safety. Furthermore, to make the imaging experience as comfortable as possible, NMTs employ various strategies such as using cushions, providing blankets, and maintaining a calm environment. They participate in the teamwork to adjust protocols or employ techniques to accommodate patient needs, further enhancing the overall quality and safety of the diagnostic process.

All these strategies to tailor the experience need to be done in adherence to safety protocols, including radiation safety measures and infection control practices to protect patients and staff. NMTs are the main actors in monitoring radiation doses and implement "As Low As Reasonably Achievable" (ALARA) principles to minimise exposure while ensuring diagnostic efficacy [4, 35].

It is also important to consider the scheduling of research studies, which require precise and rigorous execution times. These studies should not be programmed in situations that might conflict with potential emergencies. Careful planning is essential to ensure that the strict timing of research protocols does not interfere with urgent clinical cases. By coordinating with the clinical team and adjusting schedules accordingly, NMTs can prevent overlaps that could compromise both the integrity of the research and the quality of patient care.

Educating patients about what to expect before, during, and after the procedure helps in preparing them mentally and physically, which can improve the quality of the images obtained. Implementing support systems such as patient navigators or coordinators can help guide patients through the imaging process, ensuring they feel supported and informed at every step. In most realities, NMTs play these roles. To optimise this role, it is important to establish robust feedback mechanisms for continuous improvement based on patient experiences. This feedback should be systematically collected, analysed, and used to make evidence-based changes to practices and protocols. The changes should be assessed multidisciplinarly to ensure diagnostic accuracy and safety are not compromised. A good balance between patient's experience, diagnostic accuracy, and stakeholder satisfaction is the final aim of this process.

As NMTs take on more responsibilities in patient assessment and education, they can significantly enhance the patient experience and contribute to better clinical outcomes [5]. In reading this chapter please be aware that the scope of practice for NMTs is defined by national regulatory bodies and institutional policies.

15.3 Conventional Nuclear Medicine Imaging

15.3.1 Optimisation of Scanning Resources and Department Workflow

In daily clinical practice, it is essential to identify the specific clinical indications and urgent cases that necessitate hybrid imaging for prompt diagnosis and treatment planning. Clinical scenarios like acute pulmonary embolism and suspected malignancies with urgent staging requirements can significantly impact the operational flow of the department. Consequently, NMTs must streamline equipment workflow and exercise sound decision-making skills when encountering such critical situations.

When faced with these situations, having allocated dedicated time slots for emergency/inpatients is crucial to optimise the use of scanning resources. This ensures that emergencies can be handled promptly without disrupting the schedule for outpatient appointments. Furthermore, maintaining departmental flexibility to cater to emergency situations or additional imaging needs for existing patients is essential [5]. For instance, a ^{177}Lu post-therapy imaging patient may need an extra Single Photon Emission Computed Tomography (SPECT/CT) scan that was not originally scheduled.

The clinical scenario must be evaluated to determine the most suitable imaging protocol, considering both the urgency of the situation and the diagnostic requirements. Within the realm of

Conventional NM, a prevalent clinical scenario involves urgently staging suspected malignancies, often calling for a bone scan. For patients experiencing discomfort and pain, a crucial decision arises regarding whether to opt for a comprehensive Whole-Body bone scan, offering a thorough evaluation in cases demanding rapid assessment of widespread disease, potentially offering a quicker procedure, depending on the scanner and acquisition parameters. Alternatively, the choice may lean towards proceeding directly with SPECT/CT, offering superior resolution, and providing localised imaging essential for discerning complex or ambiguous lesions. Nonetheless, this option may entail a longer scan duration, potentially causing heightened discomfort for the patient.

15.3.2 Optimisation of Patient Tailored Care

In Conventional Nuclear Medicine, a range of scans utilising hybrid imaging techniques are conducted for various purposes, including detecting bone or other malignancies, sentinel node, inflammation, infections, neurodegenerative conditions in the brain, pulmonary embolism, and gastrointestinal bleeding, among others. Certain scans necessitate specific preparations, such as discontinuing medications (e.g. reserpine, cocaine, etc. for mIBG scans, thyroid hormones before WB scans, etc.), taking thyroid blockage tablets (e.g. mIBG, Ioflupane), H2 Blockers (e.g. Meckels) or adhering to specific dietary guidelines when required [6]. Understanding the significance of these requirements can pose challenges for some patients, potentially leading to non-compliance. Therefore, it is crucial to clearly communicate and emphasise these instructions to patients before their appointments. This proactive approach aims to minimise sameday cancellations and prevent disruptions to the department's workflow.

Additionally, it is crucial to ascertain certain key information from patients before they undergo a nuclear medicine scan. This includes assessing whether the patient is pregnant/breastfeeding, claustrophobic and inquiring about venous access. Some patients may have undergone prior procedures and could offer insights into their specific anxieties or challenges related to claustrophobia and/or venous access.

Before initiating any NM procedure, it is imperative to determine if patients of reproductive age (12–55 years old e.g.) are currently breastfeeding or potentially pregnant. If needed, a pregnancy test (urine or blood) should be conducted, as per local guidelines.

For claustrophobic patients undergoing SPECT/CT, several strategies can be implemented to help manage their anxiety and improve their comfort during the procedure, such as:

- Explaining the procedure and its purpose beforehand to alleviate their fear.
- Utilising images or videos and visual aids.
- Using distraction techniques and having a supportive presence.
- Enabling comfort items and creating a calm atmosphere during the procedure.
- Consider anti-anxiety or mild sedatives, which do not interfere with the pharmacokinetics of the tracer, in order not to modify the clinical significance of the study.
- Adaptive scanning times when feasible.

Establishing intravenous access is crucial for the safe and efficient conduct of nuclear medicine imaging, especially for outpatients or those with difficult venous access. It is vital to communicate this information beforehand so that the necessary resources such as skilled technologists/doctors/nurses and ultrasound systems can be arranged by the departments for the patients' visit.

Acquiring this vital information in advance enables technologists to prepare for the patient's visit effectively and personalise their care.

15.3.3 Impact of External Factors on Patient Care

Departments lacking internal radiopharmacy facilities often encounter external limitations regarding the availability of radiopharmaceuticals. These constraints directly affect departmental workflows, underscoring the importance of resource optimisation and its impact on patient care. To mitigate these challenges, one potential approach involves implementing recommended minimum administration activities. For instance, administering a slightly reduced dosage, <15% below the Diagnostic Reference Levels, (DRL), to compliant patients and extending scan durations, to ensure enough counts, can serve as a practical tactic to mitigate challenges without compromising image quality and avoid delays in diagnostics outcomes. These decisions should be made with the input from a multidisciplinary team (NMTs, doctors, and physicists) and consider the risk benefits. Another common scenario is diagnosing pulmonary embolism with a ventilation/perfusion test. However, there are situations where this may not be feasible. This could be attributed to the unavailability of a ventilation agent or external constraints on the supply of radiopharmaceuticals can hinder the process. In such instances, a thorough discussion becomes imperative. Depending on the patient's clinical history, a decision may be made to conduct only the perfusion component initially. Subsequently, if needed and possible (the ventilation is required for the diagnosis), the patient can return for the ventilation component on a later date. These patients may need ventilation to happen shortly after the perfusion, so proper management and engagement with referring team is required.

Depending on department policies, a similar approach may be used for pregnant patients suspected of having a pulmonary embolism. Since pulmonary disorders are rare in pregnant patients, a normal perfusion study can help rule out PE. However, in certain instances, a ventilation study may be necessary to assist in diagnosing the condition. This method can enhance the accuracy and sensitivity of the procedure. Some research suggests that after the first trimester, using the standard Ventilation/Perfusion protocol is feasible due to the minimal breast radiation exposure and its high accuracy rate [7].

Finally, in the scheduling of examinations dependent on the arrival of radionuclides, it is essential to plan procedures using various radio-tracers such as I-123, In-111. This planning should consider potential delays or cancellations of radionuclide arrivals, to allow for flexible reorganisation of the workflow with minimal disruptions. For example, by having the capability to substitute with examinations that utilise in-house available radiotracers, departments can maintain operational efficiency and reduce downtime. Mitigation should include the possibility of transferring patients who have already been injected with radiopharmaceuticals to another facility to conclude the exam in case of cameras malfunctions. This aspect will be covered more in detail in Sect. 15.4 of this chapter.

15.3.4 Tailored Scanning Protocols

In our clinical setting, it is essential to establish tailored imaging protocols to enhance patient comfort and compliance during hybrid imaging procedures. Our daily practice involves addressing a range of patient-specific challenges that necessitate individualised solutions:

- Patients frequently require personalised adaptations like scan duration, injected radiopharmaceutical dose, and acquisition parameters adjusted to their size. For instance, larger patients may necessitate adjustments such as extending acquisition times or dosage adjustments to ensure optimal image quality.
- Elderly or frail individuals may benefit from protocol adjustments, including shortened scan durations and modified positioning techniques, to improve their comfort and cooperation levels.
- In pediatric imaging, these considerations become even more critical. Tailoring imaging protocols to reduce radiation exposure is central in pediatric patients due to their increased sensitivity to radiation. More details are available in the dedicated chapter in this book.

It is crucial to prioritise optimal patient comfort during SPECT/CT scans to minimise motion interference during image acquisition. In practice, patient motion cannot be completely eliminated due to different factors (involuntary muscle movement, respiratory and cardiovascular motion, patients with dementia, etc). Technologists should put appropriate measures in place and utilise all available resources to ensure both patient's comfort and quality of the diagnostic image [8, 9].

These measurements may include patient positioning aids such as immobilisation techniques, always considering the type of patient and scan. For example, in ^{123}I-ioflupane imaging, it is crucial to secure and immobilise the head, especially as patients may shift positions. Taking extra care to ensure proper head alignment is vital, and using forehead and chin support can assist keeping the patient's head in the correct position without any movement. Some patients face difficulty lying flat and remaining still on the imaging table due to conditions like severe arthritis, back problems, or neck issues. Nonetheless, through gentle guidance and assistance, and strategic placement of pillows under the legs and lower back, it is possible to position those patients, ensuring that optimal imaging results are obtained, as observed in Fig. 15.1 [5]. Other strategies include using support under the knees, foam blocks set between the ankles when imaging the knees, and the feet supported in an appropriate support or even a box (home-made systems for immobilising the extremities) [9].

Moreover, performing a whole-body SPECT/CT or a 2/3 bed SPECT/CT is quite common for bone scans and/or post therapy scans. However, these procedures can be challenging for patients who may need to adjust for comfort. In such cases, it is advisable to opt for separate SPECT/CT scans. This approach allows the NMT to reduce the likelihood of patient movement while acquiring the necessary images.

In certain departments, the ventilation method used for lung scans could involve ^{81}Krypton. Some patients may find it challenging to breathe through a mask during the scan. It's crucial for NMTs to communicate with the patient and offer alternatives to enhance their experience. For example, switching from a mask to a mouthpiece for easier breathing or adjusting the scan dura-

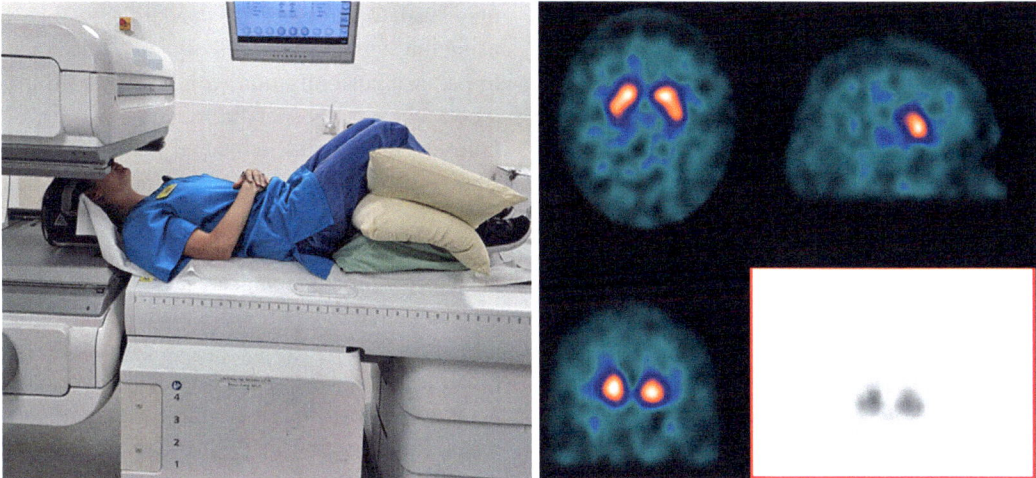

Fig. 15.1 Patient positioning with the aid of support under the knees and SPECT imaging with the correct head position

tion. If a patient struggles with SPECT/CT, the protocol should be modified for static images and breaks should be provided between images if needed. In the context of the CT component, it is recommended to employ a mid-inspiration breath-hold whenever feasible. However, if this proves impractical, utilising shallow continuous breathing is a suitable alternative [5].

NMTs should pay special attention to patients with neurological issues, who may struggle during the scan. Monitoring these patients closely will guarantee their comfort and stability throughout the procedure.

Data quality control of raw data should be performed immediately after the images acquisition before allowing the patient to leave.

15.3.5 Post-Processing

Post-processing is essential in nuclear medicine to enhance image quality and extract valuable diagnostic information, especially when dealing with suboptimal scans. Here are some solutions and techniques used in post-processing to address suboptimal scans [6]:

- Motion correction software may assist in restoring the quality and misalignment of acquired data. For example, in brain images,

reorientation of the head could be manually adjusted in the post-processing.
- Attenuation Correction (AC) vs. Non-Attenuation Correction (NAC): it's important to analyse the data with AC and NAC, as the AC image could present artefacts due to different factors, such as incorrect AC, missing tissue due to CT FOV limited radius and misalignment between SPECT and CT datasets.

15.4 PET Imaging

15.4.1 Introduction

Positron Emission Tomography (PET) imaging has revolutionised Nuclear Medicine by offering exceptional sensitivity and specificity for a broad spectrum of diagnostic applications, becoming state of the art in imaging surrogate markers for oncology application, with 18F-fluorodeoxyglucose (FDG) scanning as the workhorse. Over the years, advancements in PET technology and availability of more specific tracers have significantly enhanced image quality and diagnostic capabilities, enabling more precise detection and characterisation of diseases, as well as applications outside oncology. This section explores the optimisation of PET imaging procedures, including reconstruction parameters, tailored scanning protocols, risk management, and post-processing techniques, with a focus on the balance between customisation for individual patient needs and the standardisation of protocols to ensure consistency and reliability [10–12].

Technological advancements in PET imaging have led to the development of modern hybrid PET scanners with boosted resolution, improved sensitivity, and faster acquisition times. Evolution of technology not only refers to PET acquisition but also involves the CT or Magnetic Resonance Imaging (MRI) components that are able to provide more comprehensive anatomical and functional information.

15.4.2 Balancing Tailored Imaging and Standardisation in PET Imaging

Standardisation of PET imaging protocols ensures consistency and comparability of scans, which is essential for clinical trials, multi-centre studies, and longitudinal patient monitoring. Multiple guidelines advise on implementing standardised protocols for common clinical scenarios to ensure reproducibility and reliability across different institutions and equipment, considering the challenge of different national regulations on injected activity and clinical indications. In multicentric studies, the balance is obtained through standardised acquisition using phantoms. The use of phantoms for standardisation between technologies is fundamental in the research field. Integrating phantom calibration improves consistency between scanners, which is critical to obtaining reliable quantitative results. This practice helps achieve a balance between personalised patient care and standardised procedures, ensuring that data from different centres are comparable and that the integrity of multicentre studies is maintained. Most of international guidelines are based on standardisation projects. While advancements in PET technology enable highly detailed and patient-specific imaging, they

may lead to struggles in standardising images using the same injected activity [13]. It is crucial to balance customisation with standardised protocols, since many specific scenarios will require tailoring imaging to individual patient needs to enable sufficient diagnostic accuracy and patient care. The most common scenarios, where standardisation of procedures may clash with the need for tailored imaging, are lack of tracer, overweight patients, deteriorated patient, pathology that affects ability to stay still, extravasation, diabetes, and metabolic pathology. These scenarios need to be carefully considered in particular when quantification of PET images is required, since they can massively affect the results. Fine balance between tailored imaging approaches with standardised protocols ensures that PET imaging remains both patient-centred and consistent, ultimately improving patient outcomes and advancing the NM field.

One of such examples is related to injected activity and the acquisition time per bed position for PET and SPECT scans. These are usually optimised using metrics obtained from phantom experiments. However, delays in radiopharmaceutical delivery can compromise the available activity, significantly impacting PET due to its shorter tracer's half-life. If the available activity is insufficient for all scheduled appointments, departments might, on the advice of local clinicians and Medical Physics Experts, opt to inject less activity and proportionally increase the scan time to avoid delaying scans and patient treatment in urgent medical conditions. This tailored approach is to determine the percentage difference between the protocolled DRL and the activity injected into the patient and to increase the scan time by that percentage, as per Eq. (15.1). However, differences exceeding <15% below DRL and injections below the minimum required for the respective scan are not recommended, and appointments should be rescheduled.

Equation (15.1): Determination of tailored scan speed following an injection below established departmental protocols

$$\frac{\text{Protocol activity MBq}}{\text{Activity injected MBq}} \times \text{Protocol time per bed}(\text{min/ bed})$$

$$= \text{Tailored time per bed}(\text{min/ bed})$$

$$(15.1)$$

To provide an example, in a department that injects a standard dose of 350 MBq for patient scanning at 2.5 min/bed, in case of shortage of activity, it could be possible to inject 290 MBq and scan for 3 min/bed. Some scanners also enable the operator to select different times per bed according to the body part examined. This option can be used in these cases, to increase counts acquired in chest and abdomen areas when suboptimal activity has been injected.

15.4.3 Optimising Scanning Resources

Optimising scanning resources in PET imaging involves strategic planning and efficient utilisation of equipment and personnel to maximise throughput and diagnostic accuracy. Workflow management is also critical to maintain the balance between standardisation and adaptation to patients' needs. Scheduling of appointments should not only focus on reducing waiting times, but also on more general improvement of overall efficiency and patient experience. This involves establishing a robust triage system allowing healthcare providers to identify high-priority cases quickly and to allocate resources accordingly. As discussed above, triaging should cover clinical urgencies as well as consider the overall condition of the patient and potential extra challenges for the department, enabling an optimised use of time slots. For example, standard oncology scans might require different time allocations compared to complex neurological procedures in patients with dementia. Continuous evaluation and adaptation of these workflows, as well as strong collaboration between the clinical and the operational teams, can ensure that the imaging department remains responsive to the evolving needs of patients while operating with standardised and recognisable patterns [14]. An important aspect, already highlighted in Sect. 15.3.3 of this chapter for conventional Nuclear Medicine, is to have strong business continuity strategy for common issues like lack of tracer provision or machine malfunction. It is important to consider that backup plan is part of patient management regulations in some countries. Mitigation should include the possibility of transferring patients who have already been injected with radiopharmaceuticals to another facility to conclude the exam. Ensuring that procedures are ready for such transfers guarantees patient safety and continuity of care, even in the face of unexpected challenges. Effective coordination and communication within the multidisciplinary team are vital to implement these contingency plans seamlessly. By anticipating potential disruptions and preparing alternative strategies, nuclear medicine departments can enhance their resilience and maintain high standards of diagnostic accuracy and patient care.

15.4.4 Patient Cooperation

Key aspects include a comprehensive screen for conditions that may affect scan quality or patient safety. These include metal implants or severe obesity that could impact imaging quality. A very effective strategy is to gather advanced information on all patients coming to the department, including data related to their capability to sustain the scan. Planning of the day should be done considering all these factors to avoid delays and guarantee some time to deal with emergency situations. This effort needs to be in strong collaboration with the admin team to guarantee personalisation and effectiveness in non-standard cases. Instructions should not cover only dietary restrictions and medication adjustments but also hydration, and managing expectations during the appointment. Written guidelines and verbal explanations are crucial for patient cooperation. Special considerations are necessary for patients with conditions like claustrophobia, mobility issues, or psychiatric conditions. Sedation or relaxation techniques may be used for anxious patients, while those with mobility issues might need tailored positioning and additional support during the scan.

15.4.5 Patient Preparation

Patient preparation is a critical aspect of PET imaging that directly influences image quality, diagnostic accuracy, and patient safety. Proper preparation involves detailed instructions and may be different based on specific cases. While fasting is the most common request due to the diffusion of FDG scans, other preparation may be more complex. In particular, the preparation of patients with metabolic conditions, like diabetes, may require a massive effort in tailoring it to guarantee a safe attendance to the department together with quality scans. Classic examples are insulin and metformin, two common medications for managing diabetes, that can cause abnormal influence of FDG uptake. Unfortunately, it may prove complicated to have the patient with an adequate level of blood sugar while avoiding the medication to manage it. Flexibility in the time of the appointment may be really helpful, to ensure this balance is managed without the risk of patients feeling not well enough to sustain the scan. Also, patients should avoid strenuous physical activity for at least 24 hours before the scan. Exercise increases FDG uptake in muscles, leading to higher background noise and potentially confounding the interpretation of the scan. This effect can obscure the identification of pathological uptake, reducing diagnostic accuracy. Similarly, patients should refrain from talking excessively before and during the uptake period, especially in scans involving the head and neck regions. Talking or chewing activate muscles, increasing FDG uptake in these areas and potentially creating artefacts that complicate image interpretation. Additionally, environmental cold can affect the distribution of FDG, so is also important to ensure pleasant temperature conditions to avoid the possible pitfall.

There is no definitive data on the optimal time interval between therapy (chemotherapy or radiation therapy) and FDG PET/CT scans. Some experts recommend a minimum of 10 days after chemotherapy and 2–3 months after radiation therapy. However, in urgent clinical situations, a PET/CT scan may still be beneficial even with shorter intervals [13].

For brain FDG PET scans, it is crucial that the patient remains in a quiet and dimly lit room during both the injection of the tracer and the uptake phase [15].

In several studies, it is necessary to suspend the drugs. For example, when performing Somatostatin receptor (SSTR) imaging, it is generally recommended that patients stop taking all short-acting somatostatin analogs (SSAs) 12 hours before. Referring physicians should schedule the SSTR PET imaging just before the patient's next dose of long-acting SSAs. According to the EANM procedure guidelines for SSTR PET, there should be a 3–4 weeks interval after administering long-acting SSAs to avoid potential SSTR blockade [16].

All patients should empty their bladder just before the scan to minimise bladder activity, thereby reducing radiation exposure and image artefacts, and to ensure their comfort throughout the study.

15.4.6 Tailored Scanning Protocols and Positioning

Customising scanning protocols based on specific patient needs and clinical scenarios is essential for obtaining high-quality PET images. Examples include:

15.4.6.1 Prone PET Imaging

Prone PET imaging is a technique where the patient lies on their abdomen during the scan [36]. This position is mainly used for enhanced comfort that can lead to better compliance during the scan, reducing movement and improving image quality in patients with back pain or conditions that make lying supine difficult. However, it can offer several advantages in certain clinical scenarios, particularly in improving the detection and characterisation of lesions that might be less visible in the standard supine position. Prone positioning has proved to be particularly beneficial in breast cancer imaging [17], in particular if proper positioning is applied. A strategy could be to position the patient's breasts in a custom-built mattress made of poly foam or Plexi-glass and the patients' arms elevated above the head. This allows the breasts to hang away from the body, minimising motion and potentially improving the detection of lesions in the chest wall and upper abdomen. This positioning can provide better separation of breast tissue from the thoracic wall, enhancing image clarity and lesion detectability. Other applications aim to reduce respiratory motion, since the diaphragm and abdominal organs tend to move less with respiration compared to the supine position. For certain spinal pathologies, prone positioning can improve the visualisation of vertebral structures enabling detection of metastases or other abnormalities in the spine, where motion and anatomical overlap might obscure findings in the supine position. The NMTs' role in implementing prone PET imaging requires appropriate training and experience. Involvement will start with making a risk balanced decision to scan the patient prone and will include patient positioning, adjustment of imaging protocols, and handling the potential differences in AC calculations from CT images. Due to the shortage of scientific evidence in literature supporting the benefits of prone PET imaging, staff expertise and ability to adapt to different clinical scenarios will be needed till standardised protocols with valid findings are acknowledged.

15.4.6.2 Arms-Down Protocols

The two most commonly used positions during PET/CT imaging are standard "arms up" and "arms down". The decision on the position of the arms is determined by the indication of malignancy that is being evaluated and subsequent areas of interest being scanned, but also by overall patients' clinical conditions, since the "arms up" position may be difficult to sustain in compromised subjects. Positioning patients' arms down is mandatory in PET brain scans, to avoid artefacts and to ensure patients are comfortable and can keep their heads still for the entire duration of the exam. The nature of the pathologies

that require PET brain scans may bring a population with difficulties in complying with these requests. In these cases, if the scanner allows it, it is suggested to perform a list mode PET acquisition in addition to the traditional static scanning. This will allow the operator to "discard" some frames where movement is detected and reconstruct only frames with adequate alignment, avoiding problematic movement artefacts [15]. While in most common pathology "arms up" is preferred to minimise CT beam-hardening artefacts in the chest and abdominal area, in other indications like head and neck tumours or melanoma there is scope to perform the scan "arms down". For the reasons above, in patients with head and neck cancer it is usually preferable to perform the scan "arms down", at least at the level of the neck. In many centres, two separate scans are performed, one with data acquisition through the chest and abdomen (with or without the pelvis) while the arms are positioned up followed by a more limited second scan acquisition through the neck area with arms positioned down. Care should be taken to ensure adequate overlap of scans at the thoracic inlet, as lower neck structures can shift substantially with the change in arms position. It may be beneficial to use different CT parameters in the dedicated head and neck position to improve localisation of lesions and lymph nodes. Arms down PET scanning is also useful in patients with, for example, melanoma, sarcoma, or skin lymphoma, since the examination will require to include the arms in the field of view. A particular scenario is the choroidal melanoma indication, that requires high quality of scan in the head and neck as well as looking for potential metastasis in the liver. In this case a double acquisition is strongly indicated with both techniques used to maximise the image quality. Arms down technique is more commonly used when patients struggle to keep their arms up due to joint pain generated by their condition. In these situations, technologists need to engage in a multidisciplinary discussion about the risk balance on the decision to avoid the need for repeating the scan and extra exposure to the patient. The balance is between the risk of movement and the patient not completing the scan with arms up, versus the risk of beam hardening and CT arte-facts with arms down. Standardising these deci-sions is not feasible, so they are left to the discretion of professionals who understand the principles of protocol tailoring. When opting for the arms down technique, proper patient posi-tioning is crucial. Supports and cushions may be used to stabilise the arms and body, ensuring minimal movement during the scan. The use of straps or Velcro can help secure the arms without causing discomfort. It is fundamental to have cooperation and consent with patients and carers when using immobilisation techniques to prevent anxiety and further patient discomfort. In case the requirement is for a mandatory "arms up" position, healthcare professionals need to prop-erly engage with patients to find the best way to enable them to endure the procedure for the diag-nostic benefits. Making the patient participate in the decision-making and feel as the centre of the diagnostic process is the best strategy and has proved beneficial in multiple scenarios.

15.4.7 General Anaesthesia Scanning Protocols

15.4.7.1 Overview

Recent literature has flagged [18] the increase of diagnostic procedures in patients at the end of life, indicating that NM and PET have not received adequate consideration. More than 33% of patients in the last month of life underwent at least one high-cost imaging procedure (PET, CT, or MRI) while it is assumed that about 30% of annual Medicare costs are spent on caring for people in their last year of life. The evaluation of the number of tests performed and patients exam-ined seems to configure a form of overdiagnosis, with high costs for public health. While this is not the forum to analyse the ethics and appropriate-ness of these procedures, it is important to under-stand the impact of this trend on PET imaging procedures. One of the effects on daily practice is the increase of deteriorated patients that cannot cope with the imaging procedures, requiring gen-eral anaesthesia (GA) to perform the scan. There is a general consensus that PET scans should be conducted with the patient awake, besides some very specific scenarios that necessitate the use of GA. In these cases, the risk balance should be discussed in a multidisciplinary team to guaran-tee the diagnostic benefits outweigh the risk of the GA procedure. As mentioned above, these scenarios include not only paediatric patients, but also adult individuals with severe claustrophobia, or those unable to remain still during the proce-dure for physical or neurological conditions. The discussion needs to involve the anaesthetic team for a thorough assessment to identify potential risks associated with anaesthesia. This includes reviewing the patient's medical history, current medications, and any previous reactions to anaes-thesia. The clinical PET team plays a fundamen-tal role to identify potential abnormalities in the biodistribution of tracer following the GA proce-dure that can affect the reading of the exam. After the risk balance is analysed, a detailed anaesthe-sia plan should be developed to include the choice of anaesthetic agents, monitoring requirements, and post-procedure care. The timing of radio-tracer administration must be carefully coordi-nated with the induction of anaesthesia to ensure peak uptake coincides with the imaging window. The induction of anaesthesia should be per-formed in a controlled environment, with all nec-essary resuscitation equipment readily available, while continuous monitoring of the patient's vital signs, including heart rate, blood pressure, oxy-gen saturation, and end-tidal CO_2, is mandatory during the scan. Particular attention should be given to the consensus and discharge procedures, since they very often have to deal with compro-mised patients that require assistance and support from family or carers. In all these cases, NMTs play an important role in ensuring the benefit for the subject is at the centre of the procedure and being ready to have difficult and stressful conversations.

15.4.7.2 Paediatric PET in GA in Epilepsy

While most of the scenarios highlighted above are to be handled on a case-by-case basis, there are some clinical indications in which it is possible to have a more standardised organisation and planning [19]. In some specific paediatric neurological pathologies like epilepsy and dystonia, PET/CT and PET/MR with GA is a state-of-the-art procedure as pre-therapeutic assessment that can be standardised in advance. FDG-PET in paediatric epilepsy is indicated to assess site of surgery in cases that are resistant to medical therapies, while in dystonia it is a key factor to understand the effectiveness of treatment with Deep Stimulation Programme. The symptoms of these pathologies generate involuntary movements and inability to guarantee the stillness of the patients during the scanning procedure, making GA mandatory to obtain the necessary image quality. In this specific scenario, it is suggested to organise dedicated sessions, in collaboration with the anaesthetic team, enabling to have the necessary competent staff available for multiple patients, increasing safety and optimising resources. A potential pathway could be to organise the department to accommodate patients as a day hospital, reducing the need of paediatric patients to be admitted in the paediatric ward and also guarantee the separation of paediatric patients with adults. In this scenario, PET/MR plays an important role if available, since MRI and FDG PET are both key steps in the therapeutic pathway for these pathologies. The hybrid equipment will guarantee proper coregistration of the images, without much post-processing efforts and improving massively the diagnostic potential compared to having to coregister scans PET/CT and MRI scan happening in different time points (Fig. 15.2).

15.4.8 Technology Evolution for PCC Care: Total Body Long Axial Field of View PET Applications

The evolution of technology has always played a role in improving the ability of imaging to tailor the diagnostic potential to different types of patients and pathologies. The recent introduction of the Long Axial Field of View (LAFOV) PET is already proving to be a game-changing innovation due to the tenfold sensitivity compared to previous generation scanners. Some of the more obvious advantages of the new modality include the ability to massively reduce the injected dose, reduce scanning time, and cover all areas of interest in one single image. These advantages are not mutually exclusive, making this new modality a fantastic tool for patient-tailored care. The availability of these systems could lead to clinical decisions and diagnostic choices. Some of these particular scenarios where the advantages are shown were highlighted, for example, in the diagnostic procedures for cancer in pregnancy. These exams are challenging and preferably limited to methods without or with very limited ionising radiation. Following this approach, PET/CT is usually not considered as a suggested modality; however, experiences from Total Body PET centres start showing that individualised approaches enable scanning with an administered radioactivity dose ten times lower than the usual dose, while at the same time using specific Ultra Low Dose CT (Fig. 15.3). Another potential use is for non-compliant patients without the need of GA or repeated acquisition. The tenfold increase in sensitivity and LAFOV enables the use of list-mode protocols that cover the entire body of the patient. The whole-body coverage of the field of view in list mode allows the NMTs to retro-recon the acquisition, selecting only the timing and the images where the patient is still during the post-processing. While a systematic review is not available, case reports suggest potential applications in toddlers event with very limited activity injected [21]. In the field of brain PET imaging, the substantial increase in sensitivity, coupled with advanced deep learning reconstruction algorithms, facilitates acquisition times useful for image reconstruction from the selection of list mode post-processing data from minutes to potential few seconds to obtain a diagnostic image (Fig. 15.4), thus providing significant time efficiency or injected activity reduction [22]. This advancement is particularly beneficial for non-compliant patients, as it minimises the duration of the procedure, enhancing patient comfort and compliance.

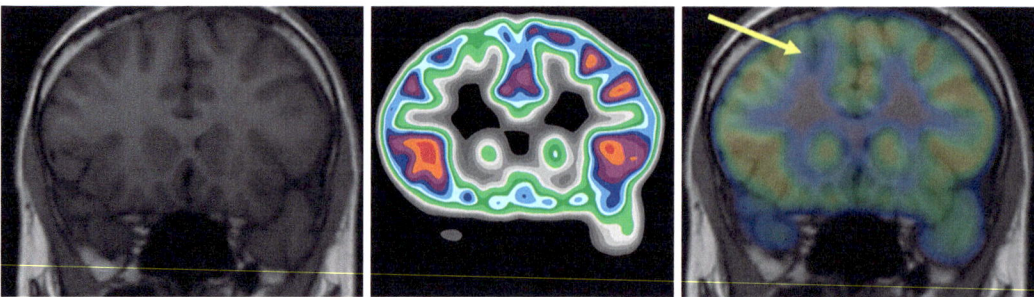

Fig. 15.2 (Courtesy of Prof. A. Hammers KCL PET Centre) PET/MR coregistration can reveal otherwise undetectable pathology causing refractory epilepsy, especially focal cortical dysplasia (FCD). Left, MRI reported as normal. Middle, FDG PET at the same position reported as normal. Right, coregistration reveals that there is little FDG uptake in the right superior frontal sulcus despite presence of grey matter (arrow). Histology showed FCD. The patient has been seizure free since the operation

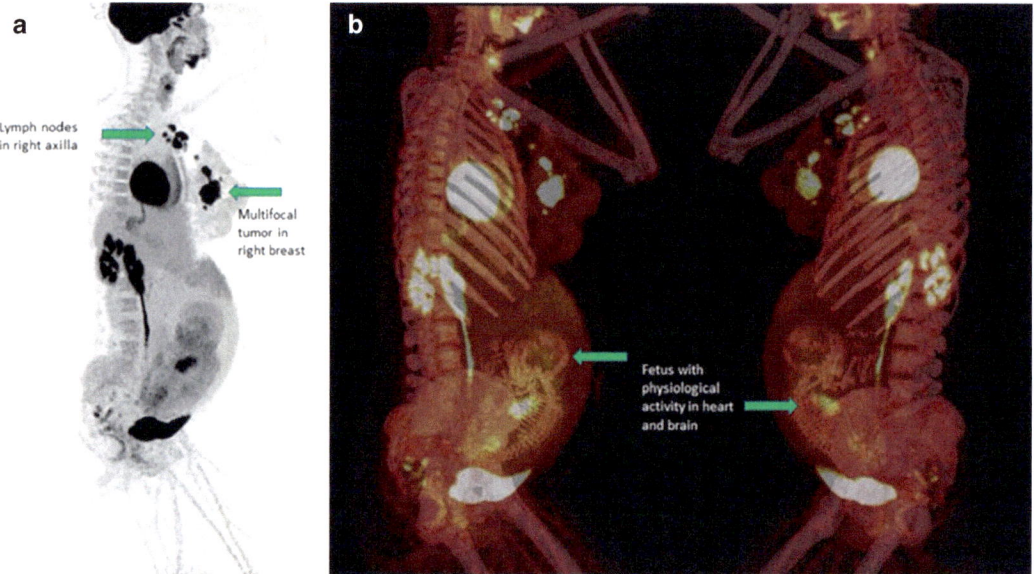

Fig. 15.3 The case in the figure shows great diagnostic accuracy in a pregnant patient with breast cancer while keeping the dose to the foetus below ~1 mSv [20]

15.4.9 Radiotherapy Planning PET

PET scanning can actively support radiotherapy (RT) planning in achieving precise targeting of tumours by highlighting metabolic activity in the lesion. Integrating PET imaging into RT planning helps delineate tumour boundaries more accurately, improving treatment efficacy and minimising damage to surrounding healthy tissues. The department may establish different methods for how the therapy PET/CT scan can be implemented in the planning process. It is quite common to use only one diagnostic whole-body therapy PET/CT scan for both staging and planning, even if unexpected results such as metastases appear, and the treatment plan must be consequently adjusted drastically. For the purposes of the chapter, we will focus on challenges and creative solutions for tailoring the treatment to patients' needs while standardising protocols for a repeatable setup [23, 24].

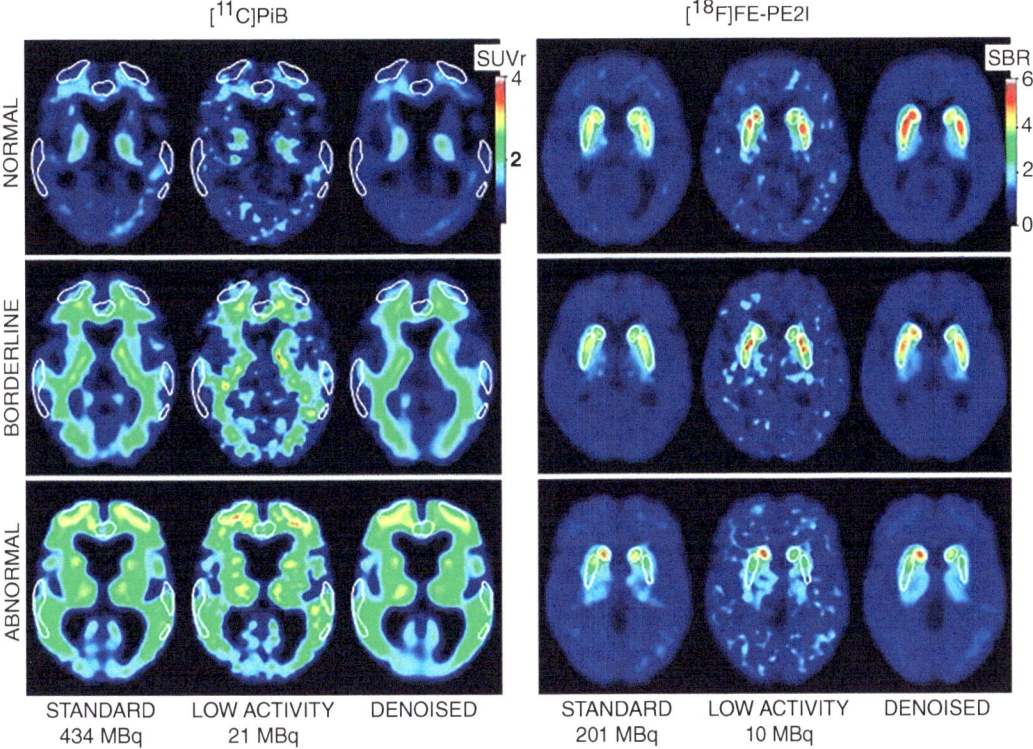

Fig. 15.4 Transverse plane PET images of the brain using [11C]PiB (left) and [18F]FE-PE2I (right) display normal (top), borderline (middle), and abnormal (bottom) scans. Each set illustrates standard-activity (left), low-activity (centre), and denoised (right) images [22]

Immobilisation is crucial in RT to ensure patient positioning is consistent across all treatment sessions, being mindful of the potential anatomical changes happening to the patients due to the effect of radiation doses. It also requires an active collaboration between the PET service and RT department with agreed standards and guidelines for the positioning technique and immobilisation options applied for the PET/CT scanner unit and treatment unit accelerators. This is especially important if the PET/CT scanner unit is geographically located in another department. All immobilisation devices must be identical and the documentation must be standardised and unambiguous.

Many factors affect the positioning and fixation of a patient. Before performing a RT planning PET/CT scan, it is important to investigate and consider what difficulties and special care need to be taken into account for each individual patient.

Some examples:

- Patient physical and mental vulnerability.
- Elderly or paediatric age.
- Overweight or very thin patients.
- Irregular respiration.
- Organ motion.
- Laser light alignment.
- Condition and placement of fixation devices.
- Incorrect original positioning or documentation.
- Skin marks from previous treatments.
- Staff competencies.
- Environment related.
- Disease progression and anatomical changes due to this.

Tailoring immobilisation devices to individual patients can enhance comfort while minimising the potential motion and misregistration. Customized masks, moulds, and cushions can be created based on the patient's anatomy and specific needs to guarantee a reproducible setup. It is also fundamental to perform regular checks and calibration of all equipment used. All these tasks are part of technologists' competencies who need to work in a multidisciplinary team to ensure the success of the modality.

Integrating PET/MR into the RT planning workflow is another approach that combines metabolic uptake from the PET side with the superior soft-tissue contrast of MRI. This hybrid imaging modality can be used in RT planning for enhanced tumour delineation in anatomical regions where it is tricky to identify tumour boundaries due to the proximity of critical structures of similar density (e.g. brain, head and neck, prostate). Integrating PET/MR into the RT planning workflow requires careful coordination. Ensuring that the immobilisation devices used for PET/MR scans are compatible with those used in the treatment setup is essential for maintaining consistency. The creativity of the NM team is important to guarantee the effectiveness of devices while not being detrimental to the image quality. Different solutions may be considered and explored to fully utilise the diagnostic potential of the modality (Fig. 15.5).

15.5 Nuclear Cardiology

This section aims to assist practitioners and operators in delivering suitable nuclear medicine care for their patients. The objective is to enhance existing nuclear cardiology practices, aligning them with current accepted standards to enhance service quality for the population across both SPECT and PET modalities. They are not rules or practice requirements and should not be used as a legal standard of care.

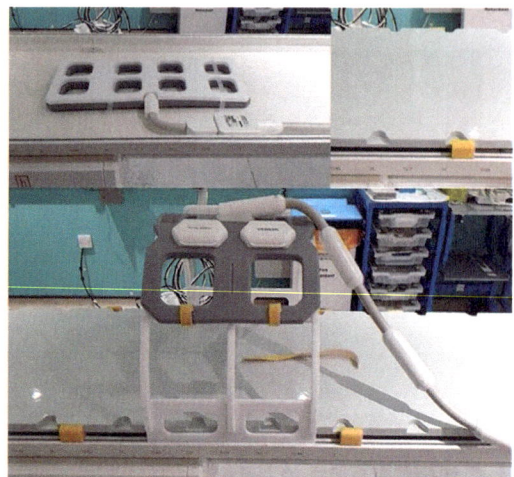

Fig. 15.5 (Courtesy of KCL PET Centre) In house made RT setup for PET/MR planning in prostate cancer. The coils in the image were designed by a teamwork of NMTs and Physicists to enable effective PET/MR using the RT table, with a coil able to be positioned between scanner bed and RT flat table. Then it was produced by the hospital workshop

15.5.1 Optimising Scanning Resources

Myocardial perfusion imaging (MPI) is one of the most common non-invasive diagnostic tests for cardiac evaluation. Various stress modalities are used in nuclear cardiology, such as exercise, vasodilators, a combination of exercise and vasodilators, and dobutamine to induce coronary vasodilation. This ensures that, upon injection of the radiotracer, its distribution within the myocardium will reveal any significant coronary stenosis through flow heterogeneity [25]. In cases where patients have low blood pressure (systolic below 90 mmHg), it is advisable to perform hand exercises using a stress ball or similar to elevate their blood pressure. Regardless of the stress modality used, it is essential to have life support equipment and emergency medications readily available for all stress studies.

All patients must be informed about the test's purpose, procedure sequence, expected duration, potential side effects and possible risks. Selecting an appropriate stress test for each patient, considering both relative and absolute contraindications, as well as the type of scan required is crucial. Adherence to local regulations mandates either a written or verbal consent [25]. Stress leads will work in collaboration with Clinical team to ensure an effective balance between the quality of the scan and patient safety.

Furthermore, it is crucial to analyse the patient's 12-lead electrocardiogram (ECG) for any pharmacological stress contraindications and ensure proper preparation. This includes suspending caffeine-containing food and drinks for at least 12 hours and stopping theophylline-containing medications at least 48 hours prior.

Establishing a secure intravenous line, such as a cannula, is crucial for administering the radiotracer and medications during or after stress [25]. It is important to ensure that the cannula can handle a flow rate exceeding the combined speeds of radiotracer and stress agent injections. While a 20G cannula is typically used, patients with challenging venous access may require a 22G cannula or the use of two cannulas. Reducing the radiotracer flow speed might be an option, according to departmental protocols. Securing an effective and stable cannula is particularly important in high-risk examinations, involving stress testing, or in patients at risk, for whom it is essential to have venous access readily available at all times.

Ensuring optimal patient comfort during cardiac imaging is crucial to mitigate motion interference during acquisition, especially since patients are typically required to have their arms positioned above their heads. Patient motion, particularly irregular breathing, can impact the frame sequence essential for extracting time-activity curves in PET and perfusion in SPECT. Thus, patients should be instructed to maintain shallow breathing and refrain from speaking during the dynamic phase, spanning a few minutes. Although respiratory gating is preferable and respiratory correction from dynamic data has been reported, it has not yet become standard practice in cardiac studies.

Activity in many subdiaphragmatic organs can interfere with evaluation of perfusion of the inferior wall [25]. To address this, some centres instruct patients to drink sparkling water immediately before scans, enlarging the stomach area and "pushing" away any other organs from the heart's inferior wall. During SPECT studies, technologists may initially position the patient on the detector's field of view to assess extracardiac activity before determining if sparkling water is necessary. Alternatively, other centres may opt to delay the scan briefly and/or request the patient to walk during uptake. If these solutions do not work, image repetition should be considered when the intensity of the extracardiac uptake matches or exceeds that of the cardiac uptake, with no distinction between the extracardiac uptake and the inferior cardiac wall when the intensity of the unwanted activity surpasses that of the cardiac uptake, provided there is a separation between it and the inferior wall of less than the thickness of one cardiac wall [26]. In case of image repetition during the workflow, the NMTs must prioritise the stress acquisition to the rest acquisition, keeping in mind the recommended imaging times of most recent guidelines.

Another challenge is claustrophobia, leading individuals to avoid situations such as undergoing SPECT or PET scans. It is crucial to inform patients about how long they will be in the scanner and explain which parts of the study will involve their head being inside the scanner ring. Suggestions such as wearing an eye mask, listening to music, or a video can help alleviate anxiety. It is necessary to reassure patients that they will be heard and can communicate with the NMTs throughout the procedure. Working closely with patients to lower their anxiety levels is imperative for a successful scan. In some rare instances, oral medication may be provided to minimise anxiety.

Besides MPI scans that involve stress tests, there are various other cardiac scans utilising hybrid imaging, such as those for myocardial viability, cardiac inflammation, or infection (e.g. amyloidosis, sarcoidosis, infective endocarditis, and myocarditis). Some of these scans require special preparation, such as adhering to a no/low-carbohydrate diet and undergoing prolonged fasting, which some patients might find difficult to comprehend and adhere to. Additionally, suspending diabetic or steroid medications may be necessary. Emphasising the importance of these preparations during appointment booking is essential to minimise cancellations and avoid business loss.

Currently, there is no specific data on the best pre-test preparation for diabetic patients undergoing PET scans for cardiac viability, inflammation or infection with FDG. Different centres use various protocols. Patients with type 1 diabetes should continue their basal insulin or may require IV insulin. In this situation, it may be necessary to admit them to a hospital ward the day before the scan to manage their blood sugar levels safely. Patients with type 2 diabetes should avoid oral diabetic medications or non-insulin injections while fasting. Given the limited data on preparing diabetic patients, the approach must be individualised and any deviations from the departmental protocols should be documented [27].

15.5.2 Tailored Scanning/Imaging Protocols

Gated studies provide simultaneous assessment of myocardial perfusion and function and are the standard in MPI. Their quality should be checked prior to commencing the acquisition. A careful assessment for a precise ECG trigger signal is conducted, in cases of relatively regular heart rhythm [25].

Consider preparing the patient's skin to improve electrode adhesion by cleaning, degreasing, exfoliating, and removing hair at the electrode site. Good electrode adhesion minimises interference and artefacts, leading to a higher quality ECG recording.

It may not be possible to place electrodes in standard positions (see Fig. 15.6) due to clinical conditions or weak ECG signal, which can prevent effective R wave triggering. This might

result in ECG triggering on both R and T waves or failure to detect the R wave, creating the appearance of an irregular heartbeat. A weaker signal is often present on patients with pacemaker, implantable cardioverter-defibrillator (ICD), or left ventricular assist device (LVAD). To address this, the following corrections can be made:

1. Change the detected lead on the scanner: Typically, lead 2 provides a stronger signal, but depending on the patient, leads 1 or 3 might offer better signals. NMTs must identify which lead has the strongest signal.
2. Repositioning the electrodes: If there is no clear differentiation of the R wave, repositioning the electrodes may enhance the ECG signal (see Fig. 15.7). Repositioning applies to either 3 or 4 leads ECG-gated imaging.

The variability in cardiac beat length during gated acquisitions, even with regular heart rhythm, has prompted the establishment of tolerances in the gating process. A beat length acceptance window of 20% (±10%) permits the accumulation of data from cardiac beats that will ensure good quality gated data. When determining the parameters for the cardiac beat length acceptance window, it is crucial to consider that a narrow window may lead to rejecting too many beats, especially in the presence of arrhythmia or gating issues. This not only hinders the assessment of cardiac function but may also compromise perfusion data. This issue can be addressed by incorporating an "extra frame" (e.g. a ninth frame in 8-frame or 17th frame in 16-frame gated imaging), where all counts rejected by the acceptance window are stored. This additional frame serves as a useful tool to assess the number of rejected counts, both globally and on a projection-by-projection basis. With an extra frame available, it is recommended to use a 20–30% beat acceptance window. In cases where no extra frame is available using a conventional camera, widening the acceptance window to 100% (±50%) or infinity is advisable to maximise the quality of the perfusion images [28] or, if feasible, acquire in list mode and retro reconstruct the bins.

Fig. 15.6 ECG lead placement [33]

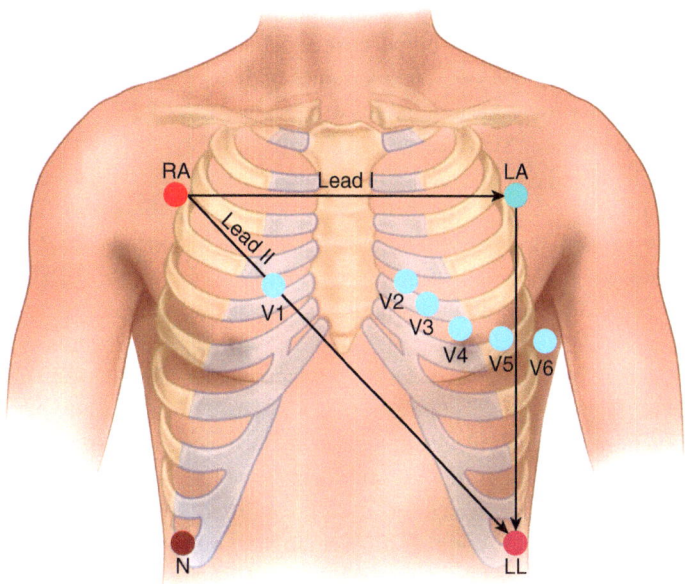

Fig. 15.7 Modified Lewis ECG lead placement [37]

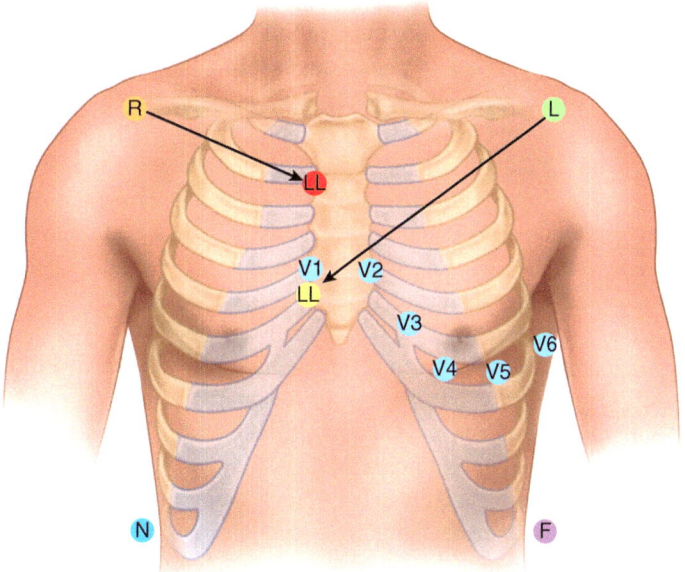

Given that ventricular contraction and thickening are often clinically useful for assessing viability, gating should be performed whenever possible [29]. However, gated volumes and ejection fraction may be unreliable in patients with atrial fibrillation, sinus arrhythmia, frequent premature beats, or intermittent or dual-chamber pacing [25].

Another highly relevant topic in nuclear medicine is attenuation and scatter correction. Photon attenuation by soft tissue in the thorax can result in a non-uniform decrease in counts from myocardial activity, potentially causing imaging artefacts. Diaphragmatic attenuation is most often seen in men, which results in a variable decrease in counts detected from the inferior wall, which may be confused with an inferior wall scar. Breast attenuation is most common in women and produces the effect of fewer photons detected from the anterior regions of the heart [25]. While prone imaging or a support around the breast region can improve image quality to some extent, these artefacts can be better minimised by using a transmission map. In hybrid imaging, these maps are generated utilising a low-dose CT (in SPECT/CT and PET/CT) or based on algorithms from MRI (in PET/MR) of the chest. Typically, these images are acquired either before, after, or simultaneously with the emission scan. If the transmission and emission images are misregistered, they need to be precisely aligned and consequently generate a new attenuation map. The high speed of CT scans freezes the heart and lungs at a specific phase of the respiratory cycle, potentially resulting in misalignment between CT-based transmission and emission scans. Respiratory misalignment between the CT image and emission data can lead to significant artefacts in myocardial segments neighbouring lung tissue. Subsequent software realignment is essential to mitigate any remaining misalignment [29].

In patients who cannot position their arms outside the camera's field of view (FOV), cardiac images should be obtained with the patient's arms resting at their sides. In such cases, the transmission scan time may need to be increased. It is crucial that the arms remain still between the transmission and emission scans to avoid artefacts. For perfusion/metabolism PET studies, maintaining a consistent patient position across both studies is imperative. In SPECT/CT or PET/CT imaging, having the arms within the FOV will cause beam-hardening artefacts on the CT-based transmission scan, typically resulting in streak artefacts on the corrected emission scans [29].

Regrettably, emission data often contain a notable percentage of scattered events. Various algorithms are available for scatter correction, but there is limited data supporting the superiority of any particular algorithm. It is advisable to refer to specific guidelines provided by each vendor's system. Scatter correction on emission data can be achieved through several methods [28]:

- Use of additional energy windows: This involves employing one or more extra energy windows to model the scatter component.
- Narrowing the primary energy window: By reducing the width of the primary energy window (e.g. from 20% to 15%), scatter can be minimised.
- Modelling scatter based on emission data: Scatter can be modelled based on the characteristics of the emission data.
- Empirical determination of an effective attenuation coefficient: While this method doesn't eliminate scatter, it involves empirically determining an effective attenuation coefficient.

15.5.3 Post-Processing

Promptly reviewing images after acquisition is crucial to identify potential sources of degradation and artefacts before the patient leaves the department [25].

First, the counting statistics need to be evaluated. If low counting statistics are detected, it is important to check the injection site for extravasation by positioning it within the detector's field of view. In myocardial blood flow (MBF) reserve on PET MPI, this is particularly critical as the radiotracer injection coincides with PET image acquisition. In MBF a time-activity curve graph should show a minimum of 1000 true counts at peak to ensure proper image quality [30].

Next, tracer biodistribution must be assessed. Abnormal tracer distribution necessitates a review of both the radiopharmaceutical's quality control and the patient's clinical information. For instance, a splenic switch-off can serve as an imaging marker for adenosine-induced myocardial blood flow response. However, it is important to note that the absence of a splenic switch-off does not necessarily indicate failed coronary vasodilatation [31, 32]. Additionally, in FDG PET imaging for cardiac infection or inflammation, extreme heart uptake requires verification that the patient followed diet and fasting instructions correctly, as these details are often overlooked at the beginning of the appointment.

Patient motion is another critical factor to review, as motion artefacts can significantly impact image quality. In conventional SPECT imaging, motion can be assessed using three parameters: cine, sinogram, and linogram, providing a thorough evaluation of any motion-related issues. On the other hand, in PET or CZT-technology imaging, motion can be analyzed by retro-reconstructing the list data into frames and examining the motion along the X, Y, and Z axes.

Moreover, extracardiac activity should be carefully examined. Focal uptake in areas such as the breast or lung could indicate malignancy, while decreased uptake in the liver or kidney might suggest the presence of cysts [25]. This assessment helps differentiate between normal and abnormal findings, guiding appropriate clinical decisions.

Missing information can often signal scanner or ECG-gated malfunctions. ECG-gated quality control is typically reflected in a narrow peak on a beat histogram. A widened peak or the presence of multiple peaks would indicate variable heart rates, frequent arrhythmias, or improper gating, which need to be addressed to ensure accurate imaging [25].

Co-registration is another crucial step, particularly in hybrid imaging. Ensuring correct overlap between SPECT/PET and CT/MR images is vital before performing attenuation correction, as misalignment can lead to significant artefacts and misinterpretations [33].

In certain cases, such as with some PET MPI radiotracers like Rubidium-82, scatter correction adjustments may be necessary due to the low number of emission photons. Changing the scatter window from relative to absolute ensures an adequate number of counts for reconstruction. It is important to document these adjustments properly, even though SUV calculations are not routinely performed on MPI.

Reconstruction processes also require careful attention. In dynamic PET imaging, if the radiotracer injection speed needs to be reduced, the static image reconstruction might be delayed. This delay, extending from 150 s to 180 or even 210 s, should follow departmental protocols to maintain image integrity.

Lastly, artefacts such as truncation are more common in cases of cardiomegaly or with some cardiac-centred cameras. These artefacts can affect the evaluation of myocardial segments, necessitating thorough checks to ensure accurate diagnosis.

By diligently evaluating these aspects, potential issues can be identified and addressed promptly, ensuring high-quality imaging and patient safety.

Attention to patient motion during image acquisition is essential to minimise motion artefacts. Vertical and transaxial displacement of the heart can occur even without chest movement, possibly due to changes in breathing patterns. This can lead to under-correction artefacts in the anterior or anterolateral regions due to the lower attenuation coefficient of overlapping lung tissue or overcorrection artefacts in the inferior region as hot spots due to the higher attenuation coefficients of overlapping sub-diaphragmatic tissues. Inspecting fused emission-transmission images for possible misalignment is crucial because such artefacts can significantly impact image interpretation. If there is patient motion, the heart does not perfectly align on the transmission and emission images. If motion degrades the transmission or emission scans during acquisition, software may fail to correct the image quality, necessitating a repeat of the scan [31].

Attention to motion correction during dynamic PET imaging is essential to minimise artefacts and ensure accurate measurement of myocardial blood flow (MBF). During the initial passage of radioactivity through the heart, first frame durations are typically set at an average time of 10 s and no less than 5 s, with incremental increases thereafter. Patient movement or changes in breathing patterns can cause frame misalignment, particularly during the early frames of the first pass, when accurate time-activity curve data is most crucial. Such misalignment can lead to significant errors in MBF quantification, compromising the quantitative results (Fig. 15.8). Therefore, utilising processing software with motion correction capabilities is crucial. If motion correction is not feasible, deleting the affected frames may be necessary to preserve the integrity of the data [34].

An important phase of cardiac processing is the reorientation of tomographic data into the natural approximate symmetry axes of an individual patient's heart. This can be performed either manually or automatically. Automated reorientation methods have been demonstrated to be at least as accurate as those performed by trained operators, often achieving greater reproducibility [25].

Images should be displayed and interpreted using a dedicated workstation and commercial cardiac image display software. Images should be presented with stress images on the top and rest images on the bottom and aligned for easy comparison. Each myocardial perfusion study should be displayed with the top of the colour scale set to the maximum count per pixel within the myocardium for each image set, using a linear colour scale, sometimes complemented by a grayscale or step scale. Removal of subdiaphragmatic activity should be attempted for quantification and the final display [25].

Quantification is an extremely valuable tool in MPI because it provides an objective assessment of the parameters under investigation, conveys the degree of severity, aids in the interpretation of results, and helps guide further appropriate action based on these results. It is also suitable for follow-up when the same software is used. Several commercially available software packages are extensively used. These methods have been extensively validated, though their use is not fully interchangeable. Quantitation software should be used as a complement to qualitative assessment, not in isolation [25].

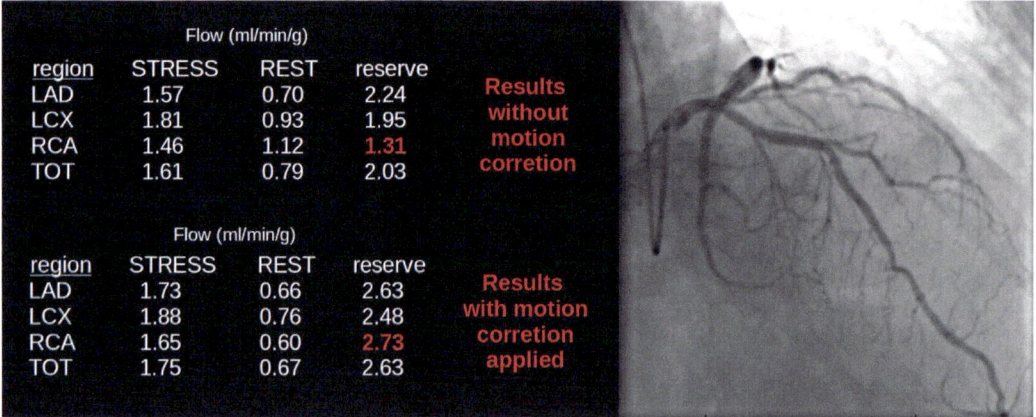

Fig. 15.8 In this 63-year-old male patient who underwent N-13 MBF PET, the figure shows myocardial blood flow (MBF) values and global reserve results both with and without motion correction. Without motion correction, a significantly reduced reserve is observed in the right coronary artery (RCA), which normalizes after motion correction is applied. This finding is consistent with the coronary angiography, which confirmed the patency of all coronary vessels (Courtesy of University of Brescia)

Effective masking is crucial to exclude extra-cardiac activity. Improper masking can lead to scaling artefacts, where structures with higher activity than the myocardium may falsely appear to have lower cardiac counts in the images [25]. In addition, alignment of the stress and rest sets of slices is essential. This involves displaying short-axis, vertical long-axis, and horizontal long-axis tomograms in a manner where each stress slice anatomically corresponds with a matching rest slice for effective comparison [25]. It is important to compare NAC and AC images when reporting to identify potential AC artefacts.

15.6 Conclusion

This chapter was not meant to provide a fully comprehensive guideline, but focused on providing a methodology to implement PCC in realistic scenarios. Most of the topics discussed are widely known and solutions are applied, but still lacking a proper systematic literature. Hope this work may help all healthcare providers and in particular NMTs to provide tailored care to patients in different scenarios and with different technologies.

References

1. European Association of Nuclear Medicine (EANM). Benchmark document for nuclear medicine technologists' competencies. London: EANM; 2018.
2. Pérez MR, Lerner CJ. Implementing patient-centered care in radiology: lessons from other disciplines. Radiographics. 2021;41(6):1741–53.
3. Champendal M, Borg Grima K, Costa P, Andersson C, Baun C, Gorga RG, Murphy S, et al. A scoping review of person-centred care strategies used in diagnostic Nuclear Medicine. Radiography (Lond). 2024;30(2):448–456. https://doi.org/10.1016/j.radi.2023.12.011
4. The College of Radiographers. Patient-centered care in nuclear medicine: scoping review and implications for practice. 2023.
5. Beckers C, Hustinx R. SPECT-CT workflow and imaging protocols. Eur J Nucl Med Mol Imaging. 2014;41:137–45.
6. Larsson Strömvall A, Rep S, Dickson J, Vukomanovic V, Ignjatovic V, Stevic M, et al. In: Mada M, Attard MC, Pietrzak A, editors. Hybrid imaging in con-

ventional nuclear medicine [internet]. London: European Association of Nuclear Medicine; 2020. https://eanm-org.staging.codecove.at/wp-content/uploads/2024/06/EANM20_TechGuide_digital.pdf.
7. Bajc M, Schümichen C, Grüning T, Lindqvist A, Le Roux PY, Alatri A, et al. EANM guideline for ventilation/perfusion single-photon emission computed tomography (SPECT) for diagnosis of pulmonary embolism and beyond. Eur J Nucl Med Mol Imaging. 2019;46(12):2429–51.
8. Livieratos L. Technical pitfalls and limitations of SPECT/CT. In: Seminars in nuclear medicine, vol. 45. Philadelphia, PA: W.B. Saunders; 2015. p. 530–40.
9. Grabher BJ. Brain imaging quality assurance: how to acquire the best brain images possible. J Nucl Med Technol. 2019;47(1):13–20.
10. EANM. Principles and practice in PET-CT part 1: a technologist guide. London: EANM; 2010. https://doi.org/10.52717/JYBK3301.
11. EANM. Principles and practice in PET-CT part 2: a technologist guide. London: EANM; 2011. https://doi.org/10.52717/NBXJ4555.
12. EANM. Advances in PET images: a technologist guide. London: EANM; 2021. https://doi.org/10.52717/PWZE5872.
13. Boellaard R, Bolton D, et al. FDG PET/CT: EANM procedure guidelines for tumour imaging: version 2.0. Eur J Nucl Med Mol Imaging. 2014;42:328. https://doi.org/10.1007/s00259-014-2961-x.
14. Cook GJR, Dickson J, Chicklore S, Dempsey M, Ferreira A, MacKewn J, Meadows A, Testenera G, Wan S. BNMS UK PET standards. Nucl Med Commun. 2024;45(1):1–15. Epub 2023 Oct 30. PMID: 37901922; PMCID: PMC10718206. https://doi.org/10.1097/MNM.0000000000001779.
15. Guedj E, Varrone A, Boellaard R, et al. EANM procedure guidelines for brain PET imaging using [^{18}F] FDG, version 3 [published correction appears in Eur J Nucl med Mol imaging. 2022 may;49(6):2100-2101. Doi: 10.1007/s00259-022-05755-3]. Eur J Nucl Med Mol Imaging. 2022;49(2):632–51. https://doi.org/10.1007/s00259-021-05603-w.
16. Hope TA, Allen-Auerbach M, Bodei L, Calais J, Dahlbom M, Dunnwald LK, et al. SNMMI procedure standard/EANM practice guideline for SSTR PET: imaging neuroendocrine tumors. J Nucl Med. 2023;64(2):204–10.
17. Nassar L, Kassas M, Abi-Ghanem AS, El-Jebai M, Al-Zakleet S, Baassiri AS, et al. Prone versus supine FDG PET/CT in the staging of breast cancer. Diagnostics. 2023;13(3):367.
18. Burroni L, Chiti A. PET/CT in senior patients: "cui prodest?". Eur J Nucl Med Mol Imaging. 2021;48:661–3.
19. Vali R, Alessio A, Balza R, Borgwardt L, Bar-Sever Z, Czachowski M, et al. SNMMI procedure standard/EANM practice guideline on pediatric 18F-FDG PET/CT for oncology 1.0. J Nucl Med. 2021;62:99–110.
20. Korsholm K, Aleksyniene R, Albrecht-Beste E, Vadstrup ES, Andersen FL, Fischer BM. Staging of breast cancer in pregnancy with ultralow dose

[18F]-FDG-PET/CT. Eur J Nucl Med Mol Imaging. 2023;50(5):1534–5. https://doi.org/10.1007/s00259-022-06076-1.

21. Reichkendler M, Andersen FL, Borgwardt L, et al. A long axial field of view enables PET/CT in toddler without sedation. J Nucl Med. 2022;63(12):1962. https://doi.org/10.2967/jnumed.121.263626.

22. Daveau RS, Law I, Henriksen OM, et al. Deep learning based low-activity PET reconstruction of [11C] PiB and [18F]FE-PE2I in neurodegenerative disorders. Neuroimage. 2022;259:119412. https://doi.org/10.1016/j.neuroimage.2022.119412.

23. Role of PET in radiotherapy planning: what are the benefits? J Nucl Med 63(1):1–12.

24. Nestle U, Weber W, Hentschel M, et al. PET for radiotherapy planning: still a challenge? Radiother Oncol. 2021;150:301–9.

25. International Atomic Energy Agency. IAEA HUMAN HEALTH SERIES No. 23 (Rev. 1) Nuclear Cardiology: Guidance on the Implementation of SPECT Myocardial Perfusion Imaging. Vienna: International Atomic Energy Agency; 2016. http://www.iaea.org/Publications/index.htm.

26. Johansen A, Lomsky M, Gerke O, et al. When is reacquisition necessary due to high extra-cardiac uptake in myocardial perfusion scintigraphy? EJNMMI Res. 2013;3(1):20. Published 2013 Mar 25. https://doi.org/10.1186/2191-219X-3-20.

27. Chareonthaitawee P, Beanlands RS, Chen W, Dorbala S, Miller EJ, Murthy VL, Birnie DH, Chen ES, Cooper LT, Tung RH, White ES, Borges-Neto S, Di Carli MF, Gropler RJ, Ruddy TD, Schindler TH, Blankstein R. Joint SNMMI-ASNC expert consensus document on the role of 18F-FDG PET/CT in cardiac sarcoid detection and therapy monitoring. J Nucl Med. 2017;58(8):1341–53. PMID: 28765228; PMCID: PMC6944184. https://doi.org/10.2967/jnumed.117.196287.

28. Verberne HJ, Acampa W, Anagnostopoulos C, Ballinger J, Bengel F, De Bondt P, et al. EANM procedural guidelines for radionuclide myocardial perfusion imaging with SPECT and SPECT/CT: 2015 revision. Eur J Nucl Med Mol Imaging. 2015;42(12):1929–40.

29. Dilsizian V, Bacharach SL, Beanlands RS, Bergmann SR, Delbeke D, Dorbala S, et al. ASNC imaging guidelines/SNMMI procedure standard for positron emission tomography (PET) nuclear cardiology procedures. J Nucl Cardiol. 2016;23(5):1187–226.

30. American Society of Nuclear Cardiology. February 2023. Cardiac PET workshop for Technologists. [Webinar].

31. Inkinen SI, Hippeläinen E, Uusitalo V. Adenosine-induced splenic switch-off on [15O]H2O PET perfusion for the assessment of vascular vasodilatation. EJNMMI Res. 2023;13(1):96.

32. Moody WE, Arumugam P. Assessment of stress adequacy with adenosine: does the answer lie in the spleen? J Nucl Cardiol. 2022;29:1215–8.

33. Krug JW, Rose G, Clifford GD, Oster J. ECG-based gating in ultra-high field cardiovascular magnetic resonance using an independent component analysis approach [internet]. J Cardiovasc Magn Reson. 2013;15:104. http://jcmr-online.com/content/15/104.

34. Sciagrà R, Lubberink M, Hyafil F, et al. EANM procedural guidelines for PET/CT quantitative myocardial perfusion imaging. Eur J Nucl Med Mol Imaging. 2021;48:1040–69. https://doi.org/10.1007/s00259-020-05046-9.

35. Kalra MK, Homayounieh F. Optimizing imaging protocols to reduce radiation dose: state of the art. Radiol Clin North Am. 2021;59(5):795–806.

36. Lee CW, Son HJ, Woo JY, Lee SH. Is prone position [18F]FDG PET/CT useful in reducing respiratory motion artifacts in evaluating hepatic lesions? Diagnostics (Basel). 2023;13(15):2539. PMID: 37568906; PMCID: PMC10417611. https://doi.org/10.3390/diagnostics13152539.

37. Huemer M, Meloh H, Attanasio P, Wutzler A, Parwani AS, Matsuda H, et al. The Lewis Lead for detection of ventriculoatrial conduction type. Clin Cardiol. 2016;39(2):126–31.

Paediatric Patient Management

16

Andrea Santos, Ana Grilo, and Domenico Albano

16.1 Introduction

"Children are not small adults". This statement highlights the important distinctions between paediatric and adult patients, particularly in medical care. This concept underscores the need for tailored approaches in diagnosing, treating and managing children's health, recognizing their unique physiological, psychological and developmental characteristics [1, 2].

There are several key points illustrating why children are not merely smaller versions of adults: physiological differences (body development and maturation, metabolism, organ sensitivity); psychological and emotional differences (communication methods differ from one age to another, different reasons for fear and anxiety related with medical interventions, different cognition and behaviour).

When it comes to ionizing radiation exposure in children, then radiosensitivity should be thought, as the rapid organ development and longer life expectancy, increase the potential for long-term effects from radiation exposure. Adhering to the ALARA (As Low As Reasonably Achievable) principle is crucial in paediatric nuclear medicine (NM). Also, dose optimization is of utmost importance, since it aims at ensuring that the applied dose is suitable for each specific medical purpose and that unnecessary radiation is avoided [3].

Regarding hybrid nuclear medicine, both modalities should be addressed, considering dose optimization. The radiopharmaceutical's administered activity should be optimal, and also the acquisition details of the CT (Computed Tomography) should be adapted to both the purpose (diagnostic and/or attenuation correction (AC)) and the patient (e.g. age, body mass index). Parisi et al. (2017) showed that typical effective dose in PET/CT procedures where CT is used for different purposes can vary considerably. This study shows that when diagnostic CT is acquired, the effective dose will vary from 2–10 mSv, and when used for AC and localization CT, the effective dose falls to 0.3–2.2 mSv. This brings us to the conclusion that the final use of the acquired CT should be carefully chosen before the examination is performed, to adapt the acquisition details [4].

A. Santos (✉)
Nuclear Medicine Department, Hospital Cuf Descobertas, Lisbon, Portugal

A. Grilo
H&TRC—Health and Technology Research Center, ESTeSL—Escola Superior de Tecnologia da Saúde, Instituto Politécnico de Lisboa, Lisbon, Portugal

CICPSI, Faculdade de Psicologia, Universidade de Lisboa, Alameda da Universidade, Lisbon, Portugal
e-mail: ana.grilo@estesl.ipl.pt

D. Albano
Department of Nuclear Medicine, University of Brescia and ASST Spedali Civili of Brescia, Brescia, Italy
e-mail: doalba87@libero.it

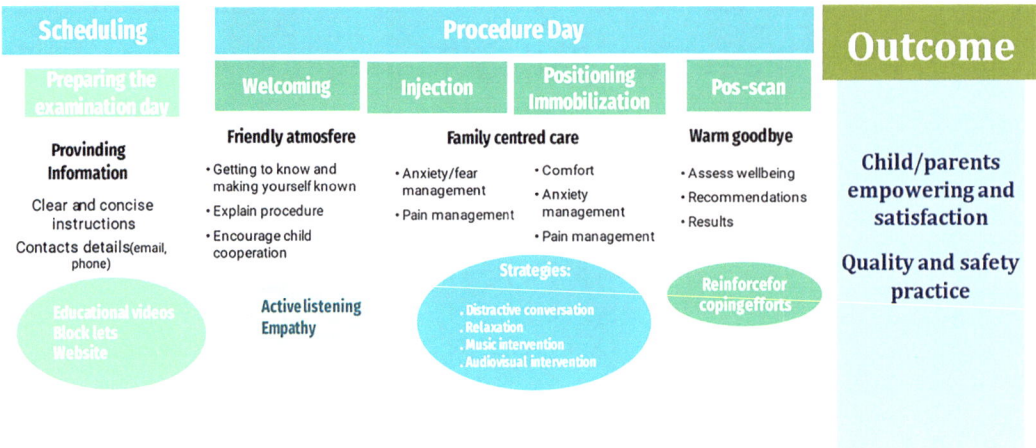

Fig. 16.1 Paediatric patient management

The capacity to manage the paediatric patient with a family-centred vision healthcare, leads to the concept of best-practice. This concept relates to the need of adaptation for each individual, considering their specific diagnostic/treatment goals and also the individual needs of each singular patient [5].

Best practices in paediatric NM focus on ensuring safety, minimizing radiation exposure, and providing compassionate, child-centred care. To be able to perform at the higher level and provide best-practice care, the NM professional should consider the patient and his/her characteristics (age, stage of development, anthropometric data, clinical and social background) as well as the parents/caregivers. All these intervenient deserve a personalized approach and an effective communication on every stage of the procedure. Figure 16.1 summarizes the various points of the entire process that will be covered in the following paragraphs.

16.2 Scheduling

Whenever a nuclear medicine procedure request is received by the department, both *Justification* and *Optimization* should be immediately considered. As with other imaging modalities, nuclear medicine procedures are required to be rigorously justified [6, 7].

When the procedure is justified—validated clinical indication and feasibility—then the procedure should be scheduled considering the best timing for performing it. The stage of disease and/or treatment should be considered and also the best date and time for the appointment, being mindful of the patient's capability of adhering to it (e.g. scheduling procedures that require fasting early in the morning). It is important to build an agenda that has time enough for doing the procedure, considering the specificities of the paediatric population and also that the human and material resources are correctly allocated [8].

NM professionals should be responsible for teaching and preparing receptionists to carry out scheduling of the appointments in an effective manner and building trust with the parents/caregivers. These interactions might happen in-person, by phone or email. Therefore, the receptionist must introduce her/himself by name and role, greet the parent/caregiver and demonstrate openness and friendliness as he/she schedules the procedure. The receptionist should show genuine interest in the child's well-being, collect necessary information for the appointment and provide clear information to parents/caregivers (e.g. fasting times, medication changes, procedure length, parking, child toys/distractions). Before the end, it is essential to check the parents'/caregivers' understanding of the information provided, clarify doubts and concerns, and express anticipation for the meeting at the MN department, showing that their presence and input are highly valued. If the appointment is made over the phone, the receptionist should continue checking for understanding and verbal agreement. When any question cannot be answered by the receptionist, then the NM Technologists or NM physicians should be notified and take time to contact these parents/caregivers and answer their questions.

16.3 Paediatric Patient and Parents/Caregivers' Education and Preparation

A comprehensive evaluation of the patient's situation before the day of the examination is advisable to have the department and the team ready on the day of the appointment. Preparing in advance for any protocol variation will prevent for delays during the day that will lead to patient increased anxiety and interfere with subsequent patient's schedules. In this sense, it is advisable to already know the indication for each patient study and to verify any special need (e.g. patient comorbidities such as autism or other characteristics that may need special logistics) [8, 9].

Time for explaining the procedure before starting it is mandatory for a family centred care approach and to capacitate the paediatric patient and their parents/caregivers to better feel during the exam and better collaborate with the nuclear medicine team [8, 10].

Pre-medication or any specific preparation (anxiolysis, analgesia, etc.) should be anticipated and planned. The venipuncture moment is a critic moment for the child, and this should be performed by skilled personnel. Injection techniques should be developed for a successful venipuncture and as a non-traumatic event (e.g. allowing caregivers to be present at the moment, adapted distraction methods and consider topic analgesia) [8].

Train et al., in a study related to ^{99m}Tc-DMSA renal scintigraphy, showed that psychological preparation, including a photo booklet and a letter providing advice to parents sent a week before the appointment decreased children's distress and the need for sedation [11].

Many options can be considered and illustrated booklets or animated educational videos that the patient and caregivers can watch together can be beneficial to provide information and for the patient and caregivers become familiar to the procedure to be done and to manage anxiety related to the unexpected [8, 12, 13].

These communication tools, including booklets, videos or other formats, should be tailored to the patient's age, considering the child's psychological development and ability to interpret and understand information. Understanding a child's cognitive development is essential in effectively communicating and reducing stress during examinations. Table 16.1 outlines the key characteris-

Table 16.1 Child main characteristics of cognitive development and sources of stress [14, 15]

	Cognitive development	Primary sources of stress
Preschool children (preoperational stage)	• Egocentric • Cannot express their feelings or emotions verbally • The adults in their lives have a significant influence on them • Concrete thinking (perceptive basis) • Magic thinking	• Separation from the mother (father/caregiver) • Separation from routines • Unfamiliar environment
School age children (concrete operational stage)	• Less egocentric behavior • Using language for expressing feelings and telling stories • Enjoy taking on responsibility. • Logical thinking about concrete events • Begin using inductive logic or reasoning from specific information to a general principle	• Fear of pain • Fear of damage resulting from the exam

tics of a child's cognitive development and the primary sources of stress that directly impact their understanding and experience of the examination. By using age-appropriate materials and approaches, healthcare professionals can significantly improve the paediatrics patient and family experience, making children feel more comfortable and parents more reassured.

Although providing written information is essential for patients and/or caregiver capacitation as discussed before, the complexity of NM examinations can confuse caregivers. In this sense, enough time must be given to understand the procedure and to answer caregivers' questions. Therefore, during scheduling, it is crucial to offer contact details (email, phone) for caregivers to raise any doubts or concerns they might have. Additionally, practical information, such as the importance of bringing the child's emotional and transitional object, if appropriate, and having objects or games that will help the child be distracted and remain still, should be included in the written information. It is essential to ensure that pregnant mothers are aware of any restrictions regarding their attendance at the department; for instance, they cannot accompany their child as a sole caregiver, and this must be communicated clearly beforehand [8, 16].

Additionally, depending on the procedure that the patient needs, preparation might be needed. A correct patient preparation is key for a successful exam, so it is important to pass the information clearly to the patient and/or parents/caregivers (depending on the patient's age) beforehand, and that the communication method is effective. Oral information should be given, with an adapted communication, but also written instructions should be provided. Additionally, a channel for caregivers to ask questions should be available [8, 9].

For example, Positron Emission Tomography (PET) with Fluorodeoxyglucose (^{18}F-FDG) can be performed for a wide variety of clinical indications, which can be related to oncological and non-oncological disease. Patients need to fast for at least 4 h before injection to reduce the glucose level and to lower circulating insulin levels, which optimize the target-to-background ratio. Blood glucose levels are measured at the start of the procedure, prior to de radiopharmaceutical administration and must be less than 11 mmol/L or 150 mg/dL. Patients are allowed to drink non-sweetened water to stay hydrated and to take any needed oral medications before arriving for the scan. If the patient is diabetic, the fasting period is discussed with the referring physician and nuclear medicine physician. Also, anti-diabetic medication should be discussed with the nuclear medicine physician, to avoid interferences in the radiopharmaceutical uptake [9, 10].

16.4 On the Day of the Procedure

16.4.1 Welcoming

When welcoming a child and caregivers for a nuclear medicine procedure, it's important to create a friendly and comforting environment to help ease any anxiety they might feel.

Creating an environment directed at a comfortable environment can help in limiting/ reducing anxiety (e.g. in the waiting area). When possible, waiting rooms should be designed using welcoming decorations and drawings. If not, the whole waiting room is possible, then a micro-environment (paediatrics' corner) should be adapted to be more friendly to children and provide distractions for the waiting time. Audiovisual tools can be considered (videos, music), materials for painting, games and toys may be available for children to be distracted while waiting. The available items should match the different age groups of patients of the day. It is important to avoid games and toys with small parts to prevent from the choking hazard risk. Also, it is important to only have washable materials, as they need to be decontaminated from biological risk after each use [8].

This special care help to indicate and make patient and/or caregiver feel the involvement, dedication and empathy of the team. Reducing the time in the waiting room is important and this relates directly with the agenda of the department, to prevent from delays in the day of the exam [8, 9, 17].

On the day of the exam, the welcome by the NM professionals should be friendly and reassuring. This can be crucial for gaining the patient's and caregivers trust and, therefore, their collaboration [8].

Although information was given beforehand, the professionals should not assume that the patient and parents/caregivers have all the information they need and that they understood it. At the beginning of the procedure, the child and the caregiver may or may not have a clear understanding of the imaging process [8]. It is important to understand that the child is often worried about any pain that he/she might experience and that caregivers are often more worried than the child [18]. Caregivers are more concerned about the exposure to radiation and possible adverse effects throughout child's lifespan, the complexity of the imaging procedure and the time to obtain scan results [8, 19].

16.4.2 Communication

Communication with the patient and their parents/caregivers is key for the success of the procedure.

An effective communication, adapted to patient's age and to the caregivers' needs should be pursued at all stages of the procedure. All patients and caregivers should be encouraged to ask any question or discuss any concerns they have. Verbal and non-verbal communication are both proven to reduce anxiety of patients performing medical examinations [9, 20]. Effective communication with paediatric patients involves a combination of verbal and non-verbal strategies to create a comfortable and trusting environment. Some of the strategies for a successful verbal communication are to use simple language (avoid medical jargon and use simple vocabulary; e.g. "picture" or "image" instead of "scan" or "acquisition"), apply positive reinforcement (praise the child when good behaviour and cooperation happens), ask open-ended questions (e.g. "how do you feel?", "do you have any question?"); give simple, clear and step-by-step instructions; do active listening (for the patient to feel heard and

their concerns addressed. As for non-verbal communication, which importance is sometimes undervalued, the professional should be always mindful of his/her non-verbal communication. A calm and open posture, warm, friendly and positive expressions, and getting into the child's eye level when speaking directly to the child. The tone of voice should be low and calm, to be less intimidating, with a variable pitch to avoid losing the child's interest [21].

The professional should be patient and reassuring, giving the child and the caregivers the time to process the information and ask questions, using a family-centred communication approach, promoting caregivers' engagement and proposing straightforward strategies in a friendly way [8, 20, 21]. It is essential that caregivers feel valued and engaged during all the NM procedures with the child [8, 20].

The AIDET® communication tool was presented by Studer Group (2005) and stands for the five key communication behaviours that create positive care interactions: *Acknowledge, Introduce, Duration, Explanation,* and *Thank You.* It can be effectively applied in a medical imaging department to improve interactions with children and their parents/caregivers. This mnemonic offers several advantages, making it especially suitable compared to other communication tools. AIDET® provides a clear and structured framework that is easy for healthcare professionals to remember and implement consistently, covering all critical aspects of effective communication, from greeting and introducing oneself to explaining and expressing gratitude. By focusing on reassurance and comfort, building trust, and reducing anxiety, AIDET® supports a family-centred approach. It emphasizes the importance of personal interaction, significantly enhancing the paediatric patient and family experience by making them feel valued and respected. AIDET's versatility allows healthcare providers to personalize their communication with each child and parent's specific concerns and needs, fostering a deeper sense of empathy and understanding. This adaptability and flexibility of AIDET® make it ideal for the varied and dynamic nature of paediatric care in Nuclear Medicine Departments.

Table 16.2 describes the AIDET® key points and illustrates its application in communicating with children and parents at the NM Department.

The use of AIDET as a tool for communicating with children must be carefully adapted based on the child's developmental characteristics. This means that every element of the communication process—from the initial meeting (*Acknowledge* and *introduce*) to the exam explanation with the proposed coping strategies (*duration* and *explanation*) and even the farewell (*thank you*)—must be tailored to align with the child's age and developmental stage. Understanding these developmental characteristics is crucial for ensuring that the child comprehends the information meaningfully and comfortably, considering their specific needs, perceptions and worries about medical procedures.

For instance, younger children may benefit from simple, straightforward explanations, visual aids or playful language. In contrast, older children might require more detailed information and the opportunity to ask questions and express concerns. Additionally, coping strategies should be age-appropriate; younger children might find comfort in holding a favourite toy or having a parent/caregiver present, while older children may benefit from deep breathing exercises, counting backwards or decision-making.

Table 16.3 outlines critical aspects to consider when explaining procedures and selecting coping strategies. It highlights the importance of adjusting communication to suit the child's cognitive and emotional development. These considerations not only help ensure the child feels understood and supported, but also empower healthcare professionals to significantly reduce anxiety and improve the child's overall experience.

In practice, it is the responsibility of healthcare professionals to use AIDET in a nuanced way. This involves being attentive and responsive to the child's verbal and non-verbal cues and continually assessing and adjusting their communication approach. By doing so, professionals can significantly enhance the child's comfort and cooperation during the NM imaging procedure, fostering a more trusting and positive relationship between the healthcare team and the family.

16.4.3 Preparation

The point 14.2 referred to the patient preparation before arrival (e.g. fasting or need to take medication for thyroid blockage), which should be confirmed by the technologist on the day of the exam, after the welcome and before starting the procedure, while this point aims at discussing the patient preparation for the exam, on the examination day.

It is important to collect all required data from the patient and caregivers. Measuring weight and height on the day of the exam, medical history, and background check (previous treatments, medication, and other pathologies). In female patients that had menarche already, the possibility of pregnancy must be considered, but it must be carefully researched during the discussion and ruled out, in case of doubt, by a urine pregnancy test before injecting the radiopharmaceutical. This can be a very sensible point of discussion considering the age of these patients but should not be disregarded [24].

Depending on the examination, some premedication or preparations are required and must be verified on a case-by-case basis. The most common examples of patient preparation on the day of the exam are:

- *Hydration and micturition*: It might be needed to ask the patient to drink water, for better hydration or, in certain cases, to provide intravenous hydration. This should be seen by the nuclear medicine physician and the correct way for hydrating the patient decided. Voiding before starting the scan (PET or SPECT) is very common and depending on the age and capability to cooperate, it can be asked to the patient directly or, instead, ask the caregiver to change diapers [8].
  Draining the bladder by administration of diuretics or with bladder catheterization is rarely advised (*except for some diuretic renal scans*) as bladder catheterization carries a risk of nosocomial infection and increases stress and discomfort [8, 24].
- *Thyroid blockage*: Many NM examinations require more specific preparations, which are

Table 16.2 AIDET® communication tool adapted to paediatric patient management in NM Department [22] Studer Group

	A Acknowledge	I Introduce	D Duration	E Explanation	T Thank you
Description	Greet the child by their name, make eye contact, smile, and acknowledge the parents or caregivers in the NM Department	Introduce yourself by providing your name, skill set, professional certification, and experience	Give an accurate time expectation for the procedure and identify all the steps	Explain what to expect next, answer questions, and let the parents/caregivers know how to access the exam results	Thank the child and parents/caregivers for their communication and cooperation, and express gratitude for the parents/caregivers' support of their child
Example with child	*Hi (name)! I'm so happy to see you today. You've got a really cool shirt on!* *Hello! I noticed that you were playing outside* with those machines. What did you think?*	*My name is (name), and I'm here to help take some memorable pictures of you today.* (younger children) *Hi, I'm (name), a Nuclear Medicine technologist. I'll be with you during your exam today to ensure everything goes smoothly.* (older children)	This will only take a few minutes, and you'll see some cool pictures at the end! *This is very quick; just about the time to supply these balls* (injection, younger children) You will need to remain in bed *a little longer*, but it's almost time to watch a video (image acquisition, older child)	*We will take some super pictures of you with this magic camera. Like a statue, you must stand still for the pictures to turn out beautifully.* (image acquisition, younger children) *We will use this special camera to take pictures of your bones/kidneys. It won't hurt, and you need to lie still like a statue.* (image acquisition, older child)	*Thank you for being such a brave and excellent patient today! You did a fantastic job I really appreciate how well you listened to the instructions. You were amazing!*

(continued)

Table 16.2 (continued)

	A Acknowledge	I Introduce	D Duration	E Explanation	T Thank you
Example with parents/caregivers	Good morning, Mr. and Mrs. (names). It's nice to meet you both Hello, welcome to our imaging department. How are you doing today?	I'm (name), a Nuclear Medicine technologist. I'll be conducting the imaging procedure today My name is Dr. (name), and I specialize in paediatric imaging. I'll be overseeing the scan today	The procedure will take about 2.5 h in total. We'll keep you updated throughout We should call (child name) back within 2 h for the scan. If there are any delays, I'll let you know immediately	To get a good image of (child's name)'s bones/kidneys, we need to inject a product that contains a small amount of radiation. It's a safe product, with far less radiation than in a CT scan. (if applicable) We're using NM equipment to obtain detailed images of your child's bones and kidneys. It's completely safe and painless Your child will need to lie still for the best pictures. We have some techniques to help them stay calm and comfortable. We will calmly analyse the best strategies for (child's name)	Thank you for bringing your child in today and for your patience during all the procedure phases We appreciate your cooperation and understanding. Please feel free to contact us if you have any questions later

Retrieved from https://www.studergroup.com/aidet

[a]Waiting room with 'miniature' NM equipment

Table 16.3 Paediatric patient communication at NM Department (based on [15, 23])

	Procedure explanation	Strategies for addressing stress and pain	Facilitators for interacting with the child
Preschool children (preoperational stage)	• Clarification of what the child should do and/or may feel (not the exam itself) • Description of a sensory and procedural approach • Use of concrete language that appeals to visible parts of the body • *Simulations typo* before the exam	• Having parents or caregivers present as mediators • Using distracting strategies facilitated by parents or professionals	• Having parents present • Creating a family/age-appropriate environment • Using affective communication • Providing both concrete and verbal reinforcement • Allowing the child to have their attachment object
School age children (concrete operational stage)	• Clarification of the exam more objectively, based on analogies from the child's world • Description of the exam through concrete methods (drawings, models, comics, videos) • Use simple effects of exams highlighting the physiological aspects • Apply reinforcement, value the child, and ask for his/her cooperation	• Using distraction techniques such as reading a book or watching a video • Practicing relaxation techniques like deep breathing	• Engaging in parent-mediated communication with the child • Employing both emotional and practical communication • Emphasizing truth-focused interaction • Respecting the child's privacy

described in detail in dedicated EANM Guidelines. A common example is thyroid blockage with a saturated solution of potassium iodide before ^{123}I-mIBG administration, to block thyroid uptake of free radioactive iodine.

• *Rest*: Depending on the procedure, the waiting time (before and after radiopharmaceutical administration) might require patient rest. When performing ^{18}F-FDG PET scan, the patient needs to comfortably rest before and after radiopharmaceutical administration. It is very important that the patient is provided with a calm room, with no stimulation and in a warm environment, to prevent for brown fat accumulation, which is very common in young patients and often hinders 18F-FDG PET interpretation [8, 10, 16, 24]. Brown fat can be significantly reduced by maintaining a warm room temperature during the uptake phase or providing a warm blanket, premedication with oral propranolol or diazepam is also effective [8, 9].

16.4.4 Radiopharmaceutical Administration

The radiopharmaceutical administration is a crucial point of the procedure, as it affects directly the quality of the exam. The correct radiopharmaceutical, the right activity and best practice administration are crucial points for a successful administration. For most of the procedures, the radiopharmaceutical is applied intravenously, and for fewer examinations, per os or respiratory intake might be used. Considering most cases, the intravenous access needs to be placed. As seen before, fear of pain is one of the most common on children, so this is very likely to be one of the most difficult moments for the child to cope, making the performance of the technologists involved even more challenging [18]. Anaesthetic cream (containing lidocaine and prilocaine) can be applied prior to venous access [8, 9, 25, 26]. In inpatients, when an intravenous cannula is already available, it should be used for tracer injection, and the line flushed with sufficient saline solution.

The venipuncture and injection are challenging for most children, so their cooperative behaviour should be reinforced [27]. The injection site should be monitored, especially in young children who cannot convey discomfort. For some children, needle-related procedures are very frightening and painful; in that situation, holding a parent/caregiver or other adult's hands could help, as squeezing the hand can help the child feel relief [17].

In a systematic review, Birnie et al. (2018) found evidence supporting the efficacy of distraction and breathing interventions for reducing children's needle-related pain or distress. In a child-centred intervention for ages 6–12, Kleye et al. (2022) demonstrated that allowing children to choose their coping strategies before cannula insertion resulted in lower distress, higher satisfaction and reduced time for the procedure. These strategies were presented to children as pictures. They included playing games, squeezing something, singing or listening to music, cuddling with a soft toy, choosing body position or focusing throughout the procedure [28, 29].

Radiopharmaceuticals are considered very safe from a pharmacological perspective and are reported to be non-toxic, non-allergenic and without adverse osmotic effect [30]. For these reasons, it is possible and safe to use radiopharmaceutical, even in the youngest. Some radiopharmaceuticals do require specific precautions, which are reported both in the summary of product characteristics and in relevant guidelines.

Administered activities should meet the ALARA principle [31, 32]. Dose optimization refers to the application of the minimum amount possible—the administered activity—guaranteeing the diagnostic accuracy of the procedure. Administered activity should follow the EANM

dosage card in its latest version. This document was first published by the EANM in 2008. Later, a consensus was reached with Society of Nuclear Medicine and Molecular Imaging (SNMMI) to harmonize activity guidelines between both groups. In 2016, the last update of the EANM Paediatric Dosage Card was issued. The Dosage Card is periodically updated [33, 34].

16.4.5 Uptake Period: Waiting

Considering the variety of the field, many different exams with different protocols can be seen. The time that the patient should wait from radiopharmaceutical administration to image acquisition can greatly vary. In the paediatric population, it is very important that this uptake period is previously thought, as to both allow the patient to fulfil what the team asks from them (e.g. rest comfortably, drink water) and to offer a patient-centred experience, in a personalized approach.

In some procedures, such as ^{18}F-FDG PET, the patient should stay in the department during the uptake period, and in a calm and warm room, being instructed to reduce muscle and brain stimulation and keep the hydration [16, 21]. For others, such as bone scans or renal scintigraphies, the patient is allowed to leave the department for the uptake period, knowing that the child should be encouraged to drink liquids and void the bladder frequently. Radioprotection concerns toward the public exposure should be passed to the patient and caregivers, and a fixed schedule for the return for imaging should be agreed upon with parents/caregivers [35].

16.5 Positioning and Immobilization

One of the most common artefacts is patient motion. Generally, the patient should be asked to remain still during image acquisition. This is especially challenging when the patient is a child. Depending on the cognitive development stage, the patient might not understand a verbal request to avoid motion, but at any age, the inability to move for a long period of time might bring anxiety and discomfort [36].

At this point, caregiver support is essential, both for bringing calmness and the sense of security to the child, and for letting the team know which are the distraction techniques that might better work for their child. Bringing a child's emotional and transitional object (such as a pacifier, blanket, toy) can help ease the anxiety. Also, by selecting the appropriate games or video, the positioning and immobilization can become less frightening.

It is recommended that the patient voids the bladder before coming into the imaging room, as seen in the previous section and that diapers should be changed before starting scans, for image quality and/or comfort and radiation protection. The caregiver should be present at the imaging room, as their reference person, to reduce children's anxiety and improve cooperation. For their presence to be effective and a source of reassurance and/or distraction for the child, it is essential that they are given clear instructions on what they can do to help the child (e.g. read a story, hold a hand). Vague instructions (e.g. *You must calm your child down*) can be interpreted as criticism and reduce the parents' sense of competence. Caregivers can be instructed to avoid patients from falling asleep in waiting times and to naturally induce their sleep immediately before the scan starts. This is only possible after venipuncture, otherwise the possible pain of the puncture and intensity of the injection moment will wake them up in distress.

Patients should be positioned in a way that meets the imaging needs (e.g. avoiding torso rotation or in frog's-leg position) but also comfortably, that should consider the time of the examination. It is quite different to do immobilization for a 5-min scan or 60 min scan. The duration of the image acquisition should be considered before immobilization devices are selected.

The term "immobilization" refers to a technique made with the consent of children and parents/caregivers, as opposed to the term "restraint" where physical force is used to hold the child still during the imaging procedure [37].

It is important to understand that babies can cry during image acquisition, and the team and the parents/caregivers should try to give them the best emotional support. Anyhow, attention should be given to the cause of the baby's cry. The professional should check if there is any possibility of the patient feeling pain or any intense discomfort due to motion constrained devices.

Parents/caregivers should not try to force the baby to stop crying but should be informed that this is natural and acceptable, as the success of the examination depends, at that point, on the absence of motion; therefore, they can try to calm and comfort the baby and, if required, help the staff with the immobilization [38].

Immobilization devices can vary from simple head rests, cushions, sandbags, sheets to vacuum mattresses or other immobilization devices. Its mandatory to not use any chest immobilizer that will block or obstruct the airway and natural breathing. It is important that whichever immobilization device is used, the child is always comfortable [37].

16.6 Distraction Techniques

The major aspect for achieving a good quality and motion-free image is applying optimal distraction techniques. Apart from the immobilization techniques which are very helpful, distraction techniques help the child to go through the procedure in an easier and calmer way. Obviously, the technique applied will differ greatly according to the age and stage of development of the child and also his/her personal preferences, as shown in Table 16.4.

Starting by the rooms, a child-friendly decor, an attractive, colourful and stimulating environment can reduce fear and anxiety. Pictures, funny things, cartoons, bubbles, starlight spinner, super looper, glitter wands, fidget cube, pinwheel, optical illusions; or for older children—challenges like riddles promote cooperation as children have things to look at that enable them to divert their minds away from the procedure [25, 29].

Other distractions methods that can be applied are to provide monitors to watch movies or short videoclips, listen to music, hear a story read by the caregiver, play games or

Table 16.4 Distraction techniques by ages

Infants under 6 months	Toddlers (6 months to 2 years)	Preschool	School age	Adolescents
• Having parents/caregivers present • Rattles or other baby toys • Rocking, stroking their face, gentle patting • Singing • Sucrose and breastfeeding	• Blowing bubbles or a windmill • Toys and books that make noise or with buttons to push • Singing the child's favourite song • Light-up toys • Reading a book	• Big belly breathing, blowing away the scary feelings or blowing away the hurt • Blowing bubbles or a windmill • Counting games • Reading a book, or a search-and-find book • Mind pictures, e.g. think about a favourite sport, family holiday, school game or activity; let your child tell a story or answer questions about what is pictured in their mind	• Big belly breathing, blowing away the nervous feelings or blowing away the hurt • Blowing bubbles and counting each one • Counting games • reading a book, or a search-and-find book • Mind pictures, e.g. think about a favourite sport, family holiday, school game or activity; let your child tell a story or answer questions about what is pictured in their mind	• Listening to music with headphones • Let them have a choice about parental presence and hand holding • Mind pictures, e.g. think about a favourite sport, family holiday, school game or activity; let them tell a story or answer questions about what is pictured in their mind • Relaxation and breathing techniques • Use humour or talk about something unrelated to their procedure • Watching a favourite movie/show or playing a game on a phone or tablet

Source: http://distraction-guide-by-childrens-hospital-at-lhsc.pdf [39]

engage in conversations in known topics of interest of the child.

The youngest children usually prefer parents to tell their favourite story, sing their favourite or familiar songs or watch their preferred songs videoclips. All these strategies help the patient to feel safe in the imaging room and that they are not left alone [9].

School-age children and adolescents should be questioned if they want to know what is happening or focus instead on an activity, as some of them want to watch the procedure as it happens.

The personal approach of these distraction methods is the reason why they should be considered from the scheduling time point, while passing information to the caregiver in the preparation for the procedure's day. The caregiver should be informed and should bring appropriate objects that will bring familiarity and calmness to the child.

16.7 Sedation

When possible, sedation should be avoided, considering the several risks associated (e.g. hypoventilation, apnoea, airway obstruction, cardiopulmonary arrest and others) [25, 40, 41]. An effective communication from the first moment is crucial to allow best practice and enable the best patient experience possible, aligned with the best immobilization devices and techniques and distraction strategies, altogether aim at achieving a good quality exam without the need for sedation.

Anyhow, the decision to sedate a child must be made on an individual basis. It depends on the child's characteristics (e.g. age and capability to cooperate) and also on the procedure requested (PET images are more likely to need sedation than for instance renal scintigraphies) due to the duration of image acquisition, physical characteristics of the bore and possibility of having the team and caregivers holding the child still [8, 40, 42].

When sedation/general anaesthesia is required, it will be administered after tracer injection and before image acquisition, especially when performing a brain ^{18}F-FDG PET/CT (PET/MR) due to the effects of anaesthesia on regional cerebral glucose metabolism [43].

This topic was developed in Chap. 15, so refer to topic 15.4.7 General Anaesthesia scanning protocols for more information.

16.8 Image Optimization

Best practices in nuclear medicine require that the image acquisition should be done in optimal conditions: the best parameter to achieve an optimal image, while respecting ALARA principles. This is especially important in paediatric patient imaging, as administered activities can vary greatly, due to the wide variety of age and weight or body mass index of the patients. In this sense, adult protocols should not be implemented in paediatric studies, but instead, an optimized version for the paediatric population [3, 5, 44].

From the first developments of hybrid imaging, the additional radiation exposure due to CT was a significant concern [8]. In fact, the addition of a CT scan to the PET or SPECT acquisition can increase the radiation burden significantly. Parisi et al. (2017), studied typical effective doses related to various applied methodologies and showed that the purpose of the CT scan (diagnostic or AC and localization CT), and consequently its acquisition details, have an impact in the effective dose of the procedure [4].

Many examples in the literature show strategies for image optimization in paediatric nuclear medicine procedures. Camoni et al. (2023), based

in the available literature, mention that the selection of the patient body volume to be investigated during the PET/CT or SPECT/CT lowers the radiation burden from CT [8, 24]. The inclusion of arms in the scanning field of view, should also be carefully selected, as in many equipments, the artefacts that lead to image quality deterioration tend to be compensated, resulting in an increase in the radiation dose [8, 45].

The optimization of hybrid imaging acquisition is mainly based on adjusting acquisition parameters and reconstruction algorithms: in conventional nuclear medicine, collimator selection acquisition matrix, energy windows, acquisition zoom, time *per* frame and imaging distance; in PET imaging, use of 2D or 3D technology, selection of matrix size, field of view, time of flight, attenuation correction, slice overlap, scatter correction and coincidence timing. In CT scans, choose appropriate tube current and voltage, slice thickness, rotation time, pitch, overlap [6].

Recently, automatic exposure control systems using automatic tube current modulation (ATCM) and automatic tube voltage selection (ATVS) have been developed. ATVS allows an automatic choice of kV and mAs settings without impairing the contrast-to-noise ratio and negligible variation when used for quantification of PET images [46].

However, exposure control settings will generally still require some weight-based classes to be defined. When the ATVS are not available, tube voltage can be manually adapted for children. Due to the small physical size of children, dose reduction can improve image contrast, rather than create the severe image noise associated with adult CT [6, 8, 46].

In image reconstruction, parameters such as the algorithm, matrix, filters, scatter correction and zoom factor also influence the image quality. Additionally, the application of appropriate image corrections (e.g. attenuation and scatter correction, and, in the case of PET systems, random correction) and, finally, the use of quantitative and qualitative capabilities, such as the generation of region of interest analysis, time–activity curve generation, image reformatting or tissue uptake ratios, specific to the clinical need [6].

Additionally, performing paediatric studies on modern cameras with high detector sensitivity (e.g. cadmium-zinc-telluride (CZT) detectors) and advanced CT scanners can reduce the effective dose by facilitating the lowering of injected activity and using the advanced paediatric CT optimization techniques [8, 47]. Similarly, SPECT or PET reconstruction with resolution recovery algorithms can improve image quality and allow reduction in the administered radiopharmaceutical activity [6, 48, 49].

With the uprise of artificial intelligence, using deep learning reconstruction, there are promising results in terms of additional dose reduction and image quality, allowing further adjustment to protocols for specific clinical cases [50–52].

It is important that the nuclear medicine technologist has a broad knowledge on the characteristics and capabilities of the equipment where the image acquisition will occur, using them for the best performance.

16.9 Patient Discharge and Final Recommendations

Before the patient leaves the department, it is important to do a quality check of the acquired raw data. If not before, then artefacts should be identified at this point and evaluated for their impact. It is important to confirm the validity of the available data for diagnostic interpretation and clinical use. One of the most common artefacts is patient motion. If present, then a motion correction software should be considered, and its results validated prior to patient discharge. If needed, the acquisition may need to be repeated [53].

It is recommended to visualize the images and check for normal biodistribution of the radiopharmaceutical. This can help to identify any attenuation artefacts caused by an external object that was inadvertently kept by the patient. In this case, if the attenuation is in the target zone, image acquisition should be repeated. Also, contamination artefacts can be identified with this procedure. Patient position should also be checked as artefacts can occur: Asymmetrical uptake can be misleading in cases where the patient is not properly positioned. In very small babies, the positioning artefacts are more likely to happen, as minor rotation may still affect the acquired image and can lead to misinterpretation. Depending on the type of image acquired (static, dynamic or tomographic), it might be possible to overcome positioning artefacts by using reorientation in the image reconstruction phase. In many cases (especially static images), it is recommended to repeat the acquisition with proper positioning.

When a hybrid image is performed, an additional point should be considered when reviewing the data: co-registration. Both emission (SPECT or PET) and transmission (CT) should perfectly overlap. When this does not happen, significant artefacts and pitfalls can occur. Software and reconstruction solutions should be used when available where manual reorientation is possible.

Image repetition in hybrid imaging should be very carefully chosen, being mindful that to repeat a CT scan is to significantly increase the radiation burden of the study.

Regarding radioprotection principles, it is recommended to teach the child and/or parents/caregivers how to naturally accelerate the radiopharmaceutical elimination. In most of the cases, renal excretion is the major elimination via, so recommending increasing oral hydration throughout the rest of the day and frequent micturition. In small children, parents/caregivers should be advised to change diapers more frequently.

After all images are checked and accepted for interpretation, radioprotection recommendations are actively communicated, then the patient and parents/caregivers should be discharged in a friendly manner, to leave a good lasting memory for the child.

Oral reinforcement of the child's cooperative behaviours is important, and it is time to offer previously agreed rewards. The rewards will vary according to the age and stage of development of the patient, and younger children are often delighted with coloured stickers, a fun activity with the caregiver, or the opportunity to put their handprint on the board of the bravest placed in the waiting room. Older children usually feel rewarded with bravery certificates or stickers, given the opportunity to take a photo of the bravest board after having written their name on it. Giving a positive reinforcement to the paediatric patient can be very beneficial to increase his/her well-being and for future examination needs. Parents should also be thanked for cooperating during the procedure and informed about examination results [8].

16.10 Tools to Support Paediatric Patient Management

For best-practice performance in the management of paediatric patients in NM, it is of utmost importance that these procedures are made by high-level skilled professionals. To have continuous improvement and professional development, it is important that the NM professionals that work with the paediatric population are updated both technically and with the best coping strategies learned and trained. This chapter provided several technical considerations that should be considered while imaging the paediatric patient, but to be continuously updated in the techniques and technologies available is mandatory.

With consideration to the psychology and behavioural level and the communication methods for better coping with the paediatric patient and their parents/caregivers, this chapter includes practical materials for developing communication, by exemplifying language to use and to avoid.

Appendix A has been developed to aid the professionals to do a self-assessment, to find opportunities for practice improvement.

16.10.1 Language to Use and to Avoid

Professionals may have varying levels of contact with children in their daily lives, and those with less experience interacting with children (e.g. those without children, younger siblings, or nephews) may find communication with paediatric patients and their parents more challenging. This can lead to the use of less appropriate expressions in an attempt to secure the child's quick cooperation, such as during a radiopharmaceutical injection or while trying to keep the child still during the image acquisition. Research on children undergoing venipuncture/immunization has shown that using critical expressions and reassuring and empathizing with the child are associated with distress (Cohen 2008; Pedro et al. 2009). Apologies and giving children excessive control can also generate or deepen anxiety (Cohen et al. 2006). Conversely, strategies like distraction (proposed by health professionals, parents or parents/caregivers before a child already shows signs of distress) and encouraging coping skills have been demonstrated to help reduce a child's distress during medical procedures (Cohen et al. 2006; Pedro et al. 2009). Table 16.5 provides examples of recommended

Table 16.5 Language for nuclear medicine practitioners (Cohen [23] adapted)

USE (appropriate language)	INSTEAD OF USING (avoid language)
Welcoming	
• *What did you do in school yesterday /during the weekend?* (distraction/ show interest)	• *Hello, I know you're very courageous, and you won't cry* (negative focus)
• *You have a lovely teddy.* What's it called? (distraction/ show interest)	• *I like your teddy. Can I keep it/play with it?* (threat—Removing a comfort object)
• *What's your favourite colour, cartoon or game?* (distraction/ show interest)	• *I see you like blue a lot* (avoids the child's conversation)
• *Did you play outside with the toys in the waiting room? What do you think?* (distraction/ show interest)	• *You don't have to be afraid. It is not difficult* (vague, negative focus)
• *Do you know what you're doing today?* (show interest)	• *Mom/dad explained what you're doing today? (questioning that generates anxiety)*
• *We're going to take some very lovely pictures* (positive focus)	• *This won't hurt anything* (vague, negative focus)
Radiopharmaceuticals injection	
• *First, I will clear your arm, you will feel the cold pad, and next...* (sensory and procedural information)	• *I will give you a shot* (vague information, negative focus)
• *It might feel like a pinch/the point of a sharp pencil on your arm* (sensory information)	• *It will feel like a bee sting* (negative focus)
• *You can stay on mom's lap* (positive focus, comfort)	• *The shot costs nothing/it won't hurt* (negative focus)
• *When I count to 3, you start blowing on the soap balls / you start counting from 10 to one/ filling the balloon.* (coaching to cope, distraction, limited control)	• *Tell me when you are ready* (too much control)
	• *Don't cry* (negative focus)
	• *You are acting like a baby* (criticism)
• *Keep making soap bubbles.* (distraction)	• *You must calm your child down* (parents' criticism)
• *Let's keep counting. I need your help.* (distraction)	• *I can't inject the radiopharmaceutical if (child's name) stays agitated like this* (parents' criticism)
• *Mrs/Mr (name) I ask you to show this book to (child's name)* (parents' cooperation/distraction)	• I'm sorry. I know it hurts. (apologize, negative focus)
• *Mrs/Mr (name), Can you hold up this poster and count with (child's name) how many red capes there are?* (parents' cooperation/distraction)	• It is over (negative focus)
	• *I'm done. It hurt more because you moved your arm* (criticism, negative focus)
• *You were very brave* (praise)	
• *That's it. It's over. You did a great job holding your arm still* (labelled praise)	
• *You can pick a* sticker (reinforcement)	
Image acquisition/positioning	
• Now, let's take the pictures. I'll show you what you must do to make the photos look great (positive focus)	• *You will be okay; there is nothing to worry about* (reassurance, lack of empathy)
• The pictures will be shorter than ... (positive focus)	• *The procedure will last as long as...* (negative focus)
• *You must stand still like a statue. Let's play the statue game (distraction, positive focus)*	• *All you must do is lie still and not move* (negative focus)
• *Some children like to imagine they're in a spaceship. What do you think?* (distraction, positive focus)	• *Yesterday, a kid younger than you stayed quiet the whole time* (blame, criticism)
• *Would you rather listen to your mother tell a story, watch a video or play the statue game?* (child-centred intervention, positive focus)	• *I know it's hard. You must hold on a little longer* (negative focus)
	• *I am sorry* (apologizing)
• *You are being very brave. Keep holding still* (praise, encouragement)	• If you move, I (mom/daddy) will *be disappointed* (blame, negative focus)

(continued)

Table 16.5 (continued)

USE (appropriate language)	INSTEAD OF USING (avoid language)
Post-scan	
• *That was hard, I am proud of you* (praise)	• *It's over.* (devaluing)
• *Tell me what it was like to be a statue for so long?* (questioning, showing interest)	• *It didn't cost anything.* (devaluing)
• *You did an excellent job holding still...* (labelled praise)	• *See, all you had to do was sit still* (devaluing)
• *You were very brave to stay in the room taking so many pictures* (labelled praise)	• *There was no need to be so afraid* (criticism)
• *"Give me five"* (valuing)	• *You're done!* (disregard)
• *Nice to meet you. Have a good day!* (appreciation/valuing)	• *Goodbye!* (disregard)

language and phrases that should be avoided, highlighting their impact on the child and the parents/caregivers. This is a practical guide for NM practitioners to refine their communication techniques, ensuring they are supportive, calming and effective in helping children cope with the NM procedures [23, 54, 55].

Appendix 1: NM Practitioners Self-Evaluation Communication Checklist

Maintaining a checklist for health professionals to assess their communication with children and parents in imaging departments is vital for promoting a culture of excellence and continuous improvement in paediatric patient care. Table 16.6 demonstrates that these tools guarantee that all healthcare professionals uphold the same high communication standards, covering all critical aspects from initial greetings to detailed explanations and expressions of gratitude. This consistency aids communicate important information clearly, reducing the risk of errors and improving the overall efficiency of the NM department. Additionally, regular use of self-assessment checklists allows Nuclear Medicine Practitioners to reflect on their communication skills, identify areas for enhancement and actively work on them. Finaly, this checklist can also be employed in training programs, ensuring all NM staff have the necessary skills for effective communication with children and parents. New staff can use them as a guide to understand expected communication standards, while for experienced staff, they are helpful to maintain and enhance their skills.

Table 16.6 Checklist for self-assessment of nuclear medicine practitioners' communication in a paediatric field

	Yes/no/some	Observation
Welcoming		
I greet the child and parent/caregiver with genuine warmth, introducing myself by name and role		
I used the information gathered at the scheduling office to establish a relationship and a friendly and caring atmosphere		
I consciously tried to connect with the child playfully and engagingly, using toys, for example, to create a fun and stimulating environment		
Build up and maintain rapport		
I watched and listened attentively to the child and parents/caregivers		
I learned the child's preferences, toys, physical condition, fears and previous experiences		
I asked open-ended questions to understand the parent/caregiver's concerns		
I empathized with and validated the parents'/caregivers' concerns and feelings		
I was attentive to signs of child distress and addressed them promptly		
I respect the child and parents'/caregivers' cultural, religious and personal preferences		
Explaining the procedure		
Provided sensory and procedural information on the examination suitable for the child's development		
I provided the necessary information that answered the parents'/caregivers' needs and expectations		
I encouraged the parents/caregivers to ask questions and express concerns		
I involved both the child and parents/caregivers in decisions about the procedure when appropriate (e.g. informed consent)		
I checked that the child and parents/caregivers had understood the information provided		
Together with the child and parents/caregivers, I found strategies that will enhance adherence to the procedure		
Injection		
I described scan details, providing sensory and processual information suitable for the child's development		
I actively involved the child and the parents/caregivers in decisions about the coping strategies to use during the injection. (e.g. sitting on the mother's lap or blowing soap bubbles)		
I praised the child's cooperation at the end of the injection		
I provided clear instructions on the rest period		
Scan		
I was interested in how the waiting period went (child and parents/caregivers)		
I checked the procedures before the scan (e.g. bladder emptying)		
I described scan details, providing sensory and processual information suitable for the child's development		
I checked that the child and the parents/caregivers understood the information provided regarding positioning		

(continued)

Table 16.6 (continued)

	Yes/no/some	Observation
I involved the child and the parents/caregivers in decisions about the coping strategies to use during the scan (e.g. listening to music, standing like a statue, watching a video, listening to the mother/father reading a story and offered pillows, blankets or other comfort measures as needed)		
I checked and reinforced the child's skills to apply mutually agreed strategies		
Post-scan		
I informed the parents how to obtain the procedure results and what care to take with the child after discharge		
I invited the child (if appropriate) to provide feedback on his/her experience		
I thanked the child and reinforced his/her cooperation		
I said a friendly goodbye to the child and the parents/caregivers		

References

1. Colson ER, Foster LH. Children are not small adults. J Virus Erad. 2015;1:133. https://doi.org/10.1016/S2055-6640(20)30511-2.

2. Spiegler BJ. Kids are nor small adults: here's why. J Int Neuropsychol Soc. 2011;17(4):753–4. https://doi.org/10.1017/S1355617711000762.

3. Prior JO, Mirzaei S, Gnesin S, Lalonde MN. Dose optimisation in pediatric studies: why it is important and how it can benefit every nuclear medicine department. J Nucl Med. 2021;62(4):568–9. https://doi.org/10.2967/jnumed.120.254193.

4. Parisi MT, Bermo MS, Alessio AM, Sharp SE, Gelfand MJ, Shulkin BL. Optimisation of pediatric PET/CT. Semin Nucl Med. 2017;47(3):258–74. https://doi.org/10.1053/j.semnuclmed.2017.01.002.

5. McCoubrey B, Ryder H, Vara A. Best practice in nuclear medicine—Part 1. London: European Association of Nuclear Medicine; 2006. https://doi.org/10.52717/WPAO3671.

6. I. S. Reports. Radiation Protection in Paediatric Radiology. In: Series No. 71, ISBN 978-92-0-125710-9; 2012, pp. 71–8.

7. The 2007 Recommendations of the International Commission on Radiological Protection. ICRP publication 103. Ann ICRP. 2007;37(2–4):1–332. https://doi.org/10.1016/j.icrp.2007.10.003.

8. Camoni L, Santos A, Luporsi M, et al. EANM procedural recommendations for managing the paediatric patient in diagnostic nuclear medicine. Eur J Nucl Med Mol Imaging. 2023;50:3862–79. https://doi.org/10.1007/s00259-023-06357-3.

9. McQquattie S. Pediatric PET/CT imaging: tips and techniques. J Nucl Med Technol. 2008;36(4):171–80.

10. Hamblen S, Lowe VJ. 18F-FDG oncology patient preparation techniques. J Nucl Med Technol. 2003;31:3–7.

11. Train H, Colville G, et al. Paediatric 99mTc-DMSA imaging: reducing distress and rate of sedation using a psychological approach. Clin Radiol. 2006;61(10):868–74. https://doi.org/10.1016/j.crad.2006.05.009.

12. Williams G, Greene S. From analogue to apps—developing an app to prepare children for medical imaging procedures. J Vis Commun Med. 2015;38(3-4):168–76. https://doi.org/10.3108/17453054.2015.1108285.

13. Szeszak S, Man R, Love A, et al. Animated educational video to prepare children for MRI without sedation: evaluation of the appeal and value. Pediatr Radiol. 2016;46(12):1744–50. https://doi.org/10.1007/s00247-016-3661-4.

14. Piaget J, Cook M. The origins of intelligence in children. New York: International University Press; 1952.

15. Bibace R, Walsh M. Development of Children's concepts of illness. Pediatrics. 1980;66(6):912–7.

16. Zucchetta P, Mansi L. Practical pediatric PET imaging. Eur J Nucl Med Mol Imaging. 2007;34:1886. https://doi.org/10.1007/s00259-007-0515-1.

17. Kleye I, Hedén L, Karlsson K, et al. Children's individual voices are required for adequate management of fear and pain during hospital care and treatment. Scand J Caring Sci. 2021;35(2):530–7. https://doi.org/10.1111/scs.12865.

18. Fahey F, Treves S, Adelstein S. Minimizing and communicating radiation risk in pediatric nuclear medicine. J Nucl Med Technol. 2012;40(1):13–24. https://doi.org/10.2967/jnumed.109.069609.

19. Schanmugham J. Educational intervention to increase parental knowledge and acceptance of pediatric imaging. J Pediatr Neonatal Care. 2018;8:00302. https://doi.org/10.15406/jpnc.2018.08.00302.

20. Borgwardt L, Larsen H, Oedersen K, et al. Practical use and implementation of PET in children in a Hospital PET Centre. Eur J Nucl Med Mol Imaging.

2003;30(10):1389–97. https://doi.org/10.1007/s00259-003-1263-5.

21. Green M. The nuclear imaging technologist and the pediatric patient. New York: Springer; 2006.

22. Huron. AIDET Patient Communication [Online]. https://www.studergroup.com/aidet. Accessed 15 Jun 2024.

23. Cohen L. Behavioral approaches to anxiety and pain management for pediatric venous access. Pediatrics. 2008;122(Suppl 3):S134–9. https://doi.org/10.1542/peds.2008-1055f.

24. Vali R, Alessio A, Balza R, et al. SNMMI procedure standard/EANM practice guideline on pediatric (18)F-FDG PET/CT for oncology 1.0. J Nucl Med. 2021;62(1):99–110. https://doi.org/10.2967/jnumed.120.254110.

25. Gelfand M, Clements C, MacLean J. Nuclear medicine procedures in children: special considerations. Semin Nucl Med. 2017;27(2):110–7. https://doi.org/10.1053/j.semnuclmed.2016.10.001.

26. Kohli M, Vali R, Amirabadi A, et al. Procedural pain reduction strategies in paediatric nuclear medicine. Pediatr Radiol. 2019;49(2):1362–7. https://doi.org/10.1007/s00247-019-04462-w.

27. Karlsson K, Englund A, Enskär K, et al. Parents' perspectives on supporting children during needle-related medical procedures. Int J Qual Stud Health Well Being. 2014;9:24. https://doi.org/10.3402/qhw.v9.23759.

28. Birnie K, Noel M, Chambers C, et al. Psychological interventions for needle-related procedural pain and distress in children and adolescents. Cochrane Database Syst Rev. 2018;10(10):CD005179. https://doi.org/10.1002/14651858.CD005179.

29. Kleye I, Sundler A, Karlsson K, et al. Positive effects of a child-centered intervention on children's fear and pain during needle procedures. Paediatr Neonatal Pain. 2023;5(1):23–30. https://doi.org/10.1002/pne2.12095.

30. Schreuder N, Koopman D, Jager P, et al. Adverse events of diagnostic radiopharmaceuticals: a systematic review. Semin Nucl Med. 2019;49(5):382–410. https://doi.org/10.1053/j.semnuclmed.2019.06.006.

31. Matusiak K, Wolna J, Jung A, et al. Impact of the frequency and type of procedures performed in nuclear medicine units on the expected radiological hazard. Int J Environ Res Public Health. 2023;20(6):5206. https://doi.org/10.3390/ijerph20065206.

32. Lassmann M, Treves S. Pediatric radiopharmaceutical administration: harmonization of the 2007 EANM paediatric dosage card (version 1.5.2008) and the 2010 north American consensus guideline. Eur J Nucl Med Mol Imaging. 2014;41(8):1636. https://doi.org/10.1007/s00259-014.2817-4.

33. Lassmann M. The new EANM paediatric dosage card. Eur J Nucl Med Mol Imaging. 2008;35(9):1748. https://doi.org/10.1007/s00259-007-0572-5.

34. Lassmann M, Eberlein U, Lopci E, et al. Standardization of administered activities in paediatric nuclear medicine: the EANM perspective. Eur J Nucl Med Mol Imaging. 2016;43(13):2275–8. https://doi.org/10.1007/s00259-016-3474-6.

35. Van den Wyngaert T, Strobel K, Kampen W, et al. The EANM practice guideline for bone scintigraphy. Eur J Nucl Mes Mol Imaging. 2016;43(9):1723–38. https://doi.org/10.1007/s00259-016-3415-4.

36. Munn Z, Jordan Z. The patient experience of high technology medical imaging: a systematic review of the qualitative evidence. JBI Libr Syst Rev. 2011;9(19):631–78. https://doi.org/10.11124/01938924-201109190-00001.

37. Ng J, Doyle E. Keeping children still in medical imaging examinations—immobilisation or restraint: a literature review. J Med Imaging Radiat Sci. 2019;50(1):179–87. https://doi.org/10.1016/j.jmir.2018.09.008.

38. Gordon I. Issues surrounding preparation, information and handling the child and parent in nuclear medicine. J Nucl Med. 1998;39(3):490–4.

39. V. H. Foundation. Distraction Guide - a break down for different ages [Online]. http://distraction-guide-by-childrends-hospital-at-lhsc.pdf. Accessed 16 Jun 2024.

40. Koch B. Avoiding sedation in pediatric radiology. Pediatr Radiol. 2008;38(Suppl2):225–6. https://doi.org/10.1007/s00247-008-0807-z.

41. Mandell G, Majd M, Shalaby-Rana E, et al. Society of Nuclear Medicine Procedure Fuideline for Pediatric Sedation in Nuclear Medicine—version 3.0. In: Society of Nuclear Medicine Procedure Guidelines Manual; 2003. p. 173–7.

42. Mohammed A. Review of pediatric sedation and anesthesia for radiological diagnostic and therapeutic procedures. J Radiat Res Appl Sci. 2024;17:100833.

43. Juengling F, Kassubek J, Martens-Le Bouar H, et al. Cerebral regional hypometabolism caused by propofol-induced sedation in children with severe myoclonic epilepsy: a study using fluorodeoxyglucose positron emission tomography and statistical parametric mapping. Neurosci Lett. 2002;335(2):79–82. https://doi.org/10.1016/s0304-3940(02)01060-1.

44. Alessio ABE, Brusa A, et al. Radiation protection and dose optimization. Londin: European Association of Nuclear Medicine; 2016. https://doi.org/10.52717/CIGE6278:.

45. Inoue Y, Nagahara K, Kudo H, et al. CT dose modulation using automatic exposure control in whole-body PET/CT: effects of scout imaging direction and arm positioning. Am J Nucl Med Mol Imaging. 2018;8(2):143–52.

46. Piwowarska-Bilska H, Hahn L, Birkenfeld B, et al. Optimisation of lowdose CT protocol in pediatric nuclear medicine imaging. J Nucl Med Technol. 2010;38(4):181–5. https://doi.org/10.2967/jnmt.109.073486.

47. Gregoire B, Pina-Jomir G, Bani-Sadr A, et al. Four-minute bone SPECT using large-field cadmium-zinc-telluride camer. Clin Nucl Med. 2018;43(6):389–95. https://doi.org/10.1097/rlu.0000000000002062.

48. Shkumat N, Vali R, Shammas A. Clinical evaluation of reconstruction and acquisition time for pediatric (18)F-FDG brain PET using digital PET/CT. Pediatr Radiol. 2020;50(7):966–72. https://doi.org/10.1007/s00247-020-04640-1.

49. Chicheportiche A, Goshen E, Godefroy J, et al. Can a penalized-likelihood estimation algorithm be used to reduce the injected dose or the acquisition time in (68)Ga-DOTATATE PET/CT studies? EJNMMI Phys. 2021;8(1):13. https://doi.org/10.1186/s40658-021-00359-6.

50. Greffier J, Hamard A, Pereira F, et al. Image quality and dose reduction opportunity of deep learning image reconstruction algorithm for CT: a phantom study. Eur Radiol. 2020;30(7):3951–9. https://doi.org/10.1007/s00330-020-06724-w.

51. Singh R, Digumarthy S, Muse V, et al. Image quality and lesion detection on deep learning reconstruction and iterative reconstruction of submillisievert chest and abdominal CT. AJR Am J Roentgenol. 2020;214(3):566–73. https://doi.org/10.2214/ajr.19.21809.

52. McLeavy C, Chunara M, Gravell R, et al. The future of CT: deep learning reconstruction. Clin Radiol. 2021;76(6):407–15. https://doi.org/10.1016/j.crad.2021.01.010.

53. Poli G, Torres L, Coca M, et al. Paediatric nuclear medicine practice: an international survey by the IAEA. Eur J Nucl Med Mol Imaging. 2020;47(6):1552–63. https://doi.org/10.1007/s00259-019-04624-w.

54. Cohen L, MacLaren J, Fortson B, et al. Randomized clinical trial of distraction for infant immunization pain. Pain. 2006;125(1–2):165–71.

55. Pedro H, Barros L, Moleiro C. Brief report: parents and nurses' behaviors associated with children distress during routine immunization in a Portuguese population. J Pediatr Psychol. 2009;35(6):602–10.

Patient Engagement in Hybrid Imaging

17

Carla Abreu, Ana Monteiro Grilo, and Luísa Roldão Pereira

17.1 Introduction

Firstly, it is crucial to reflect on the diversity of procedures carried out in a Nuclear Medicine department, which means that these specialist healthcare professionals will inherently interact with very different cohorts of patients, some of whom fear the possibility of malignant diagnosis, disease progression and assessment of response to a recent treatment, others may be monitoring benign yet chronic diseases, and even some who may still be facing the uncertainty of a diagnosis. All these patients are individuals with multifactorial needs. While these needs may be difficult to assess in the short timeframe of an imaging procedure, a good Nuclear Medicine technologist embodies a holistic approach to enable the best experience for that person. To achieve this, it is essential to establish a tacit connection with the patient, creating a sense of safety, openness and cooperation between all involved—this is possible through a respectful, responsive and proportionate communication style, encouraging the patient's meaningful contribution to their care and combining it with the necessary technical aspects of the scan.

Angela Coulter (2011) [1], a prominent reference in the field of patient engagement, defines this concept as the commitment to empowering patients with the necessary information, skills and support to enable them to actively participate in their healthcare. This definition requires patients to be knowledgeable about their health conditions, treatment options and impact on quality of life to make informed decisions. It also includes developing the confidence and skills they need to take control of their health and healthcare, fostering collaborative partnerships with healthcare providers and ensuring a supportive environment. Such an environment is characterized by policies, practices and systems that facilitate and value patient participation—essential for effective patient engagement. According to Coulter, patient engagement is crucial for improving health outcomes and the overall quality of care, which is applicable to the multiple diagnostic procedures that patients experience during their journey. The World Health Organization (WHO) [2] has emphasized the importance of patient engagement in fostering

C. Abreu (✉)
Nuclear Medicine and PET/CT Department, Royal Marsden NHS Foundation Trust, London, UK
e-mail: Carla.abreu1@nhs.net

A. M. Grilo
H&TRC—Health and Technology Research Center, ESTeSL—Escola Superior de Tecnologia da Saúde, Instituto Politécnico de Lisboa, Lisbon, Portugal

CICPSI, Faculdade de Psicologia, Universidade de Lisboa, Alameda da Universidade, Lisbon, Portugal
e-mail: ana.grilo@estesl.ipl.pt

L. R. Pereira
Nuclear Medicine, Maidstone and Tunbridge Wells NHS Trust, Maidstone, UK
e-mail: luisa.roldaopereira@nhs.net

© The Author(s), under exclusive license to Springer Nature Switzerland AG 2025
L. Camoni, L. Mansi (eds.), *Nuclear Medicine Hybrid Imaging for Radiographers & Technologists*,
https://doi.org/10.1007/978-3-031-86228-1_17

mutual responsibility and understanding between patients and healthcare professionals. Engaged patients are more confident in making informed decisions about their health and in reporting their experiences with healthcare services. Consequently, patient engagement enhances learning and health outcomes while reducing adverse events [3, 4]. In addition, increasing evidence shows that engagement is linked to improvements in healthcare costs and patient safety [5].

With the input of patients and family representatives, Carman et al. [6] developed a model that views engagement as a continuum. This continuum is characterized by the extent of information exchange between patients and healthcare providers, the degree of shared power and responsibilities, involvement in decision-making within healthcare organizations and participation in policymaking. The literature identifies various factors that influence patient engagement, including patients' characteristics, such as demographics, health status, health literacy, and the desire and motivation to be involved [2, 7], tasks, health care setting and health professions [2]. Knowing that patients' preferences for engagement may vary substantially [2], healthcare professionals should allow patients to participate in their care, considering the appropriate level of engagement for each patient and situation [8].

In Nuclear Medicine, patient engagement is implicitly connected to higher compliance with preparation instructions, radiation protection advice and acquisition of better higher quality imaging. Thus, it is increasingly recognized as crucial for delivering safer and more effective care [9, 10]. It is important to note that successful engagement enhances patient experiences during a time when they are more vulnerable and it leads to overall greater satisfaction. Several key aspects influence their perception of care while attending a Nuclear Medicine department, namely effective communication and interaction, ~~comprehensive~~ patient education and information, ensuring patient comfort and a positive experience, maintaining patient safety and demonstrating cultural sensitivity. Departments should demonstrate an active effort to obtain feedback and meaningfully act on the findings [2, 10, 11].

In this chapter, the authors will focus on how general concepts around the patient engagement theme apply to Hybrid Imaging, delving into the pragmatic, day-to-day service implications.

17.2 Patient Education and Information

Most patient engagement interventions focus on informing or educating patients [2, 12]. Nevertheless, for it to be effective, it is critical to firstly understand the term "limited (functional) health literacy" which is a person's ability to read and comprehend information and instructions in health settings [13, 14]. In Hybrid imaging, patients must understand the procedure, its purpose, the risks, and what to expect [14]. To ensure this understanding, healthcare professionals, among which are the Nuclear Medicine Practitioners (NMP) should provide comprehensive pre-procedure information. Educational videos and leaflets are useful tools for this purpose. Both provide a standardized method of conveying information, ensuring all patients receive the same quality of information [12]. Additionally, they can be supplied in multiple languages and formats to serve diverse patient populations, and complex medical jargon can be elucidated or changed into simpler terms as well as explained visually, aiding those with lower literacy levels.

Videos and leaflets should use clear, simple terminology to ensure comprehension across different patient literacy levels and to address various issues to ensure patients are well-informed and adequately prepared [12]. It should also include visual aids (diagrams, images and infographics) to enhance understanding and engagement, and provide contact information so that the patient can reach the department in case of any questions, or to share with the imaging teams if needs for adjustments are anticipated. The NMP should consider how to best accommodate these needs to optimize the imaging process.

Ultimately, these tools should help patients answer the following questions:

- What test will I undertake?
- What is the purpose of the test?
- Do I need any specific preparation?
- What will happen on the day of the exam?
- What do I have to do?
- What care do I need to take after the exam?
- Are there any side effects?

Table 17.1 presents a detailed outline of the topics they should integrate.

Adopting videos or leaflets for patient education and information requires considering the potential and limitations of each tool. Educational videos [15] are beneficial due to accessibility and convenience. They can be delivered quickly through online platforms, and patients and their relatives can watch them at their convenience, allowing them to re-examine the information as needed. Procedure understanding is enhanced as video can illustrate complex procedures (e.g. radiopharmaceutical) by combining narration, visual and animation sources. Patients can see step-by-step what to expect during imaging procedures and get familiar with the facilities, reducing anxiety and increasing compliance. A recent systematic review and meta-analysis suggest that educational videos effectively reduce anxiety and increase the satisfaction of patients undergoing diagnostic procedures. Patients understanding, comfort, tolerance and adherence were also improved with this tool [15]. Compared to reading tools alone, visual and auditory components of educational videos facilitate memory retention, and the interactive content (e.g. animations, voiceovers and patient testimonials) makes the content more engaging and significant [16–18].

To know more about educational videos see Ab Hamid et al. 2021; Dettmer 2005; Shortman et al. 2018 [16–18]

On the other hand, leaflets are inexpensive, can be produced in large quantities or tailored to specific conditions, populations (e.g. diabetic patients) or situations (e.g. leaflets distributed after imaging acquisition, with discharge recommendations) and are easily updated with new information. They are also easy to distribute in healthcare settings and do not require special technology, making them accessible to the majority of patients, including those who may not have access to digital devices or the internet (e.g. during patient booking). However, they could also be sent to patients by online platforms. Likewise, patients can easily carry leaflets and refer to them whenever needed. Leaflets that include a space for notes allow patients to feel more engaged, write on them, and bring their notes or questions to imaging services [19, 20].

To know more about leaflets see Lampert 2016 and Hasanica 2020 [19, 20].

Both the videos and the leaflets have limitations, and it is worth highlighting that they are passive learning tools (leaflets more than videos), providing general information that may be difficult to understand by patients with low literacy levels and not allow immediate interaction, feedback or doubts clarification leading to a build-up of anxiety. To maximize the potential and mitigate the limitations of educational videos and leaflets in medical imaging procedures, NM services can combine both and use other resources, such as personalized phone calls, phone/email messages with relevant information before the procedure or even interactive elements like quizzes to cater to different preferences and learning styles and promote active engagement [21]. Moreover, quality assurance should incorporate methods for patients to provide feedback not only on the videos and leaflets but about the overall process [22, 23] even during the various phases

Table 17.1 Essential topics to include in leaflets and videos regarding hybrid imaging diagnostic procedures

Procedure overview

Purpose: Explain why the hybrid imaging procedure is being performed and what it aims to diagnose or monitor

Process: Provide a step-by-step explanation of what the patient can expect during the procedure and inform how long the procedure will take from start to finish

Preparation instructions

Pre-procedure guidelines: Detailed instructions on how to prepare, including dietary restrictions, medication adjustments, fasting requirements, physical exercise restrictions; documents required for the procedure day and parking information

Clothing and accessories: Recommendations on what to wear and what not to bring (e.g. jewellery, electronic devices)

Clarify if the person can be accompanied (e.g. should not be accompanied by pregnant individuals or children—otherwise, the scan may be cancelled)

Procedure day

Department arrival: Advise the patient how to get to the NM department and what to do as soon as they arrive at the imaging service (e.g. go to reception, hand in documents)

First steps in the NM department: For instance, explain that an anamnesis will be carried out, vital signs checked/glucose levels will be determined and informed consent will be obtained

Administration of the radiopharmaceutical: Describe the purpose of the radiopharmaceutical and indicate ways of performing the administration

Post-administration guidance: e.g. continue life as normal (bearing in mind radiation protection restriction), ability to eat/drink, explain the need for a rest period after the injection and indicate its duration

Images acquisition

   Duration: Indicate the approximate time of acquisition, including the possibility of longer slots, if deemed helpful (e.g. patients with mobility constraints which require use of manual handling aids).

   Positioning and movement: Instructions on the specific position required during the imaging and need to remain still.

   What to expect: Describe the sensations or experiences (e.g. sounds, discomfort) that the patient might encounter

Post-procedure instructions

Aftercare: Guidelines on what to do immediately after the procedure/in between procedures, including hydration and activity restrictions regarding radiation-safe behaviours

Results timeline: Information on when and how patients will receive their results

Potential side effects: Common side effects and signs of complications to watch for, along with instructions on when to contact a healthcare provider (e.g. post-administration of furosemide or captopril)

Additional information

FAQs: Answers to frequently asked questions, particularly regarding concerns about radiation exposure or tailored information for patients with chronic conditions that might affect the procedure

Comfort measures: Provide tips on how to stay comfortable and calm during the procedure, including breathing techniques and the availability of sedatives if necessary.

Glossary: Include a glossary of medical terms to help patients understand complex language

Additional information: Added QR codes or links to online resources where patients can find additional information or watch explanatory videos. A visit to the department ahead of the scan day may be possible to be organized, which would allow for assessment of the conditions and more tailored adaptations (e.g. for patients who suffer from claustrophobia, a visit to trial the positioning in the equipment may help to determine the patient's ability to carry out the procedure. This is particularly important to be ascertained before the administration of any radiopharmaceutical)

of development of the videos or leaflets [18, 23]. This feedback can guide future improvements [12], as NM services should establish a routine for regularly reviewing and updating each tool to ensure accuracy and relevance [12].

The National Institute of Health Research highlights the value of embracing all forms of

feedback (consisting of formal and informal comments, complaints and unsolicited feedback), creating a healthy culture of learning and sharing such learning among peers (e.g. in team meetings) [24]. It also indicates that not all patients experience data needs to be numerical and sometimes "one-off" events, or qualitative and unrepresentative intelligence may provide rich insights on the patients' views. Patient feedback can be collected spontaneously by leaving feedback cards and anonymous boxes in the waiting rooms, or by emailing/messaging feedback links after the appointment. A good way to encourage patients' input is by demonstrating that the department takes it seriously and acts on it (e.g. a poster in the waiting area with "You said"/ "In response, we did" and give examples of improvement measures based on what has been said)— this will be especially uplifting for patients who return to their department for follow-up scans. More and more often, healthcare providers have access to Patient Groups whose role is to review patient documentation, checking if it is in in "lay language" and who simulate the patient journey in hospital, ideally being involved in designing new services (e.g. if the department or a room is being redesigned) [25, 26].

17.3 Communication and Interaction

A supportive environment that encourages and facilitates friendly and empathetic interaction with healthcare professionals is crucial for effective patient experience [27] and engagement [2, 10, 21]. The communication model that promotes meaningful involvement is the well-known "patient-centred model" [10, 28]. In the mid-twentieth century, psychoanalyst Michael Balint proposed the patient-centred model as an alternative to models centred on the disease or on the healthcare professional themselves (Balint 1969). This model, which can be defined as "care that respects and responds to the needs, wishes, and preferences of the patient and ensures that the patient's values guide all decisions" (Institute of Medicine 2001, p. 3), underpins patient involvement from the healthcare professional's perspective. The patient-centred approach requires solid and perceptive communication skills [9, 29]. In recent decades, many medical schools have recognized the impact of communication skills and have used guidelines to teach and assess these competencies during undergraduate studies [30].

More recently, it has been possible to establish a consensus regarding learning objectives for a core communication curriculum in healthcare professions [31]. The European consensus states 11 core communication objectives [31].

In the context of the imaging departments, it is essential to highlight the following:

1. Building up and upholding rapport.
2. Gathering of patient's bio-psycho-social information.
3. Provision of information to the patient in a timely, comprehensive and meaningful manner.

To note that point 1 can prove to be difficult in the context of hybrid imaging due to the brief nature of the contact with the patient. Nonetheless, the attitude and behaviour of the NMP can foster trust, therefore contributing to more productive results in points 2 and 3.

17.4 Building Up and Upholding Rapport

17.4.1 Invest in the First Moments of the Meeting

Many contacts with patients start coldly and distantly, ignoring the formation of impressions [32, 33] occurs in the first moments of the encounter. Professionals typically confirm the patient's name and date of birth, often immediately transitioning to the explanation of the technical procedures, without establishing a rapport. However, these initial interactions are structuring factors for the positive atmosphere established during the encounter, which is vital for the patient's comfort, well-being and engagement [23, 32, 34]. Sometimes there are several members of staff involved in the procedure (e.g. the person doing the administration is different than the person positioning for the scan, who is different of the person who finalizes the procedure) which breaks the continuity of the care. To address this, it is important that the NMP hands over relevant information to their colleagues, instead of gener-

Table 17.2 Examples of first interaction NMP-patient

Good morning Mr. YYY. I am XXX, the professional who will be accompanying you for this examination/treatment. (adequate non-verbal communication, with eye contact)

Before we begin, please can you confirm your personal details? Can you give me your full name, date of birth and address?

Thank you very much. It's important that we confirm we have the right person for the right scan! Now that we have confirmed the details, how would you like us to call you (Mary, Miss Smith)?

So, let's get started. How are you feeling today?

ating duplication of questions to the patient. With less time, there are simple ways to enhance the start of the meeting by always introducing themselves and including open confirmation of the patient's details (Table 17.2), always remembering that people using the service should be addressed in the way they prefer [21, 29] (whether this is by mentioning or omitting a title (Miss/ Mrs./ Ms., Mr), using the chosen pronouns (she/ he/they)). Notably, communication should be first and foremost directed at the patient, with simultaneous consideration to the accompanying people but with primacy given to the patient.

17.4.2 Listen and Show Empathy and Compassion

To build a connection with the patient, it is essential that he/she feel attended to and listened to, and that healthcare professionals show empathy and compassion. Active listening allows healthcare professionals to better understand patients' concerns, fears and questions, providing personalized care tailored to each patient's needs [23, 34, 35]. In Hybrid Imaging, patients might express concerns about radiation exposure. Listening attentively enables the provider to understand the patient's circumstances and address these specific worries more effectively [35]. Demonstrating empathy can also reduce patients' anxiety, making the procedure more accessible and comfortable. For example: "*I understand that this can be overwhelming. I am here to help you through every step. This scan is a routine and safe procedure*". Empathy makes the patient feel understood and supported, helping build trust between the patient and the healthcare provider [36]. Additionally, being

compassionate reassures patients that their emotional and physical well-being is a priority, enhancing their overall experience [38]. For instance, understanding when a patient expresses fear of needles and offering to use a numbing cream suggesting applied tension or breathing exercises can make the patient feel cared for and respected [39]. Furthermore, although a high pace can characterise imaging departments, it is vital that the patient feels that compassion is reflected in the environment of the department and not feel rushed [32, 38].

17.4.3 Be Aware of Non-Verbal Communication

What is conveyed non-verbally (e.g. eye contact, gestures, facial expressions, posture) determines the quality of the communication, qualifying it (i.e. connoting it emotionally), helping to clarify it (e.g. the use of facial expressions of concern in coherence with verbalizations of the same type by the patient) and even organizing it (e.g. the use of hand movements to reinforce a sequence of information). In addition to paying attention to their non-verbal communication, the professionals must show awareness of the patient's non-verbal communication and respond to them appropriately [31, 34, 36]. Trying to keep an appropriate distance from the patient (personal space), maintaining eye contact, which is a critical element in establishing a connection, and look at him/her gently and in a friendly manner. It is important to avoid talking solely at the relatives or carers and focusing first and foremost on the patient. In this way, health professionals transmit non-verbally that they are available for patients. To this demonstration of interest, patients tend to respond with less anxiety and a greater willingness to collaborate with the professional and the procedure.

17.5 Gathering of Patient's Bio-Psycho-Social Information

It is at times feared that the focus on technology may divert healthcare professionals' attention from the soft skills needed to gather information properly [29, 34]. This is a complex process which involves two fundamental aspects:

1. The health professional's ability to explore the context, using appropriate communication strategies, collecting the information needed to make a diagnosis, refer the patient to a pathway, assess the suitability of therapy, etc.
2. The patient's willingness/motivation to collaborate in sharing information. This last point depends partially on the healthcare professional, but establishing a relationship of trust, in which the professional presents themselves as available and interested in the patient, certainly facilitates this process [40]. A dissatisfied patient who feels that he or she is not being listened to or even that he or she is being "pushed around" is a less collaborative patient who may omit symptoms/complaints and even doubts that are very relevant to his or her process. Therefore, the professional's first task is to invest in the relationship with the patient [41]. Availability, trust, respect and a positive emotional tone and disposition are the factors that stand out most in this dynamic process, which constitutes the health professional-patient interaction. Unfortunately, the practice has highlighted the gradual devaluation of these aspects in the health professional-patient encounter [42]. It is paramount that the NMP sees the contact with the patient as a significant moment, and gathers information mindfully, thoughtfully and in a non-judgemental manner, and not approach this part of their duties as an impersonal tick-box questionnaire.

17.5.1 Elicit All the Patient's Concerns

It is essential to enable the patient to verbalise their complaint/concerns without interruption and facilitate the expression of the patient's afflictions by appropriately using open and closed questions [34, 43]. The former allows health professionals to introduce the topic without focusing on specific content [23]. The patient is thus encouraged to "tell their story," allowing the professional to get to know the patient's genuine perspective. Closed questions should not be devalued but only used when access to more specific information is necessary [34, 44]. They usually make it possible to answer in just one or two words or simply Yes/No [34] (Table 17.3).

Another aspect to consider when engaging with the patient is to ensure their dignity is always maintained [23]. When intimate or personal care are being provided, the team must make reasonable efforts to regard people's preferences about who delivers their care [21]. This may involve requesting staff of a specified gender/sex or offering a chaperone [45], for procedures such as breast or gynaecological sentinel node, cystograms, or for patients who need assistance using the toilet.

17.5.2 Value the Opinions of the Patient/Family

Emphasize the importance of valuing the opinions of the patient and their family, as it not only demonstrates empathy but also aids in better understanding of the patient's perspective [21, 23, 29]. Show sincere interest in the patient. Get to know their ideas (e.g. "*How do you feel about the lightening during the exam...*"), beliefs (e.g. "*I see you have some doubts about the use of radiation*") and experiences (e.g. "*You told me you have had this exam before, and it did not go well. Would you like to tell me a bit about it?*").

One aspect to be mindful of is the patient's right to privacy. This expectation extends to the

Table 17.3 Questionnaire for collecting information

Questions	Examples
Open	*How do you feel today?*
	What do you know about this scan?
	What questions do you have about the scan?
More specific, but still open	*How did the previous scan go?*
	What do you feel that went wrong with your previous scan?
	How did you feel listening to music during your last scan?
	I have a record here of back pain. How is it today?
Close	*At what time did you last eat?*
	Did you go to the toilet before entering the scan room?

involvement of the family, which should be only done with the patient's consent. It is important not to make assumptions. It is good practice to ask "*Who did you bring with you to this procedure? Would you like them to be present for this initial explanation?*"

While most family members are typically considered supportive and patients appreciate their presence, the NMP should always be attentive for cases of abuse, safeguarding, and negligence, particularly with fragile, older, or debilitated patients. As such, the team should be trained to discern if family and caregivers act as a positive supportive system, and prudently mediate when red flags are identified.

17.5.2.1 Managing the Level of Support Offered by Comforters and Carers

Radiation exposure concerns all individuals in radiology and NM, including carers and comforters. "Carers and comforters" mean individuals knowingly and willingly incurring an exposure to ionizing radiation by helping, other than as part of their occupation, in the support and comfort of individuals undergoing or having undergone an exposure [46]. Comforters and carers provide this care voluntarily and separately from their occupation, so it is essential to take precautions to protect their health. It is important to consider carers' age in radiation risk communication [47],

as it might impact their understanding and perception of risk. The exposure level can be reduced by applying the principles of time, distance and shielding [48]. For example, increasing the distance from the radiation source and reducing exposure time can help lower the dose carers receive.

The use of shielding can be considered, and it may reduce radiation exposure. However, it is essential to note that the shielding efficiency decreases as the radionuclide energy increases, and in some cases, the dose might increase [49].

Some carers are family members and may have a close relationship with the patient, however this should never be assumed, and it is always best to check with the patient if they consent to the carer being present during the procedure. This is of utmost importance as they may have my best interests at heart or conversely their actions may remove patients' control.

17.5.3 Look for Quality in the Information Collected

Collecting information requires excellent care and attention on the part of the healthcare professional. They should strive to clarify ambiguous and imprecise information, and avoid misinterpretations and assumptions [23] (examples provided in Table 17.4).

Table 17.4 Clarification of ambiguous/unclear information provided by the patient

Terms	Example	Possible misunderstanding	Clarification request
Ambiguous (uncertain/doubtful meaning)	*I don't think I'll be able to do the PET/CT scan*	NMP assumes the patient is referring to equipment and fears a claustrophobic reaction In fact, he/she may be referring to the positioning or the timing, for example	*What makes you say you won't be able to take the scan?*
Unclear (lack of accuracy)	*Fasting was not easy for me*	Assume that the patient has complied with the fast (even with difficulty)	*What were your difficulties in keeping the fast? (...) What time did you eat last night?*

17.6 Giving Information to the Patient in a Timely, Comprehensive and Meaningful Manner

The transmission of information is one of the most important and most difficult components of the communication process. It includes the contents the patient should retain and use to their advantage. Quality information transmission is fundamental to patient involvement, patient education and the promotion of patient safety [23, 36]. Although information must be adapted to the patient's level of understanding, language and preferences [31] ("one size does not fit all"), when providing information, it is essential to consider.

17.6.1 The 4Cs (Clear, Complete, Concise, Concrete)

The 4C aid the NMP to guide their speech in a consistent, coherent and congruent manner, effectively equipping the patient to be able to give valid, informed consent after receiving appropriate and sufficient information [23, 37]. It is important to acknowledge that this process starts before entering the hospital premises. In fact, it begins with the materials they received prior to their appointment, explanation upon arrival and their ability to discuss any remaining queries culminating in feeling competent to make the decision to proceed voluntary. Patients should always know that they are able to change their minds and withdraw consent. To note

though, that radiology departments and their staff uphold the standard of providing images of optimum quality whilst keeping patients safe from unnecessary ionizing radiation as per defined by ALARA (as low as reasonably achievable) principles [50]. Consequently, the NMP has to be aware that administering radiation without being able to then obtain a diagnostic result is, across several services, deemed as a radiation incident, and it should be suitably recorded (and in some countries, may be reportable to a national agency). This relates to the fact that the patient had radiation exposure for no actual benefit.

17.6.1.1 The Information Must Be Clear

Clear information is information that the patient can understand, is well structured and does not include ambiguous content [32]. The clarity of the message includes coherence between what is transmitted verbally and non-verbally.

Ambiguity in the message is a source of misunderstandings and errors in decoding the content transmitted [51]. Concern about ambiguity is even more relevant when health professionals want to involve patients in their care. To reduce ambiguity, pay special attention when using adverbs of quantity and intensity (e.g. a lot, a little, some, a lot) or when referring to individual subjective aspects (e.g. emotions, sensations) of the patient. For example, instead of saying at the end of the test, "*You should drink plenty of water*", say, "*For the next X hours, it is important that you drink YY amount of water, as the radiopharmaceutical is excreted by the kidneys/urine!*"

The transmitted message must also be well structured, presenting the most important content at the beginning and then moving on to complementary information or the development of what has already been transmitted. It is harder for the patient to picture what they will be going through if the NMP's speech is disorganized and jumps between phases of the procedure.

17.6.1.2 The Information Must Be Complete

The information must be complete, i.e. including all content units that empower the patient with all the information they require and/or consider relevant and available to provide all the significance information for the patient's effective collaboration in their procedure [32]. Information considered pertinent to the patient sometimes differs from what health professionals perceive as relevant. For instance, patients value aspects that are often considered minor by professionals, such as the advantage of bringing comfortable clothes (as much as possible without metal parts, or accessories, indicating the need to remove them or to change to hospital gowns—and if so, provide changing facilities), parking and the possibility of being accompanied during the scan.

17.6.1.3 Information Must Be Concise

The information should be complete but concise; for instance, health professionals should use as few words as necessary for the patient to understand. Long speeches and ancillary content are often the cause of patient distraction, loss of motivation to continue listening and errors in understanding the message [34].

Information should be conveyed from the most basic to the most relevant in the interaction with the patient. What is more, when the patient says that he/she has not understood the information provided, it is important not to show upset, and to avoid explaining it in more words and in an even more complicated way [34].

17.6.1.4 Information Must Be Concrete

Information should be specific and accurate [32]. Correctly conveying information using objective language (as opposed to the use of abstraction), comparing complex concepts with a relatable daily basis issue and including tools that can help the patient realize what they are hearing (e.g. use diagrams and models; refer to examples [34]. Examples can be found in work from Ozgur 2021 [52].

It is vital not to be dismissive of the patients' worries. Lack of knowledge and misconceptions about radiation persist in society and patients may be alarmed about the potential dangers [53, 54]. These worries must be considered and the NMP should strike a balance between being cautious (and therefore emphasizing the patient's necessary compliance with post-scan social restrictions) and being level-headed about patients' (possibly overestimated) fears. For instance, for patients referred for lung scintigraphy due to a risk of life-threatening pulmonary embolism, who may be pregnant or breastfeeding, it is vital to take time to explain the effects on the patient and on the foetus/baby. This will allow the patient to make plans and follow safety advice (e.g. expressing milk ahead of the appointment so that it is later available, discarding the milk on the first XX hours after the procedure and using instead the one that had been expressed and stored). They may also coordinate with another member of the staff (if still in hospital) or a relative to bottle feed the baby so that they avoid close prolonged contact during those first hours. It is not about denying the risks, but rather explaining how to mitigate them and explain how they have some degree of control through their behaviour and actions.

17.6.2 Be Honest

Hybrid imaging scans have different durations and levels of difficulty. Some will require the patient to stand, others require patients to lay flat, often relying on the patient to remain still (with resource to arm support bands, knee cushions, sand bags), and on occasion using aids to be immobilized (e.g. to keep feet or hands on specific positions, or to keep the head aligned). Patients should be advised if they can take painkillers, and if they have any ideas on how to facilitate the positioning. It is central to clarify with the patient when they can use the toilet (e.g. if they need to empty their bladder between two image acquisitions).

The NMP should explain consequences in a sincere manner. For instance, explain to the patient the inability to proceed if the preparation was not followed because it will effectively impair the results; explain the risk of complications or side effects (e.g. during a cardiac stress procedure; or related to the administration of furosemide or captopril in a renogram).

When the scan is finished, it is important to ensure the patient or carer understands how they will get the results, and the next steps to take. Again, there should be the opportunity for questions. At times, the NMP may feel that they are not being able to relieve the patient's apprehensions. It can be useful to admit so and seek support from a senior NMP. Radiation safety considerations are particularly important. Most organisations work closely with a Radiation Protection Advisor (who is a specialist in radiation protection), with whom it may be useful to consult regarding specific queries. The seminal point though is how the NMP will then convey such specific scientific advice to the patient, in a friendly, intelligible manner.

Lastly, patient advocacy is a primary moral duty of the NMP. This means being a "patient representative, defending the patient's rights and universal rights, contributing to decision-making and supporting the patient's decisions" [55]. In summary, being reliable and trustworthy, which in the context of hybrid imaging may be about recognizing difficulties (e.g. mobility difficulties; memory deficits that affect the patient's capability to remember what has just been said; not wanting to discuss pregnancy status in front of relatives) proposing solutions without causing embarrassment (offering mobility aids, such as walkers, or even shoehorn for the patient who is not able to get their shoes on when the scan has finished; providing extra written information, taking the patient to a private space under a different pretence, such as checking height and weight), and ultimately being gracious, helpful, transparent and frank when incidents happen

(e.g. if the schedule is delayed by keeping patients informed about realistic timeframes so that they can adjust their personal plans if need be; if an extravasation of the injection happened and longer image acquisition is needed or if they need additional images) [56].

17.6.3 Be Aware of the Patient's Emotional State

Despite technological progress, medical imaging procedures often induce high anxiety among patients due to several factors: the possibility of diagnosing life-threatening diseases; the first examination of patients; the body position during imaging; concerns about patients' examination results, diagnosis and potential changes in treatment plans; lack of understanding about procedures; difficulties in communicating or understanding during investigations; and, in some cases, concern about ionizing radiation and radiation exposure. In addition, the high frequency of sound noise can cause anxiety, and the small-bore size of the scanner may pose challenges for claustrophobic patients [28, 57].

This way, how the information is conveyed must take into consideration the emotional state of the patient.

- If the patient is in a state of <u>emotional shock,</u> he or she will not retain information because he or she cannot decode it. In these cases, continuing to inform the patient while ignoring the patient's expression of "absence" or "terror" will mislead the NMP into thinking that the patient knows what was said, when the patient has not processed what he has heard and is therefore unable to make good use of the information. Less time would be lost, and fewer adverse events would be happening if the NMP recognizes the patient's emotional state before continuing providing information.
- If the patient is depressed, he will tend to retain negative aspects and devalue the more positive ones. The selective retention of information and the apathy characteristic of depressive

states do not facilitate the involvement of the patient, who may be considered incompetent to collaborate; or consider that his or her situation is so serious that "nothing is worth it anymore". In these cases, the information should be accompanied by help in decoding the content in a more realistic/positive way, by identifying support resources, and by affirming the patient's competence to do what is being asked of (always taking care to adapt requests for collaboration to the patient's real capabilities).

- If anxious, the patient will tend to retain potentially threatening or difficult-to-control information. In addition, he or she will have difficulty focusing and maintaining attention. Very often, the anxious patient already has his or her representation of the information he or she is about to hear. And very often, this representation is very threatening. In these cases, it is advisable to transmit positive information quickly to reassure the patient; understand what the patient already knows or thinks about the subject and what their biggest concerns are; accompany the speech with alternatives for resolving/mitigating the problem; make very specific indications about what is asked of the patient in terms of collaboration [58].

17.6.4 Cultural Competency and Sensitivity

NMP encounter patients from a variety of racial, ethnic and socioeconomic backgrounds, and perspectives may differ very much from those held by the professionals treating them. Enhancing cultural competency and sensitivity among NMP can improve communication, access to health care and eventually health outcomes [59].

However, developing this cultural competence is an intricate process, and one that is necessary when discussing multiculturalism and diversity in today's field of diagnostic medical imaging. It requires staff to reflect on their own culture and understand the patterns of differences and commonalities between themselves and their own cultural group and the perceptions, values and practices of other cultural groups. Once recognized, these differences and commonalities that exist within the population can then be addressed for the benefit of patient healthcare.

In healthcare settings, regardless of department, cultural competency includes the following features:

1. Viewing the patient as a unique individual.
2. Understanding what the patient belief, preferences, needs and values, and respecting those things.
3. Communicating information to patients with terminology and in a way they can understand, and involving medical interpreters when needed.
4. Being aware of the biases and assumptions held by staff.
5. Encouraging patients to be participative in their own healthcare decisions.

Preferred language may be the most obvious cultural difference an NMP encounters. Language barriers could compromise quality of care and patient safety. When a patient's first language is not English or when a patient has limited English proficiency, a specially medically trained interpreter may be necessary. Ideally, interpreters should be proficient in both languages and have a mastery of medical terminology and the ability to conduct a three-way conversation. Assessing whether a patient will need interpretation services should begin when the patient, family member or referrer requests the scan, so the department can be prepared and allocate sufficient resources. If an interpreter is required, be sure you bring the interpreter up to speed on patient information, the imaging procedure itself and the steps involved, and where the interpreter should be during the procedure. Be sure that you continue to address your patient and not the interpreter. Keep your sentences simple, speak slowly and allow plenty of time for the interpreter to speak with and observe the patient's responses. Be sure to follow up with the interpreter after the procedure for feedback. Some guidelines to follow if an interpreter is needed during NMP-patient communication can be found on Table 17.5.

Table 17.5 Guidelines for the use of interpreter in patient communication

Never have a patient's adult family member or friend interpret

Avoid using bilingual/multilingual staff to interpret, unless they are officially qualified interpreters

Always ensure appropriate positioning of the patient to promote communication between the NMP, patient and interpreter

Adapted from Perry et al. [59]

Table 17.6 NMP-patient communication examples to assess faith-based needs

"What effect is this scan having on you and on those around you?"

"Do you have a religious or spiritual practice that would be helpful for us to know about for your scan?

Do you have a favourite practice that helps you feel calm? For example, some meditate others pray.

I know that sometimes female patients would prefer to be examined by a female NMP—Is that important for you?

Adapted from [34, 59]

On another related topic, faith-based needs may relate to religious or spiritual beliefs systems. Such nuances regarding care may include the patient's need for a same-sex provider, possible dietary restrictions that could impact compliance with regards to scan preparation (e.g. FDG PET/CT fasting preparation) and preferences for results communication. Listed in the table below are some examples that can be used to assess faith-based needs (Table 17.6).

17.6.5 Teach-Back

The teach-back technique ensures that patients have comprehended and retained the information provided to them. This method also enhances patient knowledge and engagement in their healthcare [60]. When utilizing the teach-back technique, healthcare professionals ask patients to repeat or summarize the given information and instructions or to recall concepts in their own words immediately after receiving the information [14, 60]. Example can be found in work from Guide to Patient and Family Engagement in Primary Care, Agency for Healthcare Research and Quality [61]. A systematic review by Yen et al. (2019) [62], which included 26 studies, confirmed the effectiveness of the teach-back method in reinforcing and verifying patient education and understanding.

For teach-back to be effective and not misinterpreted, healthcare professionals should maintain a close, non-judgmental attitude. They should explain to the patient that the procedure is a way of confirming that the information has been communicated clearly and that the responsibility for clear explanation lies with the healthcare professional, not the patient.

I know I've given you a lot of information about the scan. Can you tell me what you remember?/Can you remember what the first steps are?

I see you need to remember everything about the exam. Don't worry, I'll help you, and we'll review it again.

And now, what do you remember? What precautions should you take in the next few hours?

17.7 A Communication Tool for Hybrid Imaging

McHugh, Bevans and Paradis (2020) [63] developed a communication tool, LADiBUG, to enhance patient engagement and satisfaction with imaging services. This tool was created after listening to the patient's advisor's lived experiences regarding communication during their time in the imaging department and considering the organizations patient feedback data. LADiBUG, described as an "aide-mémoire", provides practical insights into improving communication with patients and their families in imaging departments. It addresses all critical aspects of the patient-family-centered model: respect and dignity, information sharing, and patient participation and collaboration. The LADiBUG tool is a communication framework that stands for Listen, Acknowledge, Discuss, (i) Be Understanding, and Give Information. This tool can be particularly useful in Nuclear Medicine procedures to improve patient communication, reduce anxiety, and enhance patient experience. Table 17.7 shows how to effectively apply each component of LADiBUG in the context of nuclear medicine diagnostic procedures.

Table 17.7 LADiBUG communication tool, description, skills and examples (adapted)

		Description	Communication skills	Examples
L	Look and Listen	Introduce yourself (name and role), confirm the patient's reason for the visit and prevent unnecessary steps in their visit. Observe nonverbal cues, assess the patient's condition and note the patient's appearance and well-being	Active listening Questioning (open/end questions) Be mindful of the surroundings—e.g. politely introduce colleagues who may enter the room during the patient's procedure	*Good morning, Mrs. Smith. My name is VVVV, and I'll assist you with your nuclear medicine scan today. Who is with you?* *My name is XXX, and I am a certified nuclear medicine technologist. I'll be conducting your PET/CT scan today.* *I'm here to ensure everything about your upcoming scan is clear. Could you tell me how you feel today?"* *Can you tell me more about your concerns regarding this scan procedure?*
A	**Acknowledge**	Acknowledge the patient's preferences and respect who they include in their care. Verbally acknowledge what the patient has seen or heard and adjust the following steps to accommodate the patient's and family's needs	Active listening Empathy Questioning (open/end questions)	*If you wish, y our partner /so n can stay with you during...* *I understand your concern, Mr. YYY. Many patients feel the same way. The amount of radiation used in this procedure is minimal and is considered safe. The benefits of the scan in diagnosing your condition far outweigh the risks.* *I understand that you might be feeling anxious about the procedure. It's completely normal to feel this way. I'm here to help answer any questions and make this as comfortable as possible for you.* *If you need me or any of my colleagues to repeat any explanation, do not hesitate to ask. We know it is a lot of new information and are happy to go through the details again.* *During the scan, we will always consider your back pain and look for ways to make the examination as comfortable as possible. How do you lie in bed at night? Where do you position the pillows?*

(continued)

Table 17.7 (continued)

		Description	Communication skills	Examples
D	Duration	Provide patients with an estimated timeframe for the procedure to give them a sense of control. Keep the patient and their family informed to create a "meaningful wait". If there is time before the procedure, offer a warm blanket, a magazine or Wi-fi connection. Inform them promptly of any changes or delays	Explaining Clarification	*This procedure will take about 2 h, including radiopharmaceutical injection and resting time. The image acquisition will last around 20 min. I'll be with you throughout the process, behind this window/ screen. There is always someone close by*
I	Inform and involve	Depending on the procedure, involve the patient or family member in the exam when possible. These interactions help staff understand the patient's expectations and clarify questions or concerns. Continuously inform and involve the patient throughout the procedure to reduce anxiety and fear. Make sure you respond to what matters to the patient	Explaining and planning Active listening Reflexion	*Did you have an opportunity to see the video regarding the procedure?* *During the procedure, we will inject a small amount of radioactive liquid into your body. This material will help us get detailed images of your body working in real time. The injection might cause a slight pinch, but it should not be painful.* *During the scan, you'll need to lie still on the table while the machine takes images of your body. Please let me know instantly if you are uncomfortable or need a break. Would you like me to explain each step as we go along?* *This is a clever machine which works like a 2 in 1, it does two scans, a 3D one (which is the one obtained from moving slowly around you) and a CT scan, which is when you enter the donut on the back. It does one scan after the other, and all you need to do is stay in the same position for both. We will let you know when it is over, but until then, we need you to stay still. How does that sound?*
B	"Burning questions"	Keep communication open and provide time and space to make patients comfortable for asking questions	Open questions	*Do you have any specific questions or concerns about the scan that we can address before we begin? It's essential that you feel fully informed and comfortable*

(continued)

Table 17.7 (continued)

		Description	Communication skills	Examples
U	Understanding	Assess the patient for signs of uncertainty, especially after giving instructions, to ensure they understand the information. Be aware of language barriers, hearing or speech impediments, and distractions that could affect comprehension. Use appropriate strategies or tools to assist. Check patient understanding	Open questions Teach back technique Clarification	*To ensure I've covered everything, tell me what you understand about the procedure and what to expect? I want to make sure I haven't missed any details*
G	Going forward/ goodbye	Review the next steps of care and inform the patient about how and when to follow up with their physician. Thank the patient for their time and trust. Help patients and companions exit the department or hospital	Summarizing Clarification	*The scan is over. You can eat and do your normal activities. Ensure you drink XX glasses of water in the next few hours and stay away from children and pregnant women today.* *Your doctor will review and discuss the results with you during your next appointment. If anything comes up or if you have any further questions, don't hesitate to contact our department*

17.8 Professionals' Engagement Self-Assessment

Given the relevance of engagement to the quality of care and the patient experience in Nuclear Medicine departments and the need for improvements [11, 27, 64], professionals need a way to assess the adequacy of their attitudes and behaviour towards patient engagement. A checklist is the answer, as it ensures that all professionals are evaluated using the same criteria, promoting consistency in patient engagement practices. This systematic approach covers all key aspects of patient engagement, ensuring no critical area is overlooked. By regularly using a checklist for self-assessment, such as the one provided in Table 17.8, NMPs are encouraged to reflect on their practices, identify patterns or issues and implement targeted quality improvement initiatives. This aspect is particularly important, as it encourages professionals to proactively address potential problems. Overall, a checklist is a practical tool that supports the continuous enhancement of patient engagement in Nuclear Medicine departments. It also serves as a tool for providing

constructive feedback to colleagues or the rest of the team, facilitating open communication between supervisors and staff regarding patient engagement practices.

To conclude, the NMP should be keen and proficient in fostering an environment conducive to patients' engagement, by communicating in a way that validates their feelings, often under challenging circumstances, while being able to ease their discomfort and optimizing their cooperation by being flexible and thoughtful, warranting physical and psychological safety and avoiding information overload. They should be patient in face of patient's frustration or confusion, whilst remaining assertive in relation to the need to conform to radiation protection guidance, ultimately safeguarding the best interest of other members of the team and the public.

As a cornerstone of their professional conduct, the NMP should always be aware of their impact in the patient's wellbeing and how their knowledgeable and sensitive posture can be substantially reassuring at a time of great complexity.

Table 17.8 Checklist for Nuclear Medicine Practitioners' self-evaluation regarding patient engagement

	Yes/no	Observation
Greeting and introduction:		
I greet the patient warmly and introduce myself by name and role?		
Did I make eye contact and use the patient's name?		
Build up and maintain rapport		
I listen attentively without interrupting		
I ask open-ended questions to understand the patient's needs and concerns		
I show empathy and acknowledge the patient's concerns and feelings		
I attentive to signs of distress and did I address them promptly		
I show kindness and understanding, especially if the patient was anxious or in pain		
I validate the patient's feelings and offer reassurance as needed		
I respect the patient's cultural, religious and personal preferences		
Procedure		
I provided information that I wanted and that met the patient's needs		
I was aware of and I did accommodate any language to literacy barriers		
I encourage the patient to ask questions and express concerns		
I involve the patient in decisions about the procedure when appropriate (e.g. inform consent)		
I respect and support the patient's choices and autonomy		
Have I checked that the patient has understood the information provided?		
Together with the patient, I have found strategies that will enhance adherence to the procedure		
I provide pillows, blankets or other comfort measures as needed		
I check and reinforce the patient's skills to apply mutually agreed strategies (e.g. distraction during positioning)		
I adjust equipment and room temperature for the patient's comfort		
I ensure the patient's privacy and modesty during the examination		
Post-procedure		
I explain what will happen after the procedure and any follow-up steps		
I invite the patient to provide feedback on their experience		
I say a friendly goodbye to the patient and thanked him/her for his/her cooperation		

References

1. Coulter A. Engaging patients in healthcare. New York: McGraw Hill Professional; 2013.
2. WHO.Patient Engagement. Technical Series on Safer Primary Care. ISBN 978-92-4-151162-9. 2016.
3. Greene J, Hibbard J. Why does patient activation matter? An examination of the relationships between patient activation and health-related outcomes. J Gen Intern Med. 2011;27(5):520–6.
4. Simmons LA, Wolever RQ, Bechard EM, Snyderman R. Patient engagement as a risk factor in personalized health care: a systematic review of the literature on chronic disease. Genome Med. 2014;6(2):16.
5. Coulter A, Ellins J. Effectiveness of strategies for informing, educating, and involving patients. BMJ. 2007;335(7609):24–7.
6. Carman KL, Dardess P, Maurer M, Sofaer S, Adams K, Bechtel C, Sweeney J. Patient and family engagement: a framework for understanding the elements and developing interventions and policies. Health Aff (Millwood). 2013;32(2):223–31.
7. Maurer M, Dardess P, Carman KL, Frazier KL, Smeeding L. Guide toPatient and family engagement: environmental scan report. AHRQPublication no. 12–0042-EF. Agency for Healthcare Research and Quality: Rockville, MD; 2012.
8. Grilo AM, Santos MC. Engaging patient: Let's talk about how health providers can do it right. JOJ Nurse Health Care. 2017;5(1):555655.
9. England A, Beardmore C, Cunha A, Executive EFRS, Board. The EFRS patient centred care awards: supporting the identification, promotion and propagation of high-quality care across Europe. Radiography (Lond). 2023;29(Suppl 1):S3–4.
10. Meertens R, Hancock A, Hyde E. Editorial: patient voice and the patient experience. Radiography (Lond). 2023;29(Suppl 1):S1–2.

11. Flood T, O'Neill A, Oliveira CM, Barbosa B, Soares AL, Muscat K, Guille S, McClure P, Hughes C, Mcfadden S. Patients' perspectives of the skills and competencies of therapy radiographers/radiation therapists (TRs/RTTs) in the UK, Portugal and Malta; a qualitative study from the SAFE Europe project. Radiography. 2023;29(Suppl 1):S117–27.

12. Rockall AG, Justich C, Helbich T, Vilgrain V. Patient communication in radiology: moving up the agenda. Eur J Radiol. 2022;155:110464.

13. Public Health England. Local action on health inequalities [Internet]. 2015. https://assets.publishing. service.gov.uk/media/5a7f46f240f0b6230268e865/4a_Health_Literacy-Full.pdf. Accessed 13 Jul 2024.

14. Goguen J. Health literacy and patient preparation in radiology. J Med Imaging Radiat Sci. 2016;47(3):283–6.

15. Grilo A, Ferreira AC, Pedro Ramos M, Carolino E, Filipa Pires A, Vieira L. Effectiveness of educational videos on patient's preparation for diagnostic procedures: systematic review and meta-analysis. Prev Med Rep. 2022;28:101895.

16. Ab Hamid MR, Mohd Yusof NDB, Buhari SS, Abd Malek K, Noor MH. Development and validation of educational video content, endorsing dietary adjustments among patients diagnosed with hypertension. Int J Heal Promot Educ. 2021;62:1–12.

17. Dettmer P. New blooms in established fields: four domains of learning and doing. Roeper Rev. 2005;28(2):70–8.

18. Shortman RI, Hoath J, Osadolor T, Inga P, Roper L, Bomanji J, et al. Development of PET/CT and PET/MRI patient-information videos in collaboration with patients previously treated for cancer. J Nucl Med Technol. 2017;46(1):26–8.

19. Lampert A, Wien K, Haefeli WE, Seidling HM. Guidance on how to achieve comprehensible patient information leaflets in four steps. International J Qual Health Care. 2016;28(5):634–8.

20. Hasanica N, Ramic-Catak A, Mujezinovic A, Begagic S, Galijasevic K, Oruc M. The effectiveness of leaflets and posters as a health education method. Mater Sociomed. 2020;32(2):135–9.

21. Higgins T, Larson E, Schnall R. Unraveling the meaning of patient engagement: a concept analysis. Patient Educ Couns. 2017;100(1):30–6.

22. Ribeiro AS, Lee M, Oyen WJG. EANM commitment towards involvement and engagement of patients and the public: learning from the UK experience. Eur J Nucl Med Mol Imaging. 2019;46(11):2218–9.

23. Robinson L, Goodwill G, Harris R, et al. Patient Public and Practitioner Partnerships within Imaging and Radiotherapy: guiding Principle guiding_principles_final_proofed_1 (sor.org). 14 July 2023. SoR.

24. National Institute For Health and Care Research. Improving care by using patient feedback [internet]. National Institute for Health and Care Research; 2020. https://evidence.nihr.ac.uk/collection/improving-care-by-using-patient-feedback/. Accessed 13 Jul 2024.

25. Regulation and Quality Improvement Authority— Regulation and Quality Improvement Authority Northern Ireland | Work with RQIA [Internet]. Rqia.org.uk. 2024. https://www.rqia.org.uk/who-we-are/get-involved/lay-assessors/#:~:text=A%20lay%20assessor%20is%20a,Infection%20prevention%2Fhygiene%20inspections. Accessed 31 Jul 2024.

26. Chinn D, Brickley K, Power A. Involvement of lay assessors in the inspection and regulation of public services: a systematic review. Health Soc Care Community. 2024;2024:1–22.

27. Kwee R, Kwee T. Communication and empathy skills: essential requisites for patient-centered radiology care. Eur J Radiol. 2021;140:109754.

28. Champendal M, Borg Grima K, Costa P, Andersson C, Baun C, Gorga RG, Murphy S, Kedves A, Santos A, Geao A. A scoping review of person-centred care strategies used in diagnostic nuclear medicine. Radiography. 2024;30(2):448–56.

29. Itri JN. Patient-centered radiology. Radiographics. 2015;35(6):1835–46.

30. Windover AK, Boissy A, Rice TW, Gilligan T, Velez VJ, Merlino J. The REDE model of healthcare communication: optimizing relationship as a therapeutic agent. J Patient Exp. 2014;1(1):8–13.

31. Bachmann C, Abramovitch H, Barbu CG, Cavaco AM, Elorza RD, Haak R, Loureiro E, Ratajska A, Silverman J, Winterburn S, Rosenbaum M. A European consensus on learning objectives for a core communication curriculum in health care professions. Patient Educ Couns. 2013;93(1):18–26.

32. Pollard N, Lincoln M, Nisbet G, Penman M. Patient perceptions of communication with diagnostic radiographers. Radiography (Lond). 2019;25(4):333–8.

33. Rimondini M, Mazzi MA, Busch IM, Bensing J. You only have one chance for a first impression! Impact of Patients' first impression on the global quality assessment of Doctors' communication approach. Health Commun. 2019;34(12):1413–22.

34. Silverman J, Kurtz S, Draper J. Skills for communicating with patients. 3rd ed. Boca Raton, FL: CRC Press; 2013. https://doi.org/10.1201/9781910227268.

35. EFRS. EFRS statement on the importance of patient engagement and the patient voice within radiographic practice. EFRS Statement on the Importance of Patient Engagement and the Patient Voice within Radiographic Practice. 2021.

36. McIntosh J. Communication and patient care in radiography. S Afr Radiogr. 2022;60(1):25–31.

37. Department of Health. Reference guide to consent for examination or treatment [Internet]. 2009. https://assets.publishing.service.gov.uk/media/5a7abdcee5274a34770e6cdb/dh_103653__1_.pdf. Accessed 7 Jul 2024.

38. Hancock A, Bleiker J. But what does it mean to us? Radiographic patients and carer perceptions of compassion. Radiography. 2023;29(S1):S74–80.

39. Alsbrooks K, Hoerauf K. Prevalence, causes, impacts, and management of needle phobia: an international

survey of a general adult population. PLoS One. 2022;17(11):e0276814.

40. Doyle C, Lennox L, Bell D. A systematic review of evidence on the links between patient experience and clinical safety and effectiveness. Br Med J Open. 2013;3(1):1–18.

41. Yang LY, Manhas DS, Howard AF, Olson RA. Patient-reported outcome use in oncology: a systematic review of the impact on patient-clinician communication. Support Care Cancer. 2018;26(1):41–60.

42. Blanch-Hartigan D, Chawla N, Moser RP, Finney Rutten LJ, Hesse BW, Arora NK. Trends in cancer survivors' experience of patient-centered communication: results from the health information National Trends Survey (HINTS). J Cancer Surviv. 2016;10(6):1067–77.

43. Robinson JD, Heritage J. Physicians' opening questions and patients' satisfaction. Patient Educ Couns. 2006;60(3):279–85.

44. Mazor KM, Roblin DW, Greene SM, et al. Toward patient-centered cancer care: patient perceptions of problematic events, impact, and response. J Clin Oncol. 2012;30(15):1784–90.

45. Intimate Examinations and Chaperone Policy [Internet]. SoR. https://www.sor.org/learning-advice/professional-body-guidance-and-publications/documents-and-publications/policy-guidance-document-library/intimate-examinations-and-chaperone-policy. Accessed 13 Jul 2024.

46. Department of Health and Social Care. Ionising Radiation (Medical Exposure) Regulations 2017: guidance [Internet]. GOV.UK. 2018. https://www.gov.uk/government/publications/ionising-radiation-medical-exposure-regulations-2017-guidance. Accessed 13 Jul 2024.

47. Badawy MK, Anderson A. Radiation protection for comforters and carers in radiology and nuclear medicine. J Med Radiat Sci. 2023;70:103–5.

48. Gains JE, Walker C, Sullivan TM, Waddington WA, Fersht NL, Sullivan KP, Armstrong E, D'Souza DP, Aldridge MD, Bomanji JB, Gaze MN. Radiation exposure to comforters and carers during paediatric molecular radiotherapy. Pediatr Blood Cancer. 2015;62:235–9.

49. Deb P, Jamison R, Mong L, U P. An evaluation of the shielding effectiveness of lead aprons used in clinics for protection against ionising radiation from novel radioisotopes. Radiat Prot Dosimetry. 2015;165(1–4):443–7.

50. Hasaneen M, AlHameli N, AlMinhali A, Alshehhi S, Salih S, Alomaim MM. Assessment of image rejection in digital radiography. J Med Life. 2023;16(5):731–5.

51. Schuster P, Nycolin L. Communication for nurses: how to prevent harmful events and promote patient safety. Philadelphia, PA: F.A Davis; 2010.

52. Ozgur DJ. How much radiation do you get from dental X-rays? [internet]. Toronto Smile Design. 2021. https://www.torontosmiledesign.ca/cosmetic-dentist-in-toronto/how-much-radiation-do-you-get-from-dental-x-rays. Accessed 13 Jul 2024.

53. Pandit M, Vinjamuri S. Communication of radiation risk in nuclear medicine: are we saying the right thing? Indian. J Nucl Med. 2014;29(3):131–4.

54. Bastiani L, Paolicchi F, Faggioni L, et al. Patient perceptions and knowledge of ionizing radiation from medical imaging. JAMA Netw Open. 2021;4(10):e2128561.

55. Davoodvand S, Abbaszadeh A, Ahmadi F. Patient advocacy from the clinical nurses' viewpoint: a qualitative study. J Med Ethics Hist Med. 2016;9:5.

56. Care Quality Commission. Regulation 20: Duty of candour | Care Quality Commission [Internet]. www.cqc.org.uk. CQC; 2022. https://www.cqc.org.uk/guidance-providers/all-services/regulation-20-duty-candour. Accessed 13 Jul 2024.

57. Bradley YC, Barlow P, Osborne DR. Reduction of patient anxiety in PET/CT imaging by improving communication between patient and technologist. J Nucl Med Technol. 2014;42(3):211–7.

58. Vieira L, Pires A, Grilo A. Anxiety experienced by oncological patients who undergo ^{18}F-FDG PET CT: a systematic review. Radiography. 2021;27(4):1203–10.

59. Perry H, Eisenberg RL, Swedeen ST, Snell AM, Siewert B, Kruskal JB. Improving imaging care for diverse, marginalized, and vulnerable patient populations. Radiographics. 2018;38(6):1833–44.

60. Bodenheimer T. Teach-Back: a simple technique to enhance patients' understanding. Fam Pract Manag. 2018;25(4):20–2.

61. Agency for Healthcare Research and Quality. Teach-Back: Intervention | Agency for Healthcare Research & Quality [Internet]. Ahrq.gov. 2017. https://www.ahrq.gov/patient-safety/reports/engage/interventions/teachback.html. Accessed 13 Jun 2024.

62. Yen PH, Leasure AR. Use and effectiveness of the teach-Back method in patient education and health outcomes. Fed Pract. 2019;36(6):284–9.

63. McHugh C, Bevans K, Paradis S. LADiBUG—a communication tool for diagnostic imaging. J Med Imaging Radiat Sci. 2020;51(4S):S31–8.

64. Hyde E, Hardy M. Patient centred care in diagnostic radiography (part 1): perceptions of service users and service deliverers. Radiography. 2021;27(1):8–13.

Nuclear Medicine Department: Organization, Staffing, and Workflow Optimization

18

Elizabeth Bailey, Marta Bissolotti, and Luca Camoni

18.1 Overview

The organizational structure of a Nuclear Medicine Department incorporating hybrid imaging technologies is important when assessing ways to improve the service, develop effective teams, and collaborate with other healthcare professionals. It is important to remember, that the most valuable asset in any organization is the employees and having the most appropriate mix of staff to achieve the most efficient, high-standard of service will always result in better workflow, resource allocation, and collaborations.

The different types of organizational structure are outlined later in the chapter and identifying which type will work best for your needs will guide the staffing requirements, the role and responsibilities for the various staff, internal and external stakeholder relationships, and how these can be structured to improve workflow. Consideration of other factors such as staffing numbers, department layout, and the types of procedures to be offered are essential. This could be as simple as considering a common control room workspace adjoining multiple SPECT or SPECT/CT systems to improve workflow efficiencies.

An understanding of effective communication with patients, referrers, other healthcare professionals and departments will assist with identifying who is responsible for which tasks, how to communicate information between team members and other healthcare areas, including the patient. Providing the right tools to assist with this such as computing infrastructure for easy access to patient and study information, easy to follow protocols that are readily accessible and appropriate staff skill mix and ratios in invaluable [1].

18.2 Understanding Organizational Structure

Organizational structure is a system that outlines how specific activities are performed to fulfill a strategic mission. An organization's structure provides a framework to assist with decision making, leadership, communication, and accomplishing the healthcare facilities goals. There are four main types of organizational structure that

E. Bailey (✉)
Nuclear Medicine Department, Royal North Shore Hospital, Sydney, NSW, Australia
e-mail: elizabeth.bailey2@health.nsw.gov.au

M. Bissolotti
Supply Chain Management, Gruppo AB, Brescia, Italy

L. Camoni
Department of Nuclear Medicine, University of Brescia and ASST Spedali Civili di Brescia, Brescia, Italy
e-mail: luca.camoni@unibs.it

© The Author(s), under exclusive license to Springer Nature Switzerland AG 2025
L. Camoni, L. Mansi (eds.), *Nuclear Medicine Hybrid Imaging for Radiographers & Technologists*,
https://doi.org/10.1007/978-3-031-86228-1_18

have been defined and can apply to many different types of work environments [2]:

1. Functional is similar to a hierarchical organization but tends to focus on the roles and responsibilities of the areas rather than on professional title. For example, employees will be grouped according to the department in which they work with colleagues exhibiting a similar skill set.
2. Divisional has employees organized according to a division, product, or geographic location and they tend to have control over their own area and resources and tend to be more common in larger organizations with multiple sites or locations. In the healthcare setting, the divisional structure may be used where a group of hospitals or services are located across multiple sites that have an executive management team for all sites.
3. Flat structure aims to place all employees on the same level by removing or reducing middle management resulting in a more autonomous workforce. The employees report more closely to higher or executive level management and are empowered to take initiative and make decisions. This structure is rarely used in the healthcare setting.
4. Matrix structure is a combination of the divisional and functional structure whereby enabling multiple areas within the organization to contribute to decision making. For example, a hospital comprises multiple departments that specialize in particular patient services, however they all work together to provide comprehensive care to the patient. The main advantage of this structure is the efficient use of all resources to achieve a common goal.

There are four organizational design principles that should be considered when deciding and implementing the best organizational structure for your facility based on its strategic goals and objectives including [3–5]:

1. Planning for implementation: This includes allocating sufficient resources with the necessary skills and knowledge to achieve the core objectives, and ensuring that these goals are achievable in the allocated timeframe.
2. Assessing impacts and plan communication: This should include a change in management plan that has full consultation with all impacted stakeholders, which for the healthcare setting will include patients, referrers, and other healthcare professionals.
3. Managing talent transitions and consultation: There may be a need to assess employee roles and responsibilities and expand opportunities for professional career development to achieve efficiency improvements.
4. Optimizing on a continuous basis: Ongoing monitoring of any changes and improvements, ensuring compliance with current best practice standards.

The ideal organizational structure for a nuclear medicine department may vary depending on whether the service is part of a larger multiple site facility or a smaller workplace with limited facilities. Whichever structure is identified, there are key components to be taken into consideration so as to create a workplace that is efficient, effective, inclusive, and optimizes resource allocation.

18.2.1 Key Components of Nuclear Medicine Department Structure

The structure of a Nuclear Medicine department that includes hybrid imaging capabilities whether that be SPECT/CT or PET/CT has common key components that will influence the layout, staffing mix, workflow design, efficiencies, and the level of services that can be provided to patients and referrers. Once these components have been defined, the roles and responsibilities of the multidisciplinary workforce, workflows (including scheduling, protocol development, documentation requirements), and initiating collaborative relationships and partnerships can be established.

18.2.1.1 Role and Responsibilities of Staff

The roles and responsibilities of each member of the multidisciplinary team will depend on the number and type of hybrid imaging equipment, the number and variety of procedures that will be performed, taking into consideration teaching, ongoing professional development, and participation in research. There are readily available tools that can be used to assess the staffing needs for a nuclear medicine department that includes defining the number of different professional groups based on service provision and how to take into consideration both clinical and non-clinical needs of the service [1].

18.2.1.2 Workflows

The development and implementation of effective workflows are one of the most important contributing factors defining the structure of the department. It encompasses consideration of the roles and responsibilities of the multidisciplinary team that has been established as well as creation of detailed protocols that outline scheduling guidelines, equipment needs (including radio-pharmaceuticals), staffing, and other resources needed to perform the study or treatment. Other resources may involve cooperation with other healthcare professionals and departments that will require pre-procedural preparation and good communication.

18.2.1.3 Collaboration and Interactions Between Nuclear Medicine and Other Departments

Collaboration and teamwork in the healthcare setting has been shown to greatly improve the outcomes for patients across all services, including imaging and diagnostics [6]. There are particular characteristics inherent in the team environment that may influence these outcomes and include communication, leadership, discipline, and having a clear strategy and purpose in place [7]. This is particularly important for a hybrid imaging service where these close collaborations with other disciplines and departments in the healthcare facility are needed to optimize workflow, patient throughput, and provide a service that is compliant with current models of care and best practice.

18.3   Staffing in Nuclear Medicine

There is no general agreement on a methodology for analyzing healthcare staffing needs at the national and regional (macro) level; however, two general approaches can be identified: supply-based or demand-based [8].

Despite the variety of models for calculating staffing needs, workload-based approaches, such as the World Health Organization's Workload Indicators of Staffing Needs (WISN) method [9], are more commonly used for planning requirements. The workload-based calculation model can also be implemented in specific areas like nuclear medicine [10].

Below is an example of formula (18.1) for calculating a demand-based staffing needs based on WISN method [9].

$$\text{FTE} = \frac{\sum_{i=1}^{n} (F_i \times T_i) \times \text{CAF} + \text{IAF}}{\text{AWT}} \quad (18.1)$$

where

F_i: is the annual frequency of activities (e.g., number of exams or procedures),

T_i: is the time required to perform the activity,

CAF: is the Category Allowance Factor, which accounts for support activities common to all staff members,

IAF: is the Individual Allowance Factor, representing additional activities performed by some staff members,

AWT: is the Annual Available Working Time (after absences for holidays, illness, training, etc.).

The FTE (Full-Time Equivalent) represents the equivalent of a full-time worker.

As an example, hypothetical values are provided to apply the formula:

D = 250 working days per year,
F = 43 days of vacation,
L = 10 days of illness or leave,

$P = 3$ days of mandatory training or other specific leave,

$H = 7.2$ working hours per day,

$F_1 = 6000$ exams (annual frequency for Exam Type 1),

$T_1 = 0.3$ h (time for Exam Type 1),

$F_2 = 3000$ exams (annual frequency for Exam Type 2),

$T_2 = 1$ h (time for Exam Type 2),

$CAF = 1.1$ (10% of time dedicated to support activities),

$IAF = 100$ (100 h of time dedicated to additional individual activities).

1. Calculating Available Working Time:

$$\begin{aligned} AWT &= (D - F - L - P) \times H \\ &= (250 - 43 - 10 - 3) \times 7.2 \\ &= 194 \times 7.2 = 1396.8 \text{ working hours / year} \end{aligned}$$

2. Calculating the workload for each activity:

$$L_{Et1} = F1 \times T1 = 6000 \times 0.3 = 1800 \text{ hours / year}$$

$$L_{Et2} = F2 \times T2 = 3000 \times 1 = 3000 \text{ hours / year}$$

$$\text{Total} : \sum_{i=1}^{n} (F_i \times T_i) = 1800 + 3000 = 4800 \text{ hours}$$

3. Multiply the total activity time by the CAF:

$$\sum_{i=1}^{n} (F_i \times T_i) \times CAF = 4800 \times 1.1 = 5280 \text{ hours.}$$

4. Add the IAF to account for additional activities:

$$\sum_{i=1}^{n} (F_i \times T_i) \times CAF + IAF$$
$$= 5280 + 100 = 5380 \text{ hours.}$$

5. Calculate the Full-Time Equivalent (FTE): Divide the total required time by the available working time:

$$FTE = \frac{\text{Total Required Time}}{AWT} = \frac{5380}{1396.8} \approx 3.85$$

The example above represents a simplified application of the traditional WISN model for calculating FTE. This model considers not only the timing of clinical services but also the times defined by the Category Allowance Factor (CAF). This factor accounts for activities not directly related to the provision of clinical services but that still must be performed by all members of a staff category. The CAF is calculated as a percentage of the staff's total working time. For instance, if the category spends an average of 40 min per day on image reconstruction, reporting, and archiving, and works 210 days per year, the total time spent on this activity will be 140 h/year. If the AWT is 1400 h/year, the CAF is calculated as in formula (18.2)

$$\text{Total FTE} = \frac{\text{Total Workload} \times \left(1 + \dfrac{140 \text{ hours dedicated to non-clinical activities}}{1400 \, AWT}\right)}{\text{Annual Available Working Time} (AWT)} \tag{18.2}$$

Furthermore, the WHO has considered also the Individual Allowance Factor (IAF) is a factor used to estimate the staff required to cover additional activities performed by only some members of a staff category. These additional activities are not common to all members of the category and may include specialized tasks or specific roles, such as supervision or training. To calculate the IAF, you must list the additional activities, the number of staff members performing them, and the time they require annually. For example, formula (18.3).

Total time for additional activities
$$= \Sigma \left(\begin{array}{l} \text{Number of staff members} \\ \times \text{Annual time required for the activity} \end{array} \right) \quad (18.3)$$

By summing all the times for the additional activities, you obtain the IAF value, expressed in hours per year.

The CAF and IAF, as described in the WISN method, represent mechanisms to account for non-clinical activities performed by healthcare staff. These activities include tasks such as training, administration, and participation in meetings, all of which take time away from direct clinical work.

Non-clinical correction factors are crucial in calculating staffing needs, as they not only ensure there is enough staff to perform clinical duties but also account for the time spent on complementary tasks that support the overall functioning of the healthcare service. This principle is also applied in the model proposed by the International Atomic Energy Agency (IAEA) for calculating staffing requirements in nuclear medicine [10]. The IAEA introduces specific correction factors to account for time spent on critical non-clinical tasks, such as equipment maintenance, daily quality control, and administrative tasks like record keeping.

These factors, expressed in additional FTEs, ensure that there is enough staff to cover both direct clinical work and the operational and technical activities that maintain service efficiency. For example, the IAEA suggests adding 0.2 FTE of a nuclear medicine technician for each PET/CT or SPECT scanner installed in the service to account for non-clinical activities related to equipment use and maintenance. Furthermore, for radiopharmacy, the IAEA model recommends additional correction factors. For instance, an increase of 0.05 FTE is suggested for each dose calibrator, while the presence of a cyclotron requires an additional 3 FTEs to handle activities related to radiopharmaceutical production.

In both models, the goal is similar: to ensure that staffing requirements account not only for clinical activities but also for essential complementary tasks that are crucial to the effective operation of the service. However, while the CAF/IAF in the WISN method provides a general percentage approximation applicable to all staff, the IAEA model applies specific correction factors based on equipment and operational needs in nuclear medicine.

For further details and insights into specific correction factors and guidelines, it is recommended to consult the official IAEA document [10].

Staffing needs models can be based on either the demand or the supply of the service. Demand-based models, such as those described earlier, focus on the performance required by users, typically calculated using historical data to estimate future workloads. This approach considers past activity volumes as an indicator of expected demand, thereby determining the number of FTEs needed to meet that demand.

However, if the goal is to optimize the use of available resources, such as fully utilizing "heavy" equipment (e.g., PET/CT or SPECT scanners), a supply-based approach can be adopted. In this scenario, the calculation of FTEs is not based on historical demand or workloads but rather on the service's maximum operational capacity. This means planning the necessary staff to make the most of the available technological resources, regardless of current demand. It is important to note that, if the organization's activities and services are already optimized, the supply and demand models should result in the same FTE calculation. If they do not, it could be crucial to identify the bottlenecks preventing the organization from reaching its full supply potential.

In a supply-based model, the numerator of the formula would include various factors such as:

- The number of available equipment units.
- The daily operating hours of the imaging service.
- The number of annual operating days of the service.

Additional factors can be incorporated to refine the calculation and accurately reflect the operational capacity of the service, such as:

- The hours required for the preparation and quality control of radiopharmaceuticals, activities that demand time and specialized staff, especially in centers with an in-house radiopharmacy.
- The correction factors proposed by the IAEA for the number of equipment units, which account for the time dedicated to non-clinical tasks such as equipment maintenance and quality assurance.

These correction factors are expressed in additional FTEs per equipment unit. For example, for each PET/CT or SPECT scanner, the IAEA recommends adding 0.2 FTE to cover the necessary non-clinical activities related to equipment maintenance and quality control. It is also important to consider the time required for other operational activities, such as staff management, continuous training, and participation in operational meetings, which, if neglected, can reduce the overall efficiency of the service. An example is reported in formula (18.4).

where:

N_E = Number of equipment (e.g., PET/CT, SPECT scanners).

H_O = Daily operating hours of the service.

D_O = Annual operating days of the service.

$T_{\{Prep\}}$ = Average time for the preparation and quality assurance (QA) of radiopharmaceuticals (in hours).

$N_{\{Prep\}}$ = Number of annual radiopharmaceutical preparations.

N_C = Number of cyclotrons present.

AWT = Available Working Time (the annual available working hours per FTE).

Adjustments:

The section regarding time for preparation and QA of radiopharmaceuticals was modified to average time for preparation and QA multiplied by the number of annual preparations.

The section on IAEA correction factors was included to address non-clinical tasks.

However, while workload-based models require determining the timing for each service, a staffing model based on supply in healthcare assumes the existence of standardized and optimized imaging protocols for equipment use. This allows for the calculation of the number of exams an apparatus can perform in a day, thus determining its operational capacity. Determining the equipment's operational capacity helps better organize exams and schedule patient appointments, considering the average time for each type of exam and the preparation time between patients. Moreover, knowing the operational capacity of the equipment in a system designed to

$$\text{FTE} = \frac{\left(N_E \times H_O \times D_O\right) + \left(T_{Pred} \times N_{Prep}\right)}{\text{AWT}} + \left(N_E \times 0.2 + N_C \times 3\right) \tag{18.4}$$

maximize supply allows for estimating the number of annual radiopharmaceutical preparations, which in turn helps determine the theoretical number of working hours required by technicians in the radiopharmacy.

Determining the timing for each activity is therefore relevant in both supply- and demand-based models. Methods for establishing these timings and contextualizing the data to your specific setting include:

- Predetermined time systems (e.g., institutional guidelines, etc.)
- Direct observation and stopwatch-based time studies.
- Work sampling.
- Historical data (from electronic records or self-monitoring, classified as estimation techniques).
- Estimates based on expert judgment.

Predetermined time systems set standard times for a particular type of exam to meet specific needs, such as reducing waiting lists.

Direct observation and measurement are the most resource-intensive technique in terms of workload analysis and demands significant resources. In particularly complex settings, this approach could follow the Pareto principle, focusing, for example, on the 20% of activities that generate 80% of the workload, while a less resource-intensive approach, such as estimation, could be used for the remaining activities.

Between the two estimation approaches, historical data tends to be more accurate. Accuracy can be improved by expanding the historical data sample used.

When using estimates based on expert judgment, accuracy limitations can be mitigated by applying the Program Evaluation and Review Technique (PERT) [11], used in critical path planning in project management. The PERT process involves calculating an average time estimate for an activity based on the beta distribution. The expert must provide three estimates for each activity: Optimistic time (to); Most likely time (tm); Pessimistic time (tp).

The average estimate is calculated using the following formula (18.5).

$$Te_{(ij)} = \frac{to_{(ij)} + 4tm_{(ij)} + tp_{(ij)}}{6} \quad (18.5)$$

where:

$Te_{(ij)}$ is the average time estimate for activity i in mode j.
$to_{(ij)}$ is the optimistic time estimate,
$tm_{(ij)}$ is the most likely time estimate,
$tp_{(ij)}$ is the pessimistic time estimate.

Finally, to ensure accurate calculation of staffing requirements, it is essential to consider human factors and ergonomics, particularly the physical limitations of staff members that limit full staff utilization beyond individual allowances for additional tasks. Industrial engineering literature has long established the importance of incorporating these factors [12], since it's unrealistic to assume that staff can be utilized at 100%, and consequently recommends incorporating a utilization rate when determining the number of required FTEs. This has recently attracted attention in the healthcare sector [13]. The use of allowances for the following three categories is well-established in industrial engineering literature [12]: personal needs, breaks or fatigue, and delays. But in addition to these, especially in a healthcare environment it is also important to recognize that when some staff have physical limitations, the additional workload often falls on other workers. This not only impacts overall productivity but can also lead to fatigue and decreased job satisfaction within staff. Therefore, allowances should be adjusted to account for this additional burden, ensuring that workload is distributed fairly and service quality is maintained.

An allowance of around 15% (0.15) is considered to be at the higher end of the recommended spectrum in industrial applications [12]. Determining the appropriate allowance percentage is highly dependent on the work context and organizational culture, as well as the variability introduced by human factors, such as patient variability or a greater prevalence of staff limitations. Recent literature suggests a greater allowance may be necessary for healthcare settings [13] There are two approaches to including allowances in the literature [14, 15]: allowances can either be factored into the time allocated for each activity, or they can be applied when converting workload into FTEs by multiplying the utilization rate ($U = 1–0.10 = 0.90$) by the AWT (i.e., $U \times AWT = 0.90 \times 1400$ h) in the denominator of the previously described formulas.

By carefully integrating these considerations into staffing calculations, organizations can develop inclusive work environments that optimize performance while prioritizing worker health and safety.

The models for calculating staffing needs presented in this part offer insights into optimizing healthcare workforce planning to better understand how to develop its tailored staffing need model, especially within nuclear medicine. However, like all models, they have limitations that must be carefully considered. Both demand-driven and supply-driven models rely heavily on accurate and up-to-date data. For demand-driven models, historical data may not always reflect future trends, especially in the face of changing healthcare demands or technological advances. Similarly, supply-driven models depend on information about equipment capacity and operating times. The supply-side approach is based on the assumption of stable and predictable operating conditions and may be difficult to apply in scenarios where equipment malfunctions, unexpected downtime or sudden increases in patient load occur. Furthermore, it is highly unlikely that these models can account for the variability of human factors such as patient complexity, staff fatigue, and the actual physical limitations of people currently on duty, which can affect the actual time required for activities. While the use of correction factors is essential to a comprehensive staffing model, you risk over-reliance on correction factors. For example, if these factors are calculated inaccurately or applied too broadly, they could lead to over- or under-staffing.

18.4   Patient-Centered Scheduling

Developing a detailed and patient-centered scheduling for nuclear medicine exams is integral to the overall efficiency of the department. This agenda must account for the specific workflow and exam requirements that are unique to nuclear medicine procedures. Common nuclear medicine exams such as PET scans, cardiac stress tests, and brain imaging, each demand individualized preparation and, when required, delayed imaging procedures. So, the agenda should reflect the necessary pre-exam preparations, which may involve pharmaceuticals administration, dedicated rooms, hydration, etc. Allocating the appropriate

time for these preparations is critical as it ensures that both the patient and staff are ready for the imaging phase. Furthermore, the duration of each exam must be estimated accurately, acknowledging that while some studies may take as little as 30 minutes, others may extend over several hours due to the need for multiple imaging stages. This is particularly relevant for dynamic studies or those that require delayed imaging post-tracer administration.

In addition to patient preparation, the agenda must also account for the preparation, quality control, and handling of radiopharmaceuticals. The administration of radioactive tracers requires careful timing, coordination, and preparation to ensure the accuracy of the prepared activity and to prevent decay within the syringe, when ready. This necessitates building sufficient time into the schedule for these preparatory activities before moving forward with imaging. Additionally, scheduling efficiency can be further enhanced by grouping similar exams together. For example, if several patients require bone scans, batch preparation of radiopharmaceuticals not only reduces waiting times but also ensures better resource utilization. Such grouping also allows for more streamlined workflow management, as similar protocols can be executed sequentially without requiring frequent changes in setup or equipment.

Furthermore, the need to optimize the use of imaging equipment is equally important, ensuring that the availability of PET/CT or SPECT/CT machines is maximized. A well-constructed schedule should account for the necessary calibration, daily quality controls for emission imaging and CT and maintenance of these machines integrating these tasks and downtimes into the agenda without disrupting patient care. Avoiding overbooking is also critical; while maximizing the number of appointments may seem appealing, overloading the schedule can result in extended patient wait times, increased stress for staff, and a higher likelihood of errors. Therefore, incorporating buffer times within the agenda not only allows for potential delays or complications but also ensures that patient care remains the focal point of the service.

Overall, the creation of an effective nuclear medicine exam agenda requires a clear understanding of the procedural demands, the careful allocation of time for both patients and staff, and a commitment to ensuring that the schedule supports the operational efficiency of the department. By prioritizing patient care, leveraging group scheduling techniques, and maintaining flexibility within the timetable, the department can provide timely, accurate diagnostic services while promoting a cohesive and collaborative environment among the multidisciplinary team.

18.5 Optimizing and Enhancing Department Efficiency

The goal of any service is to maintain and improve operational efficiencies to optimize the value of the service for all stakeholders, of which the primary focus should be the patient. A nuclear medicine department relies on the smooth flow of patients that transit through the service for a procedure and there are many factors that contribute to inefficiencies in the flow of patients. Some of these factors cannot be easily improved such as department layout, available imaging equipment, and access to radiopharmaceuticals and IT infrastructure. However, consultation with staff and initiating conversations about the factors that impact on workflow efficiencies and standardization of procedures and protocols can result in significant improvements to patient flow and overall experience [16].

The first step to improve patient flow is to determine the patient, staff, and general public workflow through the department. This will include identifying how the patient will move through the department on their journey when having a procedure done. This may vary for an outpatient compared to an inpatient, a walking patient compared to someone in a wheelchair or bed bound as well as between nuclear medicine and PET. Creating a standardized workflow for each scenario will lead to optimization of workflows and efficiency gains.

Standardization provides a framework for the nuclear medicine staff to follow to reduce errors, ensure that every procedure is performed to com-

ply with best practice guidelines, and that every patient receives the best possible care. There are three ways in which the standardization of procedures can enhance efficiencies, especially in a hybrid imaging service [17]:

1. Minimizing errors: Increasing demands on healthcare services has resulted in staff feeling pressured and burnt out. Providing evidence-based guidelines on how best to complete nuclear medicine procedures improves staff confidence and informs appropriate decision making.
2. Enhancing communication: The move to digitization of healthcare records and procedures has resulted in streamlined access to all relevant documentation. The use of IT infrastructure such as a Radiology Information System (RIS) and Picture Archiving System (PACS) is recommended.
3. Increase efficiency and save money: Review and improve the better use of available resources, through simplifying scheduling of procedures, for example, booking similar or the same test consecutively to improve workflow and reduce procedural costs.

All efforts should be made to provide staff with detailed procedural protocols that are easy to follow, readily available, and are continuously reviewed.

Furthermore, the introduction of industrial optimization systems in the healthcare field marks a significant advancement in the case for efficiency, quality of care, and cost-effectiveness. Borrowed from the principles of industrial engineering, these systems are designed to streamline operations, reduce waste, and optimize resource allocation, ultimately enhancing patient outcomes. In a sector where timely and accurate service delivery is critical, the integration of optimization techniques such as workflow automation, predictive analytics, and decision support systems has transformed both clinical and administrative processes. By addressing the complexities of patient scheduling, supply chain management, and staff utilization, industrial optimization not only boosts operational productivity but also ensures a higher standard of care. This new paradigm shift is instrumental in navigating the evolving landscape of healthcare, where demand is increasing, resources are constrained, and value-based care is becoming the norm.

Any optimization is based on some basic concepts that come from the world of Lean Production [18], the most important are:

1. Focus on customer needs (Stakeholders, client, patients, etc.).
2. Organization and processes analysis.
3. Managed information and speaking data.

Without a clear definition of process, organization, function, and data management will hardly be able to optimize them.

The starting point involved the use of simple, but effective rules:

- **SIPOC mapping**: SIPOC stands for Suppliers-Inputs-Process-Outputs-Customers and is a tool of Process Management (Fig. 18.1).
  SIPOC tool creates a way of representing how the inputs are processed into outputs, which is necessary if you are to understand how to improve the processes themselves. If you want to change the output, you must either change the processes themselves or the inputs. SIPOC tells you where to look to do this.
- **Workflow and Key Process Indicators (KPI)**: Once the processes have been built, a

graphic representation is needed to guide the actors in their execution; you will also indicate the systems or databases in which to manage the information. A fundamental step is to highlight the critical steps that must be paid great attention to and to think of processing KPIs that allow monitoring their progress and potential waste. For lean thinking, every non-value activity, manual process, movement is a waste. With the workflow, redundancies are therefore noted, functions that do not generate value or with redundant activities and this therefore allows the management to review the organization based on the processes. Thinking about the organization first and the processes after is always a serious mistake: How can we understand how many people are needed and what skills they must have if we are not first clear about what they must do, what the limits and responsibilities are?

It is necessary to define the activities, what skills are needed, in what sequence, and what tools are involved precisely to better understand what type of staff needs to be hired and how many FTEs are needed. Analyzing workflows is structural to understand if there is any waste or improvements to be applied in order to limit costs. The representation of a process can also be very useful for training staff, collaborating better, and sharing information so as to be sure that activities always develop in a consistent way.

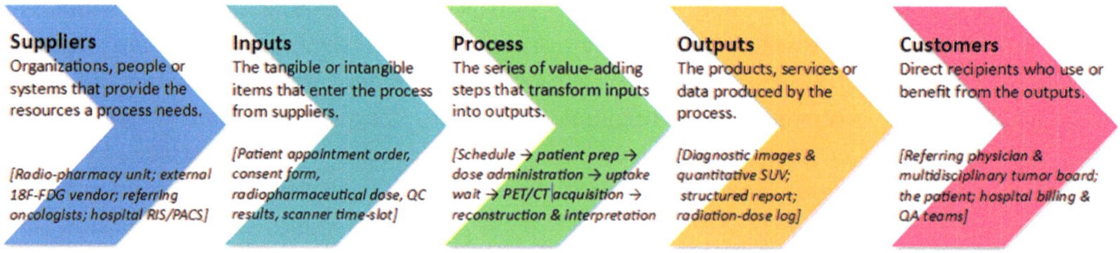

Suppliers
Organizations, people or systems that provide the resources a process needs.

[Radio-pharmacy unit; external 18F-FDG vendor; referring oncologists; hospital RIS/PACS]

Inputs
The tangible or intangible items that enter the process from suppliers.

[Patient appointment order, consent form, radiopharmaceutical dose, QC results, scanner time-slot]

Process
The series of value-adding steps that transform inputs into outputs.

[Schedule → patient prep → dose administration → uptake wait → PET/CT acquisition → reconstruction & interpretation]

Outputs
The products, services or data produced by the process.

[Diagnostic images & quantitative SUV; structured report; radiation-dose log]

Customers
Direct recipients who use or benefit from the outputs.

[Referring physician & multidisciplinary tumor board; the patient; hospital billing & QA teams]

Fig. 18.1 Colour-coded chevron diagram summarizing the SIPOC model—Suppliers, Inputs, Process, Outputs, and Customers—with each element defined in general terms and illustrated [in brackets] using a matched example from a simplified PET/CT workflow in nuclear medicine

– **Structured data**: Without numbers, it is impossible to understand how a process, an organization, or a department is going on ("Without data you're just another person with an opinion."—W. Edwards Deming). To make decisions, which are consistent with the strategies or to verify whether the cost-benefit ratio is such, any company can no longer rely on common sense, but must provide a solid information structure. Data analysis is a very powerful tool that allows you to make informed decisions. Therefore, it is necessary to build a strong data structure, which can be reworked with key parameters, and which brings value: This needs that the data is usable, scalable, and that it is the basis for concrete actions. It is useless to calculate a lot of KPIs, you need the right ones.

The three concepts mentioned above can be supported by tools derived from lean management [19], below are some examples of these tools that are most commonly used in the field to identify and reduce inefficiencies in hospital and healthcare processes. Value Stream Mapping (VSM) is a fundamental tool in lean management that allows you to visualize, analyze, and optimize the flow of value in healthcare processes. Used in hospitals, VSM helps map each phase of the patient journey, identifying activities that add value and waste (steps that do not directly contribute to improving patient health). Through VSM, it is possible to visualize the time and resources spent in each phase, highlighting areas of inefficiency or slowdowns in the process. This tool therefore allows healthcare teams to design leaner path, reduce waiting times, optimize the use of resources and improve the overall patient experience (an example is reported in box 1). To identify the values, the eight wastes could help the analysis, this method focuses on eight main types of waste: overproduction (performing unnecessary activities), waiting (dead time for patients or staff), transportation (unnecessary movements of materials or people), useless processes (activities that do not add value), excessive inventory (unused materials), superfluous move-

ments (unnecessary movements of staff), defects (errors that require corrections), and untapped human potential (employee skills not valued).

VSM is not only useful for visualizing and optimizing healthcare processes, but it is also an effective tool for identifying bottlenecks. A bottleneck is a process step where production capacity is less than demand, causing slowdowns in the entire operational flow. As literature (Eliyah Goldratt—The Goal) points out, identifying and managing bottlenecks is crucial to improving the overall efficiency of the system. In the healthcare field, identifying bottlenecks is essential to optimizing a process's takt time and takt rate, two indicators that help synchronize the operational pace with patient demand. Takt time represents the maximum amount of time that can be dedicated to each patient to meet the daily demand and is calculated by dividing the available operational time by the number of patients to be treated. Takt rate indicates the ideal pace of production of a service (for example, the number of diagnostic tests to be completed in an hour), and serves as a benchmark for process efficiency.

When a bottleneck emerges in a process—for example, an image acquisition step that takes a long time—it slows down the entire operational flow and negatively impacts the takt time and takt rate. If a step takes longer than the established takt time, the facility will not be able to meet the expected demand, leading to delays, staff overload, and patient dissatisfaction. Furthermore, the presence of a bottleneck prevents the process from maintaining a constant takt rate, as patients pile up waiting to complete the critical phase, compromising the balance of the workflow.

Analyzing bottlenecks through VSM and comparing them with the expected takt time and takt rate allows you to identify specific areas where you can intervene to reduce waiting times and improve flow. For example, you could introduce supporting technologies to speed up image acquisition times or reprogram schedules to reduce waiting times between phases. Thanks to this global optimization, you can improve service efficiency, increase operational capacity, and meet demand more effectively, maintaining the quality of care provided.

One of the analysis tools useful in process optimization in a risk management perspective (also essential to avoid worsening of the process in case of excessive simplifications in the analysis of phases that do not add value or are considered waste) and step value evaluation is FMECA (Failure Mode, Effects, and Criticality Analysis), a systematic methodology used to identify, analyze, and prevent potential failures in a process or system, evaluating the causes and effects of such failures. The main objective is to improve reliability and safety by reducing the risk of errors. Criticality then allows an analysis of criticality, classifying failures not only based on their severity but also on their probability of occurrence and the ability to be detected. A key tool in these analyses is the Risk Priority Number (RPN), a numerical index calculated by multiplying three factors: severity (S: The impact of a failure on safety, system effectiveness, or patient well-being (in the healthcare sector) is assessed. Each failure is classified based on the severity of its consequences from 1 least serious to 10 most serious), occurrence (O: Represents the probability that the failure will occur. This probability is estimated based on historical data or staff experience and classified on a scale of 1 least likely to 10 most likely), and detection (D: It is considered how easy it is to detect the failure before it causes a negative effect, on a scale of 1 high detectability to 10 high detectability. A low detectability means that the failure is difficult to detect, increasing its criticality) of the failure ($RPN = S \times O \times D$). RPNs higher than the others analyzed indicate that the failure is critical and requires priority attention. The RPN helps prioritize corrective actions, allowing healthcare organizations to focus resources on the areas with the highest risk, thus improving the effectiveness of processes also from a value perspective and patient safety.

To prioritize FMECA interventions, the Pareto principle (or 80/20 rule) can be applied. This principle suggests that 80% of the consequences (such as failures or risks in a process) are often caused by 20% of the causes. In this context, the RPN (Risk Priority Number) analysis is useful to identify those failures that contribute most to the total risk. By identifying and ranking failures with a higher RPN, the organization can focus on the 20% of high-risk causes that have the greatest impact on system reliability and safety. This

Box 18.1

To create a Value Stream Map (VSM) in healthcare, follow these steps:

Define the objective and the process to map (based on SIPOC): Choose a specific path, such as the PET patient admission and diagnosis process.

Identify the phases of the process: Break the entire path into main phases (for example, simplifying the concept: admission, medical assessment, radiopharmaceutical injection, uptake time, acquisition time, discharge). Each phase represents a specific block of the process and can be further detailed and broken down into sub-phases (for example, by adding a specific VSM for the administration room only, collecting for example the time to find the venous access).

Collect data for each phase: For each phase, collect key data, such as:

- Cycle time (time needed to complete the phase).
- Waiting time (time the patient or results wait between the phases).
- Personnel involved.
- Resources used (equipment, premises, diagnostic tools).

Draw the current VSM (Current State): On a sheet of paper or software, graphically represent each step with a box. Use arrows to indicate the flow of the process and notes to specify the times and other information for each step. Add a symbol for waiting times (for example, dotted arrows) and highlight steps that do not add value.

Identify waste: Analyze the map to find points of inefficiency or waste, such as high

(continued)

waiting times, duplication of activities, or unnecessary movements.

Draw the future VSM (Future State): Design an improved version of the process, eliminating or reducing the identified waste points. For example, you could combine steps, reorganize the flow or automate some activities to reduce waiting times.

Applied Example.

Let's imagine we want to map the management path of a patient in nuclear medicine PET:

Process steps (average times – hypothetical, not for reference):

- Admission (5 min).
- Waiting before assessment (30 min).
- Medical assessment (10 min).
- Waiting before radiopharmaceutical administration (15 min).
- Administration room (15 min).
- Waiting before imaging (60 min).
- PET imaging acquisition time (25 min).
- Waiting before discharge (20 min).
- Discharge (5 min).

Current Map: Represents each phase with average times and waits. Total path: 185 min.

Future Map (simplified): Eliminate or reduce waiting times between admission and assessment and diagnosis through better patient agenda scheduling, reduction of patient discharge time through reconstructions or faster sending of images to workstations, or support of artificial intelligence in the assessment of imaging.

approach allows for optimization of resources, significantly reducing overall risk and rapidly improving patient outcomes.

Through the application of the previous three concepts (SIPOC mapping, Workflow e Key Process Indicators (KPI), structured data), we can get to talk about Process Automation, dash-boards to support decisions and predictive analysis. Process automation is based on stable processes and information tools that are as connected as possible to avoid all those non-value activities, which we will have mapped in the workflows mentioned above.

For example, every time we find a manual or repetitive activity, automation workflows can automate it with algorithms that replicate the data digitization activities. Or reporting data from paper to the system can be made digital by modifying the device/software with which it is entered; many companies have now implemented an Artificial Intelligence system capable of reading the document and reporting the data to the system using a photo. You need to know where that data is, in which process, and who is generating it. Then, it's possible to connect Business Intelligence Dashboards that hook directly to the source databases and with simple Drag and Drop systems allow you to build reports and KPIs capable of providing the information needed by the business in real time to guide its organization. Always with the same Dashboards and trending the data, it is then simple to build statistical calculation models that hypothesize future scenarios on which to evaluate decision-making approaches. The above results in making the best use of existing technologies and optimization techniques, improving customer service, containing costs, or maintaining the same but with an increase in the effectiveness and efficiency of the different departments.

18.6 Importance of Effective Communication

Communication is a core clinical skill which can be developed and improved with practice, experience, continuous learning, mentorship, and support. Being able to effectively communicate can have a significant positive influence on all team members, and most importantly the patient. Healthcare is a dynamic and complex setting and good communication is essential for creating a safe and functional workplace and reducing the risk of errors. The multidisciplinary team in a nuclear medicine department need to be able to navigate competing priorities and problem solve issues associated with working in a patient centered, complex environment.

It is essential to consider the surrounding environment when communicating with a patient. For example, talking to a patient in a busy, noisy area with lots of people present, can be challenging and confronting for a patient. Taking the patient to a private consultation room may allow for more effective communication in a difficult situation. The use of technology should also be considered, especially if there are language, disability, or cognitive barriers, where using a translation application for example may help to put the patient at ease. Poor communication is one of the major contributing factors to teamwork failures and can result in errors, misdiagnosis, and inappropriate treatment.

18.6.1 Principles of Effective Communication

The nuclear medicine team within a hospital facility is unique and is often a service provider rather being directly involved with the care plan for patients. Therefore, communicating effectively with both internal and external stakeholders can improve efficiencies and result in better outcomes for the patients. A core set of principles that can be applied across all teams have been identified [6]:

- An understanding of who is part of the team and this must always include the person receiving the care or the patient and their relatives and family members.
- A set of shared goals of care, which in a nuclear medicine setting could be following a standardized protocol, creating a safe environment for the patient, quality assurance of all studies, and minimizing radiation exposure to patient and staff.
- Identify clear roles and responsibilities of all staff involved in performing the procedure with known expectations of each team member's function, responsibility, and accountability. This assists with optimizing efficiency and patient compliance.

- Mutual respect for all team members and most importantly the patient and their family. Undergoing a procedure can be a very difficult and stressful process, therefore being respectful, polite, and considerate will put the patient at ease and improve the overall quality of the experience.

Research has shown that ineffective communication is one of the most common complaints made about the healthcare system. Therefore, given its importance, a department should implement ongoing quality improvement through the use of tools such as audits and surveys to receive reliable and timely feedback on any successes and failures [20]. The results should be communicated to the team members to allow performance improvement and to acknowledge positive outcomes.

The ability to effectively communicate relies on a complex set of skills and the communication must occur in a structured and meaningful way. Being able to interact well with others and deal with conflict in a professional manner is essential. This becomes more important in a complex clinical situation where the use of common language without jargon is necessary when dealing with patients, however a more structured communication is needed when interacting with other healthcare professionals.

18.7 Summary

This chapter has given a brief overview of the important factors to consider when assessing ways to improve the structure and organization of the Nuclear Medicine Department. Determining the ideal structure for your department will allow improvement in workflow efficiency, a clearer understanding of your goals and strategies, and an assessment of the workforce requirements including skill mix, numbers, and roles and responsibilities. The value of effective communication between internal staff and other healthcare departments will reduce errors, improve patient compliance, and create an inclusive and productive work environment.

References

1. Paez D, Dondi M, Poli GL, et al. A model to assess staffing needs in nuclear medicine. Agency IAE; 2022.
2. Papassavas A, Chatzistamatiou TK, Michalopoulos E, Serafetinidi M, Gkioka V, Markogianni E, et al. Quality management systems including accreditation standards. In: Stavropoulos-Giokas C, Charron D, Navarrete C, editors. Cord blood stem cells medicine. Boston: Elsevier Science; 2014. p. 229–48. https://doi.org/10.1016/B978-0-12-407785-0.00017-7.
3. Morrison R. Data-driven organization design : sustaining the competitive edge through organizational analytics. London: Koganpage; 2021.
4. Morrison R. Organizational planning and analysis. London: Koganpage; 2022.
5. Morrison R, Andrew J. Strategic value creation. London: Koganpage; 2024.
6. Communicating for Safety: Improving clinical communication, collaboration and teamwork in Australian health services. In: Healthcare ACoSaQi, editor. Australian Commission on Safety and Quality in Healthcare; 2020.
7. Bosch BM, Mansell H. Interprofessional collaboration in healthcare: lessons to be learned from competitive sports. Can Pharm J. 2015;148(4):176.
8. Lopes MA, Almeida AS, Almada-Lobo B. Handling healthcare workforce planning with care: where do we stand? Hum Resour Health. 2015;13:38.
9. World Health Organization. Workload indicators of staffing need: user's manual. Geneva: World Health Organization; 2023.
10. International Atomic Energy Agency. A model to assess staffing needs in nuclear medicine. In: IAEA human health reports no. 19. Vienna: IAEA; 2022.
11. Malcolm DG, Roseboom JH, Clark CE, Fazar W. Application of a technique for Research and Development program evaluation. Oper Res. 1959;7(5):646–69.
12. Allerton LJ. Allowances. In: Zandin KB, editor. Maynard's industrial engineering handbook. 5th ed. New York: McGraw-Hill; 2001. p. 5.101–19.
13. Bam L, Cloete C, de Kock IH. Determining diagnostic radiographer staffing requirements: a workload-based approach. Radiography (Lond). 2022;28(2):276–82.
14. Smith GS. Developing engineered labor standards. In: Zandin KB, editor. Maynard's industrial engineering handbook. 5th ed. New York: McGraw-Hill; 2001. p. 5.73–5.100.
15. May JE, Hilliard K. Case study: labor controls for a bank. In: Zandin KB, editor. Maynard's industrial engineering handbook. 5th ed. New York: McGraw-Hill; 2001. p. 15.93–15.101.
16. Kruskal JB, Reedy A, Pascal A, et al. Quality initiatives: lean approach to improving performance and efficiency in a radiology department. Radiographics. 2012;32(2):573.
17. Think Research. How healthcare standardization helps improve patient safety [internet]. Think Research Canada. 2023. https://www.thinkresearch.com/ca/2023/09/27/how-healthcare-standardization-helps-improve-patient-safety/. Accessed 20 Jul 2024.
18. Lean organisation for excellence, Hoshin Kanri, value stream accounting, lean metrics e Toyota production system e lean agile scrum, Andrea Chiarini, Chiarini & Associati.
19. Burroni L, Bianciardi C, Romagnolo C, et al. Lean approach to improving performance and efficiency in a nuclear medicine department. Clin Transl Imaging. 2021;9:129–39. https://doi.org/10.1007/s40336-021-00418-z.
20. Paez D, et al. Quanum 3.0: an updated tool for Nuclear Medicine Audits, IAEA Human Health Series No. 33. Vienna: IAEA; 2021.